CELLS OF IMMUNOGLOBULIN SYNTHESIS

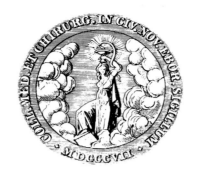

P & S BIOMEDICAL SCIENCES SYMPOSIA Series

HENRY J. VOGEL, Editor

College of Physicians and Surgeons
Columbia University
New York, New York

Henry J. Vogel (Editor). *Nucleic Acid–Protein Recognition,* 1977

Arthur Karlin, Virginia M. Tennyson, and Henry J. Vogel (Editors). *Neuronal Information Transfer,* 1978

Benvenuto Pernis and Henry J. Vogel (Editors). *Cells of Immunoglobulin Synthesis,* 1979

CELLS OF IMMUNOGLOBULIN SYNTHESIS

Edited by

BENVENUTO PERNIS
HENRY J. VOGEL

College of Physicians and Surgeons
Columbia University
New York, New York

ACADEMIC PRESS

New York   San Francisco   London   1979

A Subsidiary of Harcourt Brace Jovanovich, Publishers

599.0293
C393

ACADEMIC PRESS, INC.
111 Fifth Avenue, New York, New York 10003

United Kingdom Edition published by
ACADEMIC PRESS, INC. (LONDON) LTD.
24/28 Oval Road, London NW1 7DX

Library of Congress Cataloging in Publication Data
Main entry under title:

Cells of immunoglobulin synthesis.

(P & S biomedical sciences symposia series)
Proceedings of a symposium held at Arden House,
June 9–11, 1978.
Includes bibliographical references.
1. Immunoglobulins––Congresses. 2. B cells––
Congresses. 3. Immunogenetics––Congresses. 4. Pro-
tein biosynthesis––Congresses. I. Pernis, Benvenuto.
II. Vogel, Henry James, Date III. Series.
[DNLM: 1. Immunoglobulins––Biosynthesis––Congresses.
2. Cytology––Congresses. QW601 C393 1978]
QR186.7.C44   599'.02'93   78–20000
ISBN 0–12–551850–1

PRINTED IN THE UNITED STATES OF AMERICA

79 80 81 82   9 8 7 6 5 4 3 2 1

Contents

OPENING ADDRESS

B Lymphocyte Differentiation and the Tolerance Problem

G. J. V. NOSSAL

PART I   IMMUNOGLOBULIN GENES, MESSAGES, AND MOLECULES

Somatic Recombination and Structure of an Immunoglobulin Gene

SUSUMU TONEGAWA, CHRISTINE BRACK, MINORU HIRAMA,
AND RITA LENHARD-SCHULLER

Implications of the Assortment of Framework Segments for the Assembly of Immunoglobulin V_L and V_H Regions and the Generation of Diversity

ELVIN A. KABAT

Immunoglobulin Genes and Nuclear RNA Precursors

RANDOLPH WALL, EDMUND CHOI, MICHAEL KOMAROMY,

MAUREEN GILMORE-HEBERT, AND KATHLEEN HERCULES

Studies on mRNA Sequence and Immunoglobulin Gene Organization Using Synthetic Oligonucleotides

P. H. HAMLYN AND C. MILSTEIN

Comparative Aspects of *in Vitro* and Cellular Assembly of Immunoglobulins

SHERMAN BEYCHOK

Human Immunoglobulin Mutants

EDWARD C. FRANKLIN, BLAS FRANGIONE, AND JOEL BUXBAUM

PART II   CELLULAR IMMUNOGLOBULIN PRODUCTION

Variable and Constant Region Variants of Mouse Myeloma Cells

WENDY D. COOK, BEN DHARMGRONGARTAMA,
AND MATTHEW D. SCHARFF

Constant Region Mutants of Mouse Immunoglobulins

SHERIE L. MORRISON

Differentiation of Leukemic B Lymphocytes in Man

S. M. FU, N. CHIORAZZI, J. N. HURLEY,
J. P. HALPER, AND H. G. KUNKEL

Intracellular Events in the Differentiation of B Lymphocytes to Pentamer IgM Synthesis

RICHARD A. ROTH, ELIZABETH L. MATHER,
AND MARIAN ELLIOTT KOSHLAND

PART III   MEMBRANE IMMUNOGLOBULINS

Receptor-Mediated Triggering and Tolerance in Murine B Cells

JONATHAN W. UHR AND ELLEN S. VITETTA

Structure of Lymphocyte Membrane Immunoglobulin

A. FEINSTEIN, N. E. RICHARDSON, AND R. A. J. McILHINNEY

Role of Membrane Immunoglobulins in Lymphocyte Responses

BENVENUTO PERNIS, LUCIANA FORNI, AND SUSAN R. WEBB

PART IV   IMMUNOGLOBULINS AS REGULATORY MOLECULES

Function of Surface Immunoglobulin of B Lymphocytes

EMIL R. UNANUE

The Role of Immunoglobulin in the Induction of B Lymphocytes

J. ANDERSSON, A. COUTINHO, AND F. MELCHERS

Role of the Fc Portion of Antibody in Immune Regulation

WILLIAM O. WEIGLE AND MONIQUE A. BERMAN

Factors Affecting the Triggering of the B-Cell Repertoire

SUSAN K. PIERCE, ELEANOR S. METCALF,
AND NORMAN R. KLINMAN

PART V   LYMPHOCYTE HYBRIDS

Fusion of Immunoglobulin Secreting Cells

MARC SHULMAN AND GEORGES KÖHLER

Ontogeny of Clonal Dominance

HEINZ KÖHLER, DAVID KAPLAN, RUTH KAPLAN,
JOHN FUNG, AND JOSÉ QUINTÁNS

Anti-(T,G)-A--L Idiotypes: Initial Studies of Genetic Control and Cellular Expression

SETH H. PINCUS, ALFRED SINGER,
RICHARD J. HODES, AND HOWARD B. DICKLER

PART VII ONTOGENY OF IMMUNOGLOBULIN-SYNTHESIZING CELLS

B Lymphocyte Development and Activation: Analysis with a Mutant Mouse Strain

WILLIAM E. PAUL, BONDADA SUBBARAO, JAMES J. MOND,
DONNA G. SIECKMANN, IAN ZITRON, AFTAB AHMED,
DONALD E. MOSIER, AND IRWIN SCHER

Influence of Thymus Cells on the Ontogeny of B Lymphocyte Function

GREGORY W. SISKIND

Pre-B Cells: Normal Morphologic and Biologic Characteristics and Abnormal Development in Certain Immunodeficiencies and Malignancies

MAX D. COOPER AND ALEXANDER R. LAWTON

List of Participants

AHMED, AFTAB, Department of Immunology, Naval Medical Research Institute, Bethesda, Maryland 20014

ANDERSSON, J., Department of Immunology, Biomedical Center, Uppsala University, S-75123 Uppsala, Sweden

ANDREWS, P. W., Memorial Sloan-Kettering Cancer Center, New York, New York 10021

BERGER, CAROLE L., Department of Dermatology, College of Physicians and Surgeons, Columbia University, New York, New York 10032

BERMAN, MONIQUE A., Department of Immunopathology, Scripps Clinic and Research Foundation, La Jolla, California 92037

BEYCHOK, SHERMAN, Department of Biological Sciences, Columbia University, New York, New York 10032

BLANC, WILLIAM E., Department of Pathology, College of Physicians and Surgeons, Columbia University, New York, New York 10032

BONAGURA, VINCENT R., Department of Microbiology, College of Physicians and Surgeons, Columbia University, New York, New York 10032

BRACK, CHRISTINE, Basel Institute for Immunology, Postfach, 4005 Basel 5, Switzerland

BRANWOOD, A. MARY, Department of Pathology, College of Physicians and Surgeons, Columbia University, New York, New York 10032

BRILES, DAVID E., Department of Neurobiology, Cellular Immunology Unit, The University of Alabama in Birmingham, Birmingham, Alabama 35294

BUTLER, VINCENT P., JR., Department of Medicine, College of Physicians and Surgeons, Columbia University, New York, New York 10032

BUXBAUM, JOEL, Research Service, Veterans Administration Hospital, New York, New York 10010

CATHOU, RENATA E., Department of Biochemistry, Tufts University School of Medicine, Boston, Massachusetts 02111

CAZENAVE, PIERRE-ANDRÉ, Service d'Immunochimie Analytique, Institut Pasteur, 75724 Paris, Cédex 15, France

CHASE, MERRILL W., The Rockefeller University, New York, New York 10021

CHESKIN, HOWARD S., Department of Pathology, College of Physicians and Surgeons, Columbia University, New York, New York 10032

CHIORAZZI, N., The Rockefeller University, New York, New York 10021

CHOI, EDMUND, Department of Microbiology and Immunology, UCLA School of Medicine, University of California, Los Angeles, California 90024

CLEVELAND, W. L., Department of Microbiology, College of Physicians and Surgeons, Columbia University, New York, New York 10032

CLEVINGER, BRIAN, Department of Microbiology and Immunology, Washington University School of Medicine, St. Louis, Missouri 63110

CONE, ROBERT, Department of Pathology, Yale University School of Medicine, New Haven, Connecticut 06510

COOK, WENDY D., Department of Cell Biology, Albert Einstein College of Medicine, New York, New York 10461

COOPER, MAX D., The Cellular Immunobiology Unit of the Tumor Institute, University of Alabama, Birmingham, Alabama 35294

COSENZA, HUMBERTO, Department of Microbiology, University of Honduras, Tegucigalpa, Honduras

COUTINHO, A., Basel Institute for Immunology, Postfach, 4005 Basel 5, Switzerland

CRABEEL, MARJOLAINE, Laboratory of Microbiology, Free University of Brussels, Research Institute, C.E.R.I.A., B1070 Brussels, Belgium

CUNIN, RAYMOND, Laboratory of Microbiology, Free University of Brussels, Research Institute, C.E.R.I.A., B1070 Brussels, Belgium

DAVIE, JOSEPH M., Department of Microbiology and Immunology, Washington University School of Medicine, St. Louis, Missouri 63110

DHARMGRONGARTAMA, BEN, Department of Cell Biology, Albert Einstein College of Medicine, New York, New York 10461

DICKLER, HOWARD B., Immunology Branch, National Cancer Institute, National Institutes of Health, Bethesda, Maryland 20014

DURKIN, HELEN G., Department of Pathology, Downstate Medical College, Brooklyn, New York 11203

ECKHARDT, THOMAS, Department of Microbiology, New York University, New York, New York 10016

EDELIST, TRUDY, Department of Pathology, College of Physicians and Surgeons, Columbia University, New York, New York 10032

EISENBERG, MAX A., Department of Biochemistry, College of Physicians and Surgeons, Columbia University, New York, New York 10032

FEINSTEIN, A., A.R.C. Institute of Animal Physiology, Babraham, Cambridge, Cambridgeshire, England

FENOGLIO, CECILIA M., Department of Pathology, College of Physicians and Surgeons, Columbia University, New York, New York 10032

FINGER, IRVING, Department of Biology, Haverford College, Haverford, Pennsylvania 19041

FORNI, LUCIANA. Basel Institute for Immunology, Postfach, 4005 Basel 5 , Switzerland

FRANGIONE, BLAS, Department of Pathology, New York University Medical Center, New York, New York 10016

FRANKLIN, EDWARD C., Department of Medicine, New York University College of Medicine, New York, New York 10016

Fu, S. M., The Rockefeller University, New York, New York 10021

Fung, John, Department of Pathology, La Rabida–University of Chicago Institute, Chicago, Illinois 60649

Gates, Frederick T., III, National Institute of Allergy and Infectious Diseases, National Institutes of Health, Bethesda, Maryland 20014

Gilmore-Hebert, Maureen, Department of Microbiology and Immunology, UCLA School of Medicine, University of California, Los Angeles, California 90024

Gindes, D., Department of Microbiology, College of Physicians and Surgeons, Columbia University, New York, New York 10032

Goding, James W., Department of Genetics, Stanford University School of Medicine, Stanford, California 94305

Godman, Gabriel C., Department of Pathology, College of Physicians and Surgeons, Columbia University, New York, New York 10032

Goidl, Edmond A., Department of Medicine, Cornell University School of Medicine, New York, New York 10021

Gold, Leslie, Department of Medicine, New York University School of Medicine, New York, New York 10016

Gottlieb, Paul D., Center for Cancer Research, Massachusetts Institute of Technology, Cambridge, Massachusetts 02139

Goyert, Sanna, Department of Pathology, New York University School of Medicine, New York, New York 10016

Griffith, Rogers, Department of Microbiology and Immunology, Washington University School of Medicine, St. Louis, Missouri 63110

Habicht, Gail S., Department of Pathology, State University of New York, Stony Brook, New York 11794

Halper, James, Department of Microbiology, College of Physicians and Surgeons, Columbia University, New York, New York 10032

Halper, J. P., The Rockefeller University, New York, New York 10021

Hamlyn, P. H., MRC Laboratory of Molecular Biology, Cambridge, England

Hansburg, Daniel, Department of Microbiology and Immunology, Washington University School of Medicine, St. Louis, Missouri 63110

Harrington, William N., Department of Pathology, College of Physicians and Surgeons, Columbia University, New York, New York 10032

Henderson, Edward S., Department of Medicine, Roswell Park Memorial Institute, Buffalo, New York 14263

Hercules, Kathleen, Department of Biological Chemistry, UCLA School of Medicine, University of California, Los Angeles, California 90024

Herzenberg, Leonard A., Department of Genetics, Stanford University School of Medicine, Stanford, California 94305

Herzenberg, Leonore A., Department of Genetics, Stanford University School of Medicine, Stanford, California 94305

Hirama, Minoru, Basel Institute for Immunology, Postfach, 4005 Basel 5, Switzerland

Hodes, Richard J., Immunology Branch, National Cancer Institute, National Institutes of Health, Bethesda, Maryland 20014

HUMPHREY, RICHARD L., The Johns Hopkins Oncology Center, Johns Hopkins University School of Medicine, Baltimore, Maryland 21205

HURLEY, J. N., The Rockefeller University, New York, New York 10021

ISHIZAKA, KIMISHIGE, The Johns Hopkins University at the Good Samaritan Hospital, Baltimore, Maryland 21239

JACOBSON, ETHEL B., Merck Institute for Therapeutic Research, Rahway, New Jersey 07065

JONES, PATRICIA P., Department of Genetics, Stanford University School of Medicine, Stanford, California 94305

JOSEPHSON, ALAN G., Department of Medicine, State University of New York, Brooklyn, New York 11203

KABAT, ELVIN A., Department of Microbiology, College of Physicians and Surgeons, Columbia University, New York, New York 10032

KAPLAN, DAVID, Department of Pathology, La Rabida—University of Chicago Institute, Chicago, Illinois 60649

KAPLAN, RUTH, Department of Pathology, La Rabida–University of Chicago Institute, Chicago, Illinois 60649

KASICA, DEBORAH, Department of Pathology, College of Physicians and Surgeons, Columbia University, New York, New York 10032

KAZIN, ALICE R., Sloan-Kettering Institute for Cancer Research, Rye, New York 10580

KELSOE, GARNETT, Department of Microbiology, Harvard University, Boston, Massachusetts 02115

KINCADE, PAUL W., Sloan-Kettering Institute for Cancer Research, Rye, New York 10580

KLINMAN, NORMAN R., Department of Cellular and Developmental Immunology, Scripps Clinic and Research Foundation, La Jolla, California 92037

KNOPF, PAUL M., Division of Biology and Medicine, Brown University, Providence, Rhode Island 02912

KÖHLER, GEORGES, Basel Institute for Immunology, Postfach, 4005 Basel 5, Switzerland

KÖHLER, HEINZ, Department of Pathology, La Rabida–University of Chicago Institute, Chicago, Illinois 60649

KOMAROMY, MICHAEL, Department of Microbiology and Immunology, UCLA School of Medicine, University of California, Los Angeles, California 90024

KOSHLAND, MARIAN ELLIOTT., Department of Bacteriology and Immunology, University of California, Berkeley, California 94720

KOWALIK, SHARON, Department of Pathology, College of Physicians and Surgeons, Columbia University, New York, New York 10032

KUNKEL, H. G., The Rockefeller University, New York, New York 10021

LATOVITZKI, NORMAN, Department of Neurology, College of Physicians and Surgeons, Columbia University, New York, New York 10032

LAWTON, ALEXANDER R., The Cellular Immunobiology Unit of the Tumor Institute, University of Alabama, Birmingham, Alabama 35294

LE GUERN, CHRISTIAN, Service d'Immunochimie Analytique, Institut Pasteur, 75724 Paris, Cédex 15, France

LEISINGER, THOMAS, Mikrobiologisches Institut, Eidgenössische Technische Hochschule, Zurich, Switzerland

LENHARD-SCHULLER, RITA, Basel Institute for Immunology, Postfach, 4005 Basel 5, Switzerland

LEVINTHAL, CYRUS, Department of Biological Sciences, Columbia University, New York, New York 10027

LITWIN, STEPHEN D., Department of Medicine, Cornell University Medical College, New York, New York 10021

LOVE, PATRICIA Y., Department of Microbiology, College of Physicians and Surgeons, Columbia University, New York, New York 10032

MANGOLD, BEVERLY, Division of Biology and Medicine, Brown University, Providence, Rhode Island 02912

MARKS, PAUL A., Office of the Vice President for Health Sciences, Columbia University, New York, New York 10032

MARTINIS, JOANNE, Wistar Institute, Philadelphia, Pennsylvania 19104

MATHER, ELIZABETH L., Department of Bacteriology and Immunology, University of California, Berkeley, California 94720

MATSUUCHI, LINDA, Department of Microbiology, College of Physicians and Surgeons, Columbia University, New York, New York 10032

MCCLELLAND, KATHARINE, Department of Pathology, College of Physicians and Surgeons, Columbia University, New York, New York 10032

MCILHINNEY, R. A. J., A.R.C. Institute of Animal Physiology, Babraham, Cambridge, Cambridgeshire, England

MELCHERS, F., Basel Institute for Immunology, Postfach, 4005 Basel 5, Switzerland

MESA-TEJADA, RICARDO, Department of Pathology, College of Physicians and Surgeons, Columbia University, New York, New York 10032

METCALF, ELEANOR S., Department of Microbiology, Uniformed Services University of the Health Sciences, Bethesda, Maryland 20014

MILSTEIN, C., MRC Laboratory of Molecular Biology, Cambridge, England

MITSIALIS, S. ALEXANDER, Department of Microbiology, College of Physicians and Surgeons, Columbia University, New York, New York 10032

MOND, JAMES J., Laboratory of Immunology, National Institute of Allergy and Infectious Diseases, National Institutes of Health, Bethesda, Maryland 20014

MORAN, MARY C., Department of Pathology, College of Physicians and Surgeons, Columbia University, New York, New York 10032

MORRISON, SHERIE L., Department of Microbiology, College of Physicians and Surgeons, Columbia University, New York, New York 10032

MOSIER, DONALD E., Laboratory of Immunology, National Institute of Allergy and Infectious Diseases, National Institutes of Health, Bethesda, Maryland 20014

NEILSON, ERIC G., Department of Medicine, Allergy, and Immunology, University of Pennsylvania School of Medicine, Philadelphia, Pennsylvania 19104

NISONOFF, ALFRED, Rosenstiel Basic Sciences Research Center, Brandeis University, Waltham, Massachusetts 02154

NOSSAL, SIR GUSTAV, The Walter and Eliza Hall Institute of Medical Research, Melbourne, Victoria 3050, Australia

O'DONOVAN, GERARD A., Department of Biochemistry and Biophysics, Texas A & M University, College Station, Texas 77843

OI, VERNON T., Department of Genetics, Stanford University School of Medicine, Stanford, California 94305

OSSERMAN, ELLIOTT F., Department of Medicine, College of Physicians and Surgeons, Columbia University, New York, New York 10032

PALUCH, EDWARD, Department of Pathology, College of Physicians and Surgeons, Columbia University, New York, New York 10032

PARONETTO, FIORENZO, Department of Pathology, Mt. Sinai School of Medicine, New York, New York 10029

PAUL, WILLIAM E., Laboratory of Immunology, National Institute of Allergy and Infectious Diseases, National Institutes of Health, Bethesda, Maryland 20014

PEREIRA, MIERCIO E. A., Department of Microbiology, College of Physicians and Surgeons, Columbia University, New York, New York 10032

PERLMUTTER, ROGER M., Department of Microbiology and Immunology, Washington University School of Medicine, St. Louis, Missouri 63110

PERNIS, BENVENUTO, Departments of Microbiology and Medicine, College of Physicians and Surgeons, Columbia University, New York, New York 10032

PESTKA, SIDNEY, Roche Institute of Molecular Biology, Nutley, New Jersey 07110

PHILLIPS, S. MICHAEL, Department of Medicine, Allergy and Immunology, University of Pennsylvania School of Medicine, Philadelphia, Pennsylvania 19104

PHILLIPS, STEPHANIE, Department of Human Genetics, College of Physicians and Surgeons, Columbia University, New York, New York 10032

PIERCE, SUSAN K., Department of Biochemistry and Molecular Biology, Northwestern University, Evanston, Illinois 60201

PINCUS, SETH H., Immunology Branch, National Cancer Institute, National Institutes of Health, Bethesda, Maryland 20014

PITT, JANE, Department of Pediatrics, College of Physicians and Surgeons, Columbia University, New York, New York 10032

POLLACK, MARILYN S., Memorial Sloan-Kettering Cancer Center, New York, New York 10021

POTASH, MARY J., Division of Biology and Medicine, Brown University, Providence, Rhode Island 02912

PRAKASH, OM, Department of Biochemistry, College of Physicians and Surgeons, Columbia University, New York, New York 10032

QUINTÁNS, JOSÉ, Department of Pathology, La Rabida–University of Chicago Institute, Chicago, Illinois 60649

READ, STANLEY E., The Rockefeller University, New York, New York 10021

RICHARDSON, N. E., A.R.C. Institute of Animal Physiology, Babraham, Cambridge, Cambridgeshire, England

RIFKIND, RICHARD A., Departments of Medicine and Human Genetics and Development, College of Physicians and Surgeons, Columbia University, New York, New York 10032

ROTH, PHILIP, Department of Microbiology, College of Physicians and Surgeons, Columbia University, New York, New York 10032

ROTH, RICHARD A., Department of Bacteriology and Immunology, University of California, Berkeley, California 94720

SABBATH, MARLENE, Department of Pathology, College of Physicians and Surgeons, Columbia University, New York, New York 10032

SCHARFF, MATTHEW D., Department of Cell Biology, Albert Einstein College of Medicine, New York, New York 10461

SCHEID, MARGIT, Sloan-Kettering Institute for Cancer Research, New York, New York 10021

SCHER, IRWIN, Department of Experimental Pathology, Naval Medical Research Institute, Bethesda, Maryland 20014

SEEGAL, BEATRICE C., Department of Microbiology, College of Physicians and Surgeons, Columbia University, New York, New York 10032

SETCAVAGE, THOMAS M., Sloan-Kettering Institute for Cancer Research, Rye, New York 10580

SHARON, JAQUELINE, Department of Microbiology, College of Physicians and Surgeons, Columbia University, New York, New York 10032

SHEN, F.-W., Sloan-Kettering Institute for Cancer Research, New York, New York 10021

SHULMAN, MARC, Basel Institute for Immunology, Postfach, 4005 Basel 5, Switzerland

SIECKMANN, DONNA G., Laboratory of Immunology, National Institute of Allergy and Infectious Diseases, National Institutes of Health, Bethesda, Maryland 20014

SIEGAL, FREDERICK P., Sloan-Kettering Institute for Cancer Research, New York, New York 10021

SINGER, ALFRED, Immunology Branch, National Cancer Institute, National Institutes of Health, Bethesda, Maryland 20014

SISKIND, GREGORY W., Division of Allergy and Immunology, Department of Medicine, Cornell University Medical College, New York, New York 10021

SLOVIN, SUSAN F., Department of Clinical Research, Scripps Clinic and Research Foundation, La Jolla, California 92037

SUBBARAO, BONDADA, Laboratory of Immunology, National Institute of Allergy and Infectious Diseases, National Institutes of Health, Bethesda, Maryland 20014

SUGII, SHUNGI, Department of Microbiology, College of Physicians and Surgeons, Columbia University, New York, New York 10032

SUNG, LAMPING A., Department of Microbiology, College of Physicians and Surgeons, Columbia University, New York, New York 10032

TALAL, NORMAN, Department of Medicine, University of California, San Francisco, California 94143

TAPLEY, DONALD F., Office of the Dean, College of Physicians and Surgeons, Columbia University, New York, New York 10032

TERRES, GERONIMO, Department of Physiology, Tufts University School of Medicine, Boston, Massachusetts 02111

THEIS, GAIL A., Department of Microbiology, New York Medical College, Valhalla, New York 10595

THOMSON, JEANNE W., Department of Pathology, New York Medical College, Valhalla, New York 10595

TONEGAWA, SUSUMU, Basel Institute for Immunology, Postfach, 4005 Basel 5, Switzerland

TUNG, AMAR S., Department of Pathology, University of Pennsylvania School of Medicine, Philadelphia, Pennsylvania 19104

UHR, JONATHAN W., Department of Microbiology, University of Texas Southwestern Medical School, Dallas, Texas 75235

UNANUE, EMIL R., Department of Pathology, Harvard Medical School, Boston, Massachusetts 02115

VANDE STOUWE, ROBERT, Roosevelt Hospital, New York, New York 10019

VAN VOORHIS, WESLEY C., The Rockefeller University, New York, New York 10021

VICTOR, CAROL B., Department of Microbiology, College of Physicians and Surgeons, Columbia University, New York, New York 10032

VITETTA, ELLEN S., Department of Microbiology, University of Texas Southwestern Medical School, Dallas, Texas 75235

VOGEL, HENRY J., Department of Pathology, College of Physicians and Surgeons, Columbia University, New York, New York 10032

VOGEL, RUTH H., Department of Pathology, College of Physicians and Surgeons, Columbia University, New York, New York 10032

WALL, RANDOLPH, Department of Microbiology and Immunology, UCLA School of Medicine, University of California, Los Angeles, California 90024

WEBB, SUSAN R., Department of Microbiology, College of Physicians and Surgeons, Columbia University, New York, New York 10032

WEIGLE, WILLIAM O., Department of Immunopathology, Scripps Clinic and Research Foundation, La Jolla, California 92037

WELLERSON, RALPH, Ortho Diagnostics Inc., Raritan, New Jersey 08869

WOOD, CHARLES, Department of Microbiology, College of Physicians and Surgeons, Columbia University, New York, New York 10032

WOOD, DAVID D., Merck Institute, Rahway, New Jersey 07901

WOODWARD, KIMBALL P., Department of Pathology, College of Physicians and Surgeons, Columbia University, New York, New York 10032

Wu, ALBERT M., Department of Microbiology, College of Physicians and Surgeons, Columbia University, New York, New York 10032

YELTON, DALE E., Department of Cell Biology, Albert Einstein College of Medicine, New York, New York 10469

ZAUDERER, MAURICE, Department of Biological Sciences, Columbia University, New York, New York 10027

ZITRON, IAN, Laboratory of Immunology, National Institute of Allergy and Infectious Diseases, National Institutes of Health, Bethesda, Maryland 20014

ZUCKERKANDL, EMILE, Linus Pauling Institute of Science and Medicine, Menlo Park, California 94025

Preface

Recently, cellular immunology and related molecular and biochemical areas have seen development and increases in sophistication at an impressive rate. Particularly intriguing are certain clusters of advances associated with cells of immunoglobulin synthesis. For instance, in regard to the molecular biology of immunoglobulin synthesis, there is the emergence of the "several genes—one polypeptide" concept. Here, immunology led the way in posing the problem and provided a partial solution. In the cellular production of immunoglobulins, the use of hybrid cell lines has opened the door to the preparation of monoclonal antibodies of any desired specificity. Membrane immunoglobulins are evoking great current interest in terms of different classes of receptors and in terms of immunoglobulin triggering. As regulatory molecules, immunoglobulins impinge significantly on the tolerance phenomenon. Novel concepts of idiotype–antiidiotype interactions involving both bone marrow-derived (B) and thymus-derived (T) cells reveal the immunocyte family as an integrated complex. The recent elucidation of successive stages in the development of B immunocytes is of high utility to studies of immunodeficiency states.

With these and related advances as a backdrop, a symposium on "Cells of Immunoglobulin Synthesis" was held at Arden House, on the Harriman Campus of Columbia University from June 9 through June 11, 1978. The meeting was the third of the P & S Biomedical Sciences Symposia. The proceedings are contained in this volume.

The participants were welcomed by Dr. Donald F. Tapley, Dean of the Faculty of Medicine, who discussed some facets of the history of the College of Physicians and Surgeons (P & S), which sponsors the symposia.

Our sincere thanks go to Sir Gustav Nossal who delivered the Opening Address. The contributions of the session chairmen, Dr. Elvin A. Kabat, Dr. Matthew D. Scharff, Dr. Jan Andersson, Dr. Elliott Osserman, Dr. Henry G. Kunkel, and Dr. William E. Paul, are gratefully acknowledged.

Dr. Ruth H. Vogel's constructive role in the organization of the symposium and in the preparation of this volume is much appreciated.

Welcome financial aid was provided by a grant from the National Science Foundation.

Benvenuto Pernis
Henry J. Vogel

OPENING ADDRESS

B Lymphocyte Differentiation and the Tolerance Problem

G. J. V. NOSSAL

The Walter and Eliza Hall Institute of Medical Research
Melbourne, Victoria, Australia

Early thinking on immunological tolerance centered around two concepts, namely that tolerance was exclusively inducible in embryonic life; and that the failure of an antigen to cause an immune response was a distinctly unusual thing, requiring some special explanation. We now know that an encounter between immunocyte and antigen is by no means always followed by cell activation, and that various kinds and degrees of immunological suppression can be induced by antigen acting on both immature and mature lymphoid cell populations. We have thus had to adopt a much more pluralistic attitude to mechanisms of tolerance induction, recognizing that there exists under the broad umbrella of the term immunological tolerance a variety of distinct phenomena, and that tolerance must be viewed simply as a facet of immunological homeostasis (1). Nevertheless, it is becoming increasingly clear (2) that the original notions which placed the fields of lymphoid ontogeny and self-recognition into a linked conceptual framework (3) contained seeds of great wisdom and fascination. The purpose of this paper is briefly to review recent findings from my laboratory, pertaining to this linkage, which we believe have now placed it on a firm scientific footing, at least as far as the B lymphocyte is concerned. It is heartening to note that, following a period during which most investigators placed stress on suppressor T cells as the main factor behind tolerance and self-recognition, the recent literature has abounded with reports which show a special sensitivity of immature B cells to tolerance induction, lending credence to the clonal abortion theory of B lymphocyte tolerance (4). As is inevitable in a rapidly moving field, quite a number of apparent differences in

3

findings or interpretation have emerged from different laboratories. Where possible, I shall try to resolve or at least explain the points of contention. It is appropriate to begin with a consideration of our work in the field of B lymphocyte differentiation.

SEQUENCE OF ACQUISITION OF Ia, IgM, and IgD IN ADULT MURINE BONE MARROW

We have previously demonstrated (5,6) an interesting sequence of maturation events in lymphocytes generated in adult murine bone marrow. The small lymphocyte exits from the mitotic cycles of large and medium lymphocytes generating it lacking readily-detectable surface Ig receptors. These are added in progressively larger amounts during a critical nonmitotic maturation phase lasting about 2 days. We wished to know at what stage during this postmitotic period Ia antigens and IgD made their appearance at the cell surface. Accordingly (7,8), cells bearing various quantities of IgM from adult bone marrow were separated using the fluorescence-activated cell sorter (FACS). For IgD antigens, we made use in the second stage of labeling of the suitable congenic mouse strains and anti-δ chain allotype reagents (9) and of quantitative autoradiographic methods to determine relative amounts. For Ia, A.TH. anti A.TL. serum and CBA mice were used. It was found that even the small lymphocytes with no detectable surface Ig showed readily detectable Ia antigen in 18% of cases. Furthermore, the cohort with the least amount of detectable Ig, out of five separate Ig-positive fractions, showed 48% Ia-positive cells under the conditions used, and a low median amount. Increasingly high Ig cohorts showed increasing amounts of Ia on an increasing percentage of the cells. All cells that would have been scored IgM-positive by conventional techniques were also Ia-positive. No evidence of a lag between IgM acquisition and Ia acquisition was noted. In contrast, Ig-negative lymphocytes were uniformly IgD-negative and even those with the highest IgM density showed only 70% positivity. Intermediate fractions gave intermediate results. Thus in the marrow, IgD appears *after* IgM and as the amount of IgM increases, (but probably after a considerable lag), the amount of IgD also increases.

These findings are of some interest in relation to functional maturation of B cells. For example, we have found (7) that the capacity to respond to agar mitogens by clonal colony growth matures concurrently with increasing Ig and Ia density on marrow small lymphocytes.

The special susceptibility of adult marrow small lymphocytes to tolerance induction has also been documented (2), but we have not yet pursued this among marrow cells sorted on the basis of their Ig density.

KINETICS OF TOLEROGENESIS AMONG IMMATURE B CELLS OF VARIOUS CATEGORIES

In support of the clonal abortion theory of B lymphocyte tolerance (4) we have previously drawn attention to the fact that fetal liver stem cells repopulating irradiated mice (10), adult bone marrow cells (4) and newborn spleen cells (11,2) all can be rendered tolerant by surprisingly low concentrations of antigen. However, in our previous work, tolerance induction among the hapten-specific B cells under study involved a prolonged period of co-incubation of the cell population with tolerogenic antigen. In fact, maximal effects were seen only when tolerogen and the cell population were held together for 3 days. Over such a period, control populations not being tolerized matured considerably, increasing their capacity to give adoptive immune responses or to initiate clones of antibody-forming cells *in vitro*. The chief effect of the tolerogen was to abrogate this maturation in a hapten-specific manner. For this reason, the studies did not produce evidence for a direct effect of tolerogen on the few triggerable cells present in the immature cell population at the beginning of the culture period.

The existence of immature B cells, capable of being activated to clonal expansion and antibody formation through the action of antigen plus T cell help, yet capable of being rendered tolerant by very low concentrations of antigen in the *absence* of T cell activity, was shown by the work of Klinman's group (12,13). Their studies on the tolerizability of the immature B cell paralleled ours in several respects, but one important difference was noted. The degree of tolerance reached within 8 hr was near maximal. Clearly, the negative signal was being read by a cell that could also respond to a positive signal, not simply by the progenitor of the triggerable cell.

To solve this apparent difference in results and interpretation, we decided to attempt to isolate the immature B cell capable of behaving in this dual fashion in relatively pure form. D. W. Scott, at that time part of our group, termed these the "caught in the act of clonal abortion" experiments. If Ig-negative cells could be eliminated from consideration, there would be no contribution from pre-B cells. Furthermore, interpretation would be facilitated if cohorts of cells of relatively uniform and high avidity for the test hapten could be studied. Accordingly, a method was devised involving two-stage fractionation of hapten-specific cells (14). The hapten fluorescein (FLU) was chosen at Scott's suggestion. Spleen cells from newborn or adult mice were first fractionated on FLU-gelatin dishes by the method of Haas and Layton (15), providing 100- to 500-fold enrichment for clonable precursors of FLU-specific plaque-forming cells (PFC) as tested by an appropriate limit dilution microculture system. Then, these cells were relabeled with FLU-gelatin and sorted into cohorts of relatively homogeneous fluorescence intensity in FACS. The cohort representing the most fluorescent ten percentile of the FLU-gelatin pre-fractionated population yielded, under optimal triggering conditions, one cell in eight (in the case of adult spleen) or one cell in eleven (for newborn spleen) capable of giving a FLU-specific PFC clone within 3 days after challenge. Tolerogenesis proceeded with the cells distributed at limit dilution in microcultures. Cells from mature mice were unaffected within 24 hr by concentrations of a standard $FLU_{3.6}$ HGG tolerogen below 25–50 μg/ml. Cells from newborn mice displaying the same avidity for antigen were tolerized at 1000-fold lower concentrations. Moreover, the higher the median avidity, the lower the threshold concentration for tolerogenesis (16).

The two-stage fractionation procedure was associated with severe yield losses, and it proved more practical to study certain details of the phenomenon with FLU-gelatin fractionated cells. These showed that immature FLU-specific B cells could be tolerized to a near-maximal extent within 8 hr by 5 μg/ml of tolerogen, but if the concentration was reduced to 1 μg/ml, 16–24 hr were required for a maximal effect. Moreover, the capacity to tolerize the immature B cells was abrogated by the concomitant presence of the polyclonal B cell activator, *Escherichia coli* lipopolysaccharide (LPS). The immature B cells could receive negative signals from tolerogens, but could have these overridden by stimulatory signals from LPS or T-independent antigens such as FLU-polymerized flagellin (FLU-POL). Interestingly, tolerogen acting for 2 hr and then removed from the cultures could not cause tolerance.

Thus these studies in a T-independent system completely vindicated Metcalf and Klinman's (12,13) results in a T-dependent system. How can they be reconciled with our earlier studies (4,11)? The latter were obviously more complex in design. First, the median antigen-binding avidity of the FLU-specific cells in unfractionated populations is lower than in FLU-gelatin fractionated populations (14), and thus to tolerize all the triggerable B cells present would have required a higher antigen concentration and/or a longer time. Perhaps more importantly, with a heterogeneous starting population containing pre-B cells and stem cells as well as B cells of various degrees of Ig density, the question of the exact target for tolerance induction is rendered difficult to approach because of progressive maturation. The longer the required tolerogenesis period, the greater this problem becomes. In the present experiments, we place great emphasis on the fact that a cell population consisting exclusively of Ig-positive cells, and distributed at limit dilution, could be tolerized within 8 hr. If we add these new findings to our older ones, we reach the position shown in Fig. 1. Rather than thinking of a single, brief phase in ontogeny where clonal abortion can occur, we accept a gradation of effects—a gradual decrease in sensitivity to negative signals accompanying a gradual increase in the capacity to be triggered. In other words, we now believe that clonal abortion as such does occur, but also that immature B cells exist which can be either tolerized or triggered depending on circumstances.

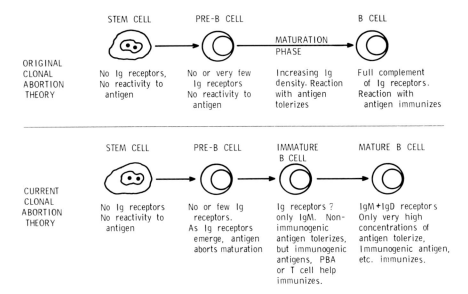

Fig. 1.   Current concepts of B cell tolerance susceptibility at various differentiation stages.

THE CAMBIER DILEMMA—DIFFERENCES BETWEEN T-INDEPENDENT AND T-DEPENDENT CELLS

Cambier *et al.* (17) have produced evidence to suggest that immature T-dependent B cells are indeed more readily tolerized than adult T-dependent cells; but that T-independent B cells show an exquisite tolerizability whether they come from immature or mature sources. In their work, hapten–protein conjugates of a much higher degree of substitution have been used. Accordingly, we tested tolerance induction with $FLU_{12}HGG$ in our limit dilution microculture system. The tolerogen was allowed to act for 24 hr before the "T-independent" challenge antigen FLU-POL was substituted for the immunogen. We did indeed find that adult spleen B cells, both unfractionated, and, to a slightly greater degree, FLU-gelatin fractionated, were much more susceptible to tolerogenesis by this conjugate than by $FLU_{3.6}HGG$. Fifty percent tolerogenesis was achieved at 1 μg/ml of antigen (16). However, immature B cells and especially the FLU-gelatin fractionated subset showed *much* greater sensitivity—0.2 μg/ml causing an 80% reduction in response. In other words, in our hands, the differential sensitivity between immature and mature B cells is maintained even with these stronger tolerogens. Moreover, we are impressed by the overall similarity of Metcalf and Klinman's tolerogenesis results (12), which we have largely confirmed (18), and those of our microculture system. As T cell help is an obligate prerequisite in the Klinman system, this suggests that overall patterns of behavior are not drastically dissimilar among T-dependent and T-independent immature B cells.

It is an attractive simplification to think of T-independent cells as being largely $IgM^+ IgD^-$, readily tolerizable perhaps because of their paucity of IgD (19,20); and T-dependent cells being largely $IgM^+ IgD^+$ and nontolerizable if mature. Unfortunately, our data do not support this view. First, in the T-independent microculture cloning system, we find FLU-gelatin-fractionated $IgM^+ IgD^+$ cells from 16–18-day-old C57 B1. Ig^e mice cloning out with a somewhat *higher* efficiency than their $IgM^+ IgD^-$ counterparts (21). There is no evidence that the $IgM^+ IgD^-$ cells are readily tolerizable. Also, we find cells from 17-day fetal mice capable of giving a T-dependent response, even though these are all $IgM^+ IgD^-$. Finally, in all our tolerance experiments, even those using fetal mice, there is a small tolerance-resistant subset and we do not believe these necessarily to be $IgM^+ IgD^+$ cells. In fact, we are not yet convinced that a subdivision of B cells into essentially T-dependent and T-independent is warranted. A relationship between surface Ig isotype expression and tolerizability is suggested in experiments where IgD is removed (19) or covered by antibody (20), and mature B cells thereby have their tolerizability threshold lowered. However, details of this relationship still require elucidation. In particular, $IgM^+ IgD^-$ cells from mature animals will have to be examined in detail.

MULTIVALENCY OF TOLEROGENS AND THE NATURE OF TOLERANCE PHENOMENA IN ADULT ANIMALS

Hapten–globulin conjugates are potent B cell tolerogens in adult animals (22). Recently, attention has been focused on this observation in terms both of the valency of the tolerogenic antigen and the degree of maturity of the target cells for tolerance induction (23,24). It has been claimed that adult hapten-specific tolerance is due, at least in part, to the production of a small amount of high affinity antibody; and that for multivalent antigens a true clonal abortion style tolerance is induced in newborn but not in adult lymphocyte populations (24,25). Curiously, univalent antigens were found to be equally potent partial tolerogens for adult and newborn B cell populations (24) by Szewczuk and Siskind.

We have approached this question by analysis of antigen-binding cells in FACS. When FLU_4HGG was injected into newborn or adult mice on a weight-adjusted basis, approximately equivalent degrees of B cell nonreactivity within the intact animal were induced (26). However, when the FLU-binding properties of the spleen cell populations were examined in FACS 1–2 weeks after tolerogen injection, major differences between newborns and adults were noted. The newborn populations contained very few cells exhibiting any residual fluorescence following the tolerogen injection, but showed a marked and consistent deficit in antigen-binding cells. The factorial reduction was avidity-related, being up to 13-fold for the most intensely FLU-binding cells, but only 2–4-fold for FLU-specific cells of low avidity. The adult cell populations showed relatively more cells with residual postinjection fluorescence, though this was of low intensity and certainly not sufficient to blockade all the receptors of FLU-specific B cells. On relabeling with FLU-protein, FACS analysis showed no consistent deficit in antigen-binding cells of any degree of avidity. In fact, on occasions a slight increase in the numbers of antigen-binding cells was noted, although it is too early to say whether this represented statistical variation among pools of adult spleen cells, or a slight degree of immunization. These findings agree with and extend the prior work of Venkataraman and Scott (25). They support the clonal abortion theory for the tolerance found in newborn mice, but do not illuminate the mechanisms of adult tolerance.

As regards the effects of univalent antigens on B cells, we have no new data to offer but would venture the comment that the findings of Szewczuk and Siskind (24) claiming an equal degree of partial tolerance with newborn and adult B cells are not entirely conclusive. Their assay of the *in vitro* tolerogenicity of bovine gamma globulin (BGG) depended on an adoptive transfer, challenge of the adoptive host with BGG in complete Freund's adjuvant, and determination of splenic anti-BGG PFC numbers 13 days later. Adoptive assays in general throw the spotlight on a small and atypical subset of primary B cells known as pre-progenitors (2); and the depot of antigen and the long delay between cell transfer and PFC assay might also have allowed stem cells and pre-B cells to have matured in the adoptive host and contributed to the final plaque number (10). That this is likely is shown by the fact that adult spleen, consisting of 50% B cells, gave no more plaques than neonatal liver, containing at most 5% B cells. Thus, in the absence of more work on the assay system, we are reluctant to regard it as a quantitative test for direct progenitor B cells as claimed. The final resolution of this matter is very important, as in physiological situations of the induction of self-tolerance, there are many cases in which the maturing immune system is presented with univalent self antigens. For such cases, the very strong highly multivalent hapten–protein tolerogens represent poor models; our standard oligovalent conjugates are better; but strictly univalent tolerogens would repay much closer study.

CONCLUSIONS

We believe that with the modifications outlined in Fig. 1, the clonal abortion theory has stood the test of time reasonably well. Clonal abortion is clearly not the only mechanism of antigen-induced hyporeactivity, though we believe it to be one of the most important. Whether the principle has equal relevance to tolerance induction among T cells remains to be determined. We attach importance to the clearcut *in vivo* vindication of clonal abortion which our FACS studies have shown. We also think that the model of tolerance induction within 8 hr in FLU-specific immature B cells of homogeneous antigen-binding avidity will present good opportunities for studying the receptor biodynamics and molecular phenomena in B lymphocyte tolerogenesis. For both preparative and analytical studies, the FACS has been an invaluable tool which will continue to add precision and elegance to the studies on the many residual puzzles remaining in the field of B cell differentiation.

ACKNOWLEDGMENTS

This brief review has touched on recent results from many colleagues in my group including: F. L. Battye, M. C. Howard, G. Johnson, T. Kay, P. K. Lala, J. W. Layton, T. Mandel, B. L. Pike, D. W. Scott, K. D. Shortman, J. Teale.

This work was supported by the National Health and Medical Research Council, Canberra, Australia and by Grant Number AI-03958 from the National Institute for Allergy and Infectious Diseases, U.S. Public Health Service.

REFERENCES

1. Howard, J. G. (1972) *Transplant. Rev.* **8**, 50.
2. Nossal, G. J. V., Shortman, K., Howard, M., and Pike, B. L. (1977) *Immunol. Rev.* **37**, 187.
3. Burnet, F. M. (1957) *Aust. J. Sci.* **20**, 67.
4. Nossal, G. J. V., and Pike, B. L. (1975) *J. Exp. Med.* **141**, 904.
5. Osmond, D. G., and Nossal, G. J. V. (1974) *Cell. Immunol.* **13**, 117.
6. Osmond, D. G., and Nossal, G. J. V. (1974) *Cell. Immunol.* **13**, 132.
7. Lala, P. K., Johnson, G. R., Battye, F. L., and Nossal, G. J. V. (1979) *J. Immunol.* **122**, 334–341.
8. Lala, P. K., Layton, J. E., and Nossal, G. J. V. (1978) *Eur. J. Immunol.* (in press).
9. Goding, J. W., Warr, G. W., and Warner, N. L. (1976) *Proc. Natl. Acad. Sci. U.S.A.* **73**, 1305.
10. Nossal, G. J. V., and Pike, B. L. (1975) *In* "Immunological Aspects of Neoplasia" (E. M. Hersh and M. Schlamowitz, eds.), p. 87. Williams & Wilkins, Baltimore, Maryland.
11. Stocker, J. W. (1977) *Immunology* **32**, 283.
12. Metcalf, E. S., and Klinman, N. R. (1976) *J. Exp. Med.* **143**, 1327.
13. Metcalf, E. S., and Klinman, N. R. (1977) *J. Immunol.* **118**, 2111.
14. Nossal, G. J. V., Pike, B. L., and Battye, F. L. (1978) *Eur. J. Immunol.* **8**, 151.
15. Haas, W., and Layton, J. E. (1975) *J. Exp. Med.* **141**, 1004.
16. Nossal, G. J. V., and Pike, B. L. (1978) *J. Exp. Med.* **148**, 1161–1170.
17. Cambier, J. C., Vitetta, E. S., Uhr, J. W., and Kettman, J. R. (1977) *J. Exp. Med.* **145**, 778.
18. Teale, J., M., Howard, M. C. and Nossal, G. J. V. (1978) *J. Immunol.* **121**: 2561–2565.
19. Cambier, J. C., Vitetta, E. S., Kettman, J. R., Wetzel, G., and Uhr, J. W. (1977) *J. Exp. Med.* **146**, 107.
20. Scott, D. W., Layton, J. E., and Nossal, G. J. V. (1977) *J. Exp. Med.* **146**, 1473.
21. Layton, J. E., Pike, B. L., Battye, F. L. and Nossal, G. J. V. *J. Immunol.* Submitted for publication.

22. Borel, Y., and Kilham, L. (1976) *Proc. Soc. Exp. Biol. Med.* **145**, 470.
23. Szewczuk, M. R., Halliday, M., Soybel, T. W., Turner, D., Siskind, G. W., and Weksler, M. E. (1977) *J. Exp. Med.* **145**, 968.
24. Szewczuk, M. R., and Siskind, G. W. (1977) *J. Exp. Med.* **145**, 1590.
25. Venkataraman, M., and Scott, D. W. (1977) *J. Immunol.* **119**, 1879.
26. Kay, T., Battye, F. L., and Nossal, G. J. V. (1978) In preparation.

PART I

IMMUNOGLOBULIN GENES, MESSAGES, AND MOLECULES

Somatic Recombination and Structure of an Immunoglobulin Gene

SUSUMU TONEGAWA, CHRISTINE BRACK,
MINORU HIRAMA, AND
RITA LENHARD-SCHULLER
Basel Institute for Immunology
Basel, Switzerland

INTRODUCTION

Is the organization of DNA sequences altered in cell differentiation? If so, an obvious implication is that such a somatic change might play a key role in cell determination. One of the best systems to which this question can be addressed is that of immunoglobulin genes. Twelve years ago, Dryer and Bennett proposed that a single immunoglobulin chain is encoded in two separate DNA segments, one for the amino terminal half (V region) and the other for the carboxyl terminal half (C region), and that synthesis of a complete chain is preceded by rearrangement of the DNA segments (1). The hypothesis was extended by Gally and Edelman to incorporate a mechanism for somatic generation of the V region diversity (2). Direct investigation into the issue became possible upon discovery of bacterial restriction enzymes. Using a restriction enzyme to digest total cellular DNA of embryo and myeloma cells, Hozumi and Tonegawa produced experimental results that were compatible with the Dryer and Bennett hypothesis (3). Development of the *in vitro* recombinant technique opened a way for further studies on this problem. This paper deals with isolation and characterization of DNA clones containing mouse λ type light chain genes. The study

15

not only provided a direct evidence for somatic recombination but also revealed a surprising feature of the structure of an immunoglobulin gene.

SCHEME FOR ISOLATION OF Ig GNES FROM CELLULAR DNA

Various steps involved in the gene cloning experiment are schematically illustrated in Fig. 1. We first digested highly polymerized total cellular DNA with restriction endonuclease *Eco*RI and fractionated the resulting DNA fragments by electrophoresis in a slab agarose gel. We then identified the DNA fragments carrying specific Ig gene sequences by hybridization. This step was carried out in two different

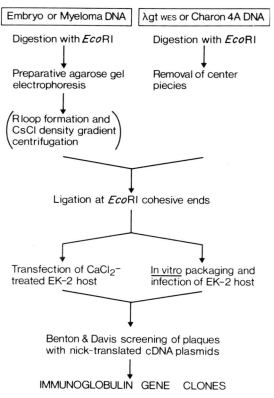

Fig. 1.   Scheme for isolation of immunoglobulin genes. See text for explanation.

ways. Earlier, we had extracted DNA fragments from the gel slices and carried out hybridization in liquid using ^{125}I-labeled, purified Ig mRNA (3). More recently, we synthesized complementary DNA on the purified mRNA template by reverse transcriptase and constructed a plasmid composed of pCRI and Ig DNA sequences. Using chimeric plasmids as the hybridization probes, we applied the blotting technique developed by Southern (4) to a strip of slab gel (5). This procedure obviated the time-consuming extraction step necessary in the liquid hybridization method. Results of the Southern gel blotting of embryo and myeloma DNA's are illustrated in Fig. 2.

The gel electrophoresis step gave 10- to 100-fold enrichment for various Ig gene-positive fragments. In some cases, we further enriched the relevant DNA fragments by incubating the duplex DNA with excess Ig mRNA in 70% formamide and subjected the mixture to equilibrium centrifugation in a CsCl gradient. Since RNA–DNA hybrids are more stable than DNA duplexes in aqueous formamide under certain conditions, one can construct a structure in which duplex DNA is partially denatured and one of the two strands is replaced by complementary RNA (R-loop stucture) (6). Such hybrid molecules are denser than either double- or single-stranded DNA, and therefore can be separated by equilibrium density gradient centrifugation (7). Efficiency of enrichment depends largely on the relative size of the DNA fragments and mRNA molecules. For 4 kb DNA fragments and ~1 kb λ chain mRNA, we obtained enrichment of about fortyfold.

As the cloning vector we used either λgt$_{WES}$ (8) or Charon 4A (9). These phages were attenuated by several genetic tricks to be used specifically in cloning of eukaryotic DNA fragments (EK-2 vectors). When digested with EcoRI, phage DNA's generate left and right arms as well as one or two DNA fragment(s) that originate from the center section of the genome and are dispensible for phage growth. The center pieces were removed by agarose gel electrophoresis. Vector and mouse DNA were mixed and ligated with T4-ligase at the EcoRI cohesive ends.

We used two different methods in generating phage plaques from recombinant DNA molecules. The first method is to transfect a CaCl$_2$-treated Escherichia coli with the naked recombinant DNA molecules (10). The second method is to package the DNA molecules in vitro into phage λ coats and to plate viable phage particles on an ordinary E. coli K12 (11).

Identification of the Ig gene sequence-positive plaques was carried out by the replica method developed by Benton and Davis (12). A plaque plate was covered with a dry nitrocellulose membrane filter to

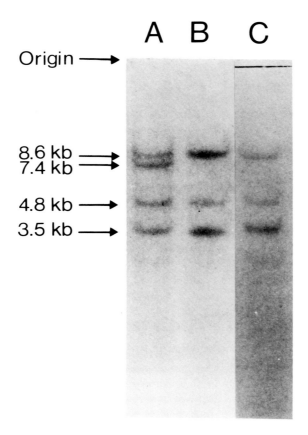

Fig. 2. λ_1 Gene sequence-containing DNA fragments in embryo and myeloma cells. High molecular weight DNA's extracted from 13-day-old BALB/c embryos (B), myelomas HOPC 2020 (a λ_1 chain producer) (A), and MOPC 321 (a κ chain producer) (C) were digested to completion with *Eco* RI, electrophoresed on a 0.9% agarose gel, transferred to nitrocellulose membrane filters, and hybridized with a nicktranslated *Hha* I fragment of the plasmid B1 DNA. This DNA fragment is 2.5 kb long and contains the full (or near full) λ_1 gene sequence (M. Hirama, G. Matthyssens, and S. Tonegawa, unpublished).

absorb the phage particles and unpackaged phage DNA in the plaques. The filter was briefly dipped in an alkali solution to disrupt the phage particles and also to denature DNA, neutralized in Tris buffer, and baked in a vacuum oven to fix the DNA. The filter was then incubated under proper conditions with a radiolabeled hybridization probe (as the probe we used ^{125}I-labeled mRNA or nicktranslated plasmid DNA's containing κ or λ gene sequences), washed extensively, and subjected to autoradiography. Phages in the plaques that gave positive autoradiographic spots were picked, purified, and propagated in an EK-2 host, *E. coli* DP50 SupF[+] (8).

The efficiency of the *in vitro* packaging method is at least one, and usually two, orders of magnitude greater than that of transfection (11). We now obtain over 10^5 plaques by packaging 0.1 μg of mouse DNA fragments (about 10 kb in length, ligated with 0.3 μg of Charon 4A or λgt$_{WES}$ DNA arms) in a standard 40 μl packaging mixture prepared from 10 ml each of the two heat-induced lysogen cultures. This scale of packaging is sufficient for the cloning of a unique mammalian gene, if the DNA preparation used is ten- to twentyfold enriched for the particular gene sequence. The simple preparative agarose gel electrophoresis, combined with Southern gel blotting using a nicktranslated cDNA clone probe, easily provides the necessary enrichment. The plaque screening method developed by Benton and Davis is easy, fast, and reliable. With a little care for controlling various factors that affect the plaque size (time of incubation, humidity of the agar plates), one can obtain as many as 10^5 distinct plaques on a single 20 × 20 cm plate, and thereby process as many plaques for *in situ* hybridization on a single sheet of membrane filter (19 × 19 cm). In summary, the combined use of preparative agarose gel electrophoresis, *in vitro* packaging, and the Benton and Davis plaque screening technique facilitates cloning of essentially any unique mammalian gene, for which hybridization probes are available, by the handling of a few micrograms of total cellular DNA, less than 100 μl of the packaging mix, and one or two large agar plate(s). Because the entire experiment is done on a relatively small scale, it is easy to contain and therefore reduce the chances of accidental escape of hypothetically hazardous clones.

DNA CLONES ISOLATED FROM EMBRYO AND MYELOMA CELLS

We have applied the gene cloning procedures described in the last section to the various DNA components from BALB/c embryos (12 days old) and from both κ-chain secreting (MOPC 321) and λ-chain secreting (HOPC 2020 and J 558) myelomas. In the present paper we

TABLE I

List of λ Chain Gene Clones

Clones	DNA source	DNA pre-enrichment steps	Approximate[a] pre-enrichment factors	Screening procedures and probes	Approximate number of plaques screened	λ Gene[b] sequences contained	References
Ig 99λ	Embryo 3.5 kb	Agarose gel R-looping (one cycle)	300	Benton and Davis (12) with nick-translated cDNA plasmid	3,000	$V_{\lambda I}$	This paper
Ig 25λ	Embryo 8.6 kb	Agarose gel	15		80,000	$C_{\lambda I}$	This paper
Ig 303λ	HOPC 2020 7.4 kb	Agarose gel	15		70,000	$V_{\lambda I} + C_{\lambda I}$	Brack and Tonegawa (16)
Ig 13λ	Embryo 4.8 kb	Agarose gel R-looping (two cycles)	360	Kramer et al. (15) with [^{125}I]λ₁ mRNA	4,000	$V_{\lambda II}$	Tonegawa et al. (7)

[a] See Tonegawa et al. (14) for the definition of the enrichment factor.

[b] This column lists the λ gene-sequences assigned to the cloned DNA's. See text for more details.

shall restrict ourselves to description and discussion of λ gene clones. Four types of λ gene clones were isolated. Three clones, Ig 25λ, Ig 13λ and Ig 99λ, are from the three DNA components visualized by Southern gel blotting of embryo DNA, while the fourth clone is from the DNA component (7.4 kb) that is present only in the myeloma (Fig. 2 and Table I).

TYPE OF λ GENE SEQUENCES CONTAINED IN THE DNA CLONES

In order to find out what kinds of λ gene sequences ($V_λ$, $C_{λI}$, or $V_λ$ plus $C_{λI}$) are contained in the isolated clones, we carried out gel blotting (Southern) experiments with *Eco*RI digested, cloned DNA, using three different λ gene sequences probes. The first probe was the plasmid clone B1 that contains essentially the whole sequence of a $λ_I$ gene. The second probe was a 470 base pair DNA fragment that was excised from the $V_{λII}$-carrying Ig 13λ DNA by restriction endonucleases *Hae*III and *Mbo*II (13). Since $V_{λI}$ and $V_{λII}$ gene sequences are extensively homologous, this DNA fragment serves as a probe for both $V_{λI}$ and $V_{λII}$ gene sequences. The third probe was an approximately 400 base long cDNA that was synthesized on a purified HOPC 2020 $λ_I$ mRNA using the oligo (dT_{12-18}) primer and was isolated by acrylamide gel electrophoresis in 98% formamide. Because of the specificity of the priming activity of the oligo(dT), and the size of the cDNA, this probe mostly contains $C_{λI}$ gene sequences.

When digested with *Eco*RI, the Ig 303λ, Ig 25λ, Ig 99λ, and Ig 13λ DNA generated, in addition to the left (21.5 kb) and right (14 kb) arms of the phage DNA, fragments of 7.4, 8.6, 3.5, and 4.8 kb, respectively. The sizes of these DNA fragments are in good agreement with those assigned to the respective DNA fragments that were visualized by the gel blotting of the total cellular DNA. These DNA fragments all hybridized with the plasmid B1 probe. The 8.6 kb, Ig 25λ fragment hybridized with the $C_{λI}$ probe but not with the $V_λ$ probe. Conversely, the 3.5 kb, Ig 99λ fragments hybridized with the $V_λ$ probe but not with the $C_{λI}$ probe. The 7.4 kb Ig 303λ fragment hybridized with both the $V_λ$ and the $C_{λI}$ probes, while the 4.8 kb, Ig 13λ fragment hybridized with the $V_λ$ probe but not with the $C_{λI}$ probe. In addition, our current nucleotide sequencing studies demonstrated that the $V_λ$ sequence contained in Ig 99λ and Ig 303λ are of the $λ_I$ type (N. Hozumi, O. Bernard, and S. Tonegawa, unpublished observations). The assigned λ gene sequences are listed in Table I.

LOCATION OF THE λ CHAIN GENE SEQUENCE IN THE DNA CLONES

The position of λ chain gene sequences in the DNA clones was determined by R-loop mapping (6). The clones Ig 303λ DNA was incubated with HOPC 2020 λ chain mRNA under the conditions for R-loop formation. Upon examination in the electron microscope, more than 50% of the molecules displayed DNA–RNA hybrid regions. However, we did not observe the single R-loop of about 1000-nucleotide length that would have been expected if the mRNA had hybridized with a stretch of DNA corresponding to contiguous V and C gene sequences. Instead, two small R-loops (460 and 380 base long) separated by a double-stranded DNA loop (1.2 kb) were observed (Fig. 3). The interpretation of such a hybrid structure is that one RNA molecule is annealed to two stretches of DNA that are separated by a duplex DNA region. In many cases the hybrid segment or R-loop generated by the longer homology had a short whisker (50–100 nucleotides) at its left end. The whisker is probably the poly(A) at the 3′ end of the mRNA. This suggests that the longer homology is composed of the C gene sequence and that the shorter one is composed of the V gene sequence. The validity of this assumption was confirmed by analysis of the heteroduplexes formed between the Ig 303λ DNA and a V_λ gene-carrying DNA fragment (16).

R-loop molecules formed with the 8.6 kb, Ig 25λ fragment displayed a double loop structure composed of a 410 nucleotide R-loop at 3.9 kb from one and, and a 1.2 kb double-stranded DNA loop (Fig. 3). This structure closely resembles the triple loop of Ig 303λ, except that the Ig 25λ hybrids have a long RNA tail (~260 bases) instead of the second, smaller R-loop. Because the Ig 25λ fragment showed homology only with $C_{\lambda I}$, but not with V_λ sequences (see above), we conclude that the 410 base pair R-loop contains the $C_{\lambda I}$ gene sequence, and that the long RNA tail corresponds to the 5′-end or V-coding part of the mRNA. A second, short RNA tail (~100 bases) observed sometimes at the other end of the R-loop would correspond to the poly(A) sequence at the 3′-end of the mRNA. The presence of the 1.2 kb DNA loop indicates that Ig 25λ DNA contains a short homology region that hybridizes to a region near the V–C junction of the mRNA molecule. This second homology, which we call the J sequence, is separated from the $C_{\lambda I}$

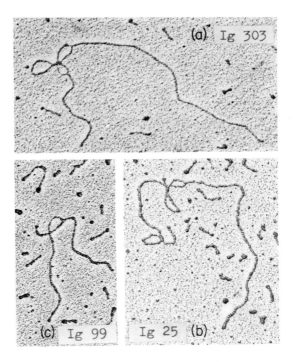

Fig. 3. R-loop molecules obtained by hybridizing HOPC 2020 λ_l mRNA with the *Eco* RI fragments of the DNA clones. (a) Ig 303λ DNA showed two R-loops corresponding to the V and C genes that are separated by the double-stranded DNA loop of about 1.2 kb. The short tail at the end of one loop is the 3′ poly(A). (b) Ig 25λ DNA displays one R-loop corresponding to the C gene, the double-stranded DNA loop, and a long RNA tail corresponding to V sequences. The short tail observed in some molecules is the 3′ poly (A) tail. (c) Ig 99λ DNA has one R-loop corresponding to V sequences, and a long RNA tail that is composed of the C gene sequences plus poly(A) tail.

sequence by 1200 base pairs. It is too short to be visualized as a separate R-loop but is strong enough to hold the double loop structure together.

The 3.5 kb, Ig 99λ fragment formed a single R-loop very similar to the one observed in Ig 13λ (7). It is 380 nucleotides long, lies in the middle of the DNA fragment, i.e., 1.65–1.66 kb from either end, and carriers a ~340 nucleotide RNA tail at one end. Since this DNA fragment contains a $V_{\lambda l}$ sequence (see above), the R-loop should contain the $V_{\lambda l}$ sequence and the RNA tail should correspond to the $C_{\lambda l}$ sequence plus the poly(A).

SEQUENCE HOMOLOGY BETWEEN THE CLONED DNA FRAGMENTS

Analysis of sequence homology between the cloned DNA fragments, both within the λ chain genes and in the adjacent regions, may be helpful in discovering the mechanism by which somatic rearrangement of immunoglobulin genes occurs. The four cloned fragments were therefore hybridized in various combinations and the heteroduplex molecules analyzed by electron microscopy. We shall describe below the observations made with various combinations of the three λ_I DNA clones Ig 99λ, Ig 25λ, and Ig 303λ. A summary of all the results is given in Fig. 4.

Ig 25λ VERSUS Ig 303λ

Ig 25λ hybridized with Ig 303λ DNA to form Y-shaped heteroduplex molecules with two single-stranded and one double-stranded arms (Fig. 5). The lengths of the three arms are: 2.87 kb (long single strand), 1.98 kb (short single strand), and 5.47 kb (double strand). The measurements indicate that the shorter single-stranded arm and one strand of the double-stranded arm correspond to the Ig 303λ DNA, whereas the longer single-stranded arm and the other strand of the double-stranded arm derive from the Ig 25λ DNA. In the entire 5.5 kb homology region we observed no local mismatchings that would indicate partial nonhomology between the two strands. R-loop mapping had

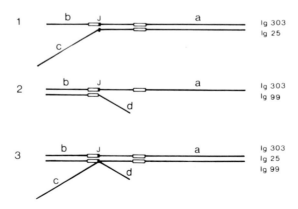

Fig. 4. Interpretation of the heteroduplex molecules. The position of V and C gene sequences (white boxes) was deduced from R-loop molecules.

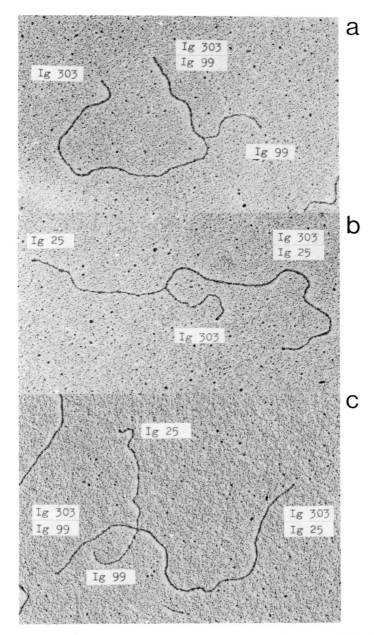

Fig. 5. Heteroduplex molecules formed by various combinations of the three λI sequence-containing cloned DNA fragments. (a) Myeloma DNA Ig 303λ versus embryo DNA Ig 99λ; (b) myeloma DNA Ig 303λ versus embryo DNA Ig 25λ; (c) combination of all three clones gave double heteroduplex structures.

shown that in both DNA fragments the $C_{\lambda I}$ gene lies between 3.8 and 4.2 kb from one end. The 5.5 kb homology region therefore contains the $C_{\lambda I}$ gene. In addition, most if not all of the 1.2 kb DNA segment separating the V and C sequences in the Ig 303λ fragment is highly homologous to the DNA segment of similar length that separates the J and C sequences in the Ig 25λ fragment. The measurements indicated that the J sequence lies very near or at the branch point of the heteroduplex.

Ig 99λ versus Ig 303λ

These two fragments also formed Y-shaped heteroduplex molecules with two single-stranded (5.48 and 1.53 kb) and one double-stranded (1.98 kb) arms (Fig. 5). The sum of the lengths of the long single-stranded arm and the double-stranded arm corresponds to the length of the Ig 303λ fragment, whereas the short single strand and the second strand of the double-stranded region belong to the Ig 99λ fragment. Again, we did not observe any local nonhomology in the double-stranded part of the heteroduplex. These results indicate that on one end of each fragment, the two DNA's are highly homologous. The V_λ sequence lies between 1.66 and 2.0 kb from one end of both Ig 303λ and Ig 99λ DNA's. Therefore the V gene is within the 2.0 kb homology region and lies near the fork of the Y-shaped heteroduplex (Fig. 5).

Ig 303, Ig 25, and Ig 99

The results described in the last two sections strongly suggest that a large part of the Ig 303 fragment (5.5 kb) is homologous to the Ig 25 DNA whereas the rest of the molecule (2 kb) is homologous to the Ig 99 DNA.

In order to confirm this, the three DNA fragments were mixed, denatured, and annealed. A low proportion of the molecules displayed a double heteroduplex structure or cruciform structure composed of the double-stranded and two single-stranded arms (Fig. 5). Measurements of the arms allowed us to assign each part of the hybrid to the three DNA fragments as illustrated in Fig. 4. The observed structure can be formed only if each of the two ends of the Ig 303 fragment is homologous to only one of the two DNA fragments Ig 99 or Ig 25. The two homology regions meet at a point which corresponds to the J sequence in Ig 25 and lies near the junction between the V sequence and the 1.2 kb intron of Ig 303 DNA. The myeloma DNA fragment, Ig 303, thus seems to be entirely composed of DNA segments that are homologous to parts of the two embryonic fragments.

EVIDENCE FOR SOMATIC REARRANGEMENT OF IMMUNOGLOBULIN GENES

The heteroduplex analysis of the three λ_I DNA clones, combined with the gel blotting analysis of the total cellular DNA's demonstrated beyond doubt the occurrence of somatic rearrangements of immunoglobulin gene sequences. The double heteroduplex structure generated by co-annealing the three cloned λ_I DNA's is incompatible with the trivial alternative interpretation (3) of the results obtained by restriction enzyme mapping of total cellular DNA. The observed heteroduplex structures can not be artifacts of DNA cloning. The length of each of the cloned DNA fragments coincides well with that of the corresponding cellular DNA fragments visualized by the gel blotting technique. Furthermore, certain restriction enzyme sites identified in the cloned DNA's are also present at corresponding positions in cellular DNA (5).

The results reported here identified a single recombination site on each of the two embryonic DNA clones. These sites were visualized as the branch point of the Y-shaped heteroduplex molecules formed between the cloned myeloma DNA (Ig 303λ) and either of the two cloned embryonic DNA's (Ig 99λ and Ig 25λ). That the branch points correspond to a single site on the Ig 303λ DNA was suggested by the double heteroduplex structure, in which two single-stranded tails, one of Ig 99λ and the other of Ig 25λ, extend from a single site on the Ig 303λ DNA. We conclude that the three cloned λ_I DNA's are related by a single recombination event as illustrated in Fig. 6. Embryonic DNA recombines at the right end of the V sequence and the left end of the J sequence to generate the sequence arrangement present in myeloma DNA. The entire 1.2 kb intron in the Ig 303λ DNA originates from the Ig 25λ DNA. Measurements of various parts of the R-loops and heteroduplex structures described in the present work are entirely consistent with this model. Further support has come from our more recent nucleotide sequencing studies (O. Bernard, N. Hozumi, and S. Tonegawa, unpublished results). These studies revealed that the Ig 303 V DNA segment codes for the polypeptide chain consecutively for a length corresponding to a complete V-region as defined by amino acid sequence studies, whereas the Ig 99λ V DNA segment ceases to

Embryo DNA

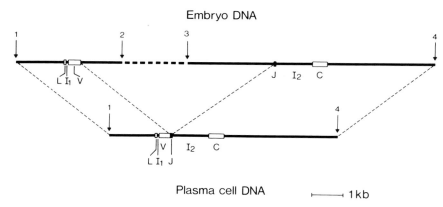

Plasma cell DNA   ⊢———⊣ 1 kb

Fig. 6. Arrangement of mouse λ_I gene sequences in embryos and λ_I chain-producing plasma cells. In embryo DNA a full κ_I gene sequence is split into two parts that lie separately on two *Eco* RI fragments. On one, the coding sequence is further split into two parts, one for most of the leader peptides (L) and the other for the rest of the leader peptides plus the variable region peptides (V). The two coding sequences are separated by a 93 nucleotide long intron (I_1) (N. Hozumi, O. Bernard, and S. Tonegawa, unpublished observation). On the second *Eco* RI fragment the coding sequence is also split into two parts by a 1250 base long intron (I_2). The two parts are for the constant region peptides (C) and about 13 residue peptides near the junction of the variable and constant regions (J). The relative orientation of and the distance between the two *Eco* RI fragments are unknown. In the DNA of a λ_I chain-producing myeloma (HOPC 2020) the λ_I gene sequence is rearranged as a result of one or more recombination(s) that involve sequences in the two embryonic *Eco* RI fragments. One recombination takes place at the ends of the V and the J sequences and brings the two sequences directly in contact. The limits of the corresponding sequences in the embryo and the myeloma DNA's are indicated by thin dotted lines. The Figure is not intended to imply that the recombination results in deletion or looping-out of the embryonic DNA sequences that lie between the V and the *Eco* RI site 2, or between the *Eco* RI site 3 and the J. It is not intended to imply that the embryo and myeloma V sequences are identical. Additional short introns may be present in the C sequences. Arrows with numbers indicate *Eco* RI sites.

code at residue 97. This suggests that the nucleotides necessary to code for the extra amino acids at the end of the Ig 303λ V region are contributed by the J sequence on the Ig 25λ DNA. Our correct sequencing study of the J region confirmed this contention.

GENE IN PIECES

The R-loop mapping demonstrated the presence of a 1.2 kb intron both on the Ig 303λ and the Ig 25λ DNA. The resolution of cytochrome spreadings will not allow detection of introns shorter than about 100 nucleotides. Indeed, the 93 base long intron near the region corresponding to the amino terminal of the Ig 13λ DNA was revealed only by nucleotide sequence determination (13). Our recent nucleotide sequencing studies (O. Bernard, N. Hozumi, and S. Tonegawa) established that both Ig 303λ and Ig 99λ DNA contain an intron equivalent to that of Ig 13λ both in length and position. These findings are incorporated into Fig. 6. It should be added that additional short introns may be revealed in the C DNA sequence by the nucleotide sequencing now in progress in this laboratory. In any case, in each of the three λ$_I$ DNA clones the protein-coding sequences are arranged in discrete pieces. For instance, the somatically rearranged, complete λ$_I$ gene in the myeloma (Ig 303λ) consists of at least three DNA segments, one coding for the leader, one for the V region, and one for the C region. The introns separating the three coding segments are present in the original mouse DNA and are not introduced during the cloning procedure. The unique restriction enzyme cleavage sites that have been identified within the introns of the cloned DNA were also demonstrated in the uncloned cellular DNA (5).

Recent studies on other genes of eukaryotes (17–22), as well as their viruses (23–26) have revealed several cases of this unexpected gene structure: informational DNA interspersed with introns (silent sequences). Introns are probably transcribed together with the informational DNA and subsequently excised during maturation of pre-mRNA. One recent experiment concerning the mouse globin β chain gene seems to support this hypothesis (27). These observations have led us to propose an additional evolutionary pathway for creation of genes in higher organisms (13). By this pathway, a new gene can be created from two or more separate DNA segments upon emergence, at the boundary of the DNA segments, of mutations that generate signals for RNA splicing. If the new polypeptide chain coded by the spliced RNA has survival value, such mutations may be fixed in evolution. As the splicing does not have to be 100% efficient, creation of the new gene need not destroy the old: usually a disadvantageous event.

We assume that RNA splicing is an intramolecular reaction. This will restrict the operation of the gene creation mechanism described above to the space of a single transcription unit. One way to enlarge the effectiveness of this gene creation mechanism is to shuffle DNA segments by introducing them into transcription units. DNA sequences thus newly introduced into a transcription unit are then available for splicing with pre-existing sequences. Actual evolutionary use of such DNA sequences depends on the emergence of mutations leading to new splicing signals at the proper positions in the transcription unit. We hypothesize that many genes in higher organisms have arisen through such evolutionary processes.

SOMATIC REARRANGEMENT AS A MECHANISM FOR GENE CONTROL IN CELL DIFFERENTIATION

Does a higher organism utilize such a gene creation mechanism in the normal process of cell differentiation? We consider that the immunoglobulin genes are the perfect example. Here, the J sequence seems to play a key role by providing a "bridge" between DNA recombination and RNA splicing. Its left half most probably contains a nucleotide sequence for a site-specific recombination with the V DNA segment, while the sequence in the right half would almost certainly be involved in the RNA splicing event that connects the V and C sequences.

When a gene is created in this manner during ontogeny only in a particular subpopulation of cells composing an organism, the recombination itself can provide a novel mechanism for gene control in cell differentiation. The somatic rearrangement involving particular immunoglobulin gene sequences seem to be restricted to a small subpopulation of cells. Arrangement of a κ chain sequence in DNA's of several nonlymphatic adult tissues was identical to that of embryo DNA when analyzed by the electrophoresis–hybridization assay (28; also M. Hirama, unpublished observation). Analogous experiments carried out using DNA from a λ_I chain-producing myeloma and a κ sequence probe and *vice versa* indicated that there is a mutual exclusion in rearrangement of κ and λ chain DNA sequences (28). The results shown in Fig. 2 gave an additional example, namely that the 7.4 kb *Eco*RI fragment carrying the rearranged full λ_I gene sequence is absent in the DNA of κ-producing MOPC 321. It should be added that presence of the 7.4 kb fragment is not peculiar to HOPC 2020 myeloma DNA. DNA's from other λ_I-producing myelomas studied (MOPC 104E and J 558) also contained this fragment. [The $V_{\lambda I}$ regions synthesized by these myelomas are identical and differ from HOPC 2020 $V_{\lambda I}$ region by two residues (29), but all $V_{\lambda I}$ regions are believed to share an identical germ line V gene (30).] Conversely, absence of the 7.4 kb fragment is not peculiar to MOPC 321 DNA. DNA's from other κ chain-producing myelomas studied (TEPC 124 and MOPC 21) gave no such fragment (M. Hirama, unpublished observations).

On the molecular level one can conceive many variations of a gene control mechanism operated by somatic DNA rearrangement. For instance, in the case of immunoglobulin genes, a V sequence-carrying DNA segment that has been transcriptionally silent may be excised and inserted into a constitutively active transcription unit containing the C sequence. Alternatively, the act of V DNA insertion itself may create a new promoter at the very site of insertion. As we previously discussed (16), a gene control mechanism directly dependent on somatic sequence rearrangement in DNA seems to fulfill most easily the "one lymphocyte clone–one light chain" rule of the immune system.

ACKNOWLEDGMENTS

We are very grateful to Dr. B. Hohn for invaluable help in the packaging experiments. We thank Dr. W. Arber, Dr. J. Carbon, Dr. R. Curtis, Dr. P. Leder, and Drs. K. and N. E. Murray for bacteria and phage strains. We also thank Dr. J. Beard, Dr. N. Hozumi, Dr. C. P. Kung, and Dr. J. Summers for enzymes, and Dr. G. Matthyssens who participated in the construction of the Bl plasmid. We are grateful to Mr. G. Dastoornikoo, Mr. A. Traunecker, and Mrs. R. Hiestand for their expert technical assistance.

REFERENCES

1. Dryer, W. J., and Bennett, J. C. (1965) *Proc. Natl. Acad. Sci. U.S.A.* **54**, 864–879.
2. Gally, J. A., and Edelman, G. M. (1970) *Nature (London)* **227**, 341–346.
3. Hozumi, N., and Tonegawa, S. (1976) *Proc. Natl. Acad. Sci. U.S.A.* **73**, 3628–3232.
4. Southern, E. M. (1975) *J. Mol. Biol.* **98**, 503–518.
5. Brack, C., Hirama, M., and Lenhard-Schuller, R. (1978) *Cell* **15**, 1–14.
6. White, R. L., and Hogness, D. S. (1977) *Cell* **10**, 177–192.
7. Tonegawa, S., Brack, C., Hozumi, N., and Schuller, R. (1977) *Proc. Natl. Acad. Sci. U.S.A.* **74**, 3518–3522.
8. Leder, P., Tiemeier, D., and Enquist, L. (1977) *Science* **196**, 175–177.
9. Blattner, F., Williams, B. G., Blechl, A. E., Denniston-Thompson, K., Faber, H. E., Furlong, L., Grunwald, D. J., Kiefer, D. O., Moore, D. D., Schumm, J. W., Sheldon, E. L., and Smithies, O. (1977) *Science* **196**, 161–169.
10. Mandel, M., and Hoga, A. (1970) *J. Mol. Biol.* **78**, 453–471.
11. Hohn, B., and Murray, K. (1977) *Proc. Natl. Acad. Sci. U.S.A.* **74**, 3259–3263.
12. Benton, W. D., and Davis, R. W. (1977) *Science* **196**, 180–182.
13. Tonegawa, S., Maxam, A. M., Tizard, R., Bernard, O., and Gilbert, W. (1978) *Proc. Natl. Acad. Sci. U.S.A.* **75**, 1488–1489.
14. Tonegawa, S., Hozumi, N., Matthyssens, G., and Schuller, R. (1976) *Cold Spring Harbor Symp. Quant. Biol.* **41**, 877–889.
15. Kramer, R. A., Cameron, J. R., and Davis, R. W. (1976) *Cell* **8**, 227–232.
16. Brack, C., and Tonegawa, S. (1977) *Proc. Natl. Acad. Sci. U.S.A.* **74**, 5652–5656.
17. Glover, D. M., and Hogness, D. S. (1977) *Cell* **10**, 167–176.
18. Wellauer, P. K., and David, I. B. (1977) *Cell* **10**, 193–212.

19. Breathnach, R., Mandel, J. L., and Chambon, P. (1977) *Nature (London)* **270**, 314–319.
20. Jeffreys, A., and Flavell, R. (1977) *Cell* **12**, 1097–1107.
21. Goodman, H. M., Olson, M. V., and Hall, B. D. (1978) *Proc. Natl. Acad. Sci. U.S.A.* **74**, 5453–5457.
22. Tilghman, S. M., Tiemeier, D. C., Seidman, J. G., Peterlin, B. M., Sullivan, M., Maizel, J. V., and Leder, P. (1978) *Proc. Natl. Acad. Sci. U.S.A.* **75**, 725–729.
23. Berget, S. M., Moore, C., and Sharp, P. A. (1977) *Proc. Natl. Acad. Sci. U.S.A.* **74**, 3171–3175.
24. Chow, L. T., Gelinas, R. E., Broker, T. R., and Robert, R. J. (1977) *Cell* **12**, 1–8.
25. Klessig, D. F. (1977) *Cell* **12**, 9–21.
26. Aloni, Y., Dhar, R., Laub, O., Horowitz, M., and Khoury, G. (1977) *Proc. Natl. Acad. Sci. U.S.A.* **74**, 3686–3690.
27. Tilghman, S. M., Curtis, P. J., Tiemeier, D. C., Leder, P., and Weissmann, C. (1978) *Proc. Natl. Acad. Sci. U.S.A.* **75**, 1309–1313.
28. Tonegawa, S., Brack, C., Hozumi, N., and Pirrotta, V. (1977) *Cold Spring Harbor Symp. Quant. Biol.* **42**, 921–931.
29. Weigert, M. G., Cesari, I. M., Yonkovich, S. J., and Cohn, M. (1970) *Nature (London)* **228**, 1045–1049.
30. Tonegawa, S. (1976) *Proc. Natl. Acad. Sci. U.S.A.* **73**, 203–207.

Implications of the Assortment of Framework Segments for the Assembly of Immunoglobulin V_L and V_H Regions and the Generation of Diversity

ELVIN A. KABAT

Departments of Microbiology, Human Genetics and Development, and Neurology
Columbia University
New York, New York
and
The National Cancer Institute
National Institutes of Health
Bethesda, Maryland

Data were recently presented (1) that the various framework segments (FR1, FR2, FR3, and FR4) of immunoglobulin V-region light (V_L) and heavy chains (V_H) could be sorted into sets, members of each FR set having an identical sequence. When each chain was traced, it was seen that members of a given set in FR1 could be associated with the same or different sets in FR2, FR3, and FR4 and these associations appeared to be random. The residues which comprise the framework (FR) and complementarity-determining regions or segments (CDR) are given in Table I. The data are given in Figs. 1–4. Of substantial significance were the findings that an FR2 segment of fifteen residues (35–49) of V_L was identical in eight rabbit, four mouse, and one human chains indicating substantial preservation of this segment over evolutionary time, of the order of 80 million years. An FR4 segment of ten residues (98–107) in V_L of human $V_\kappa I$, also oc-

33

ELVIN A. KABAT

TABLE I
**Framework (FR) and Complementarity-Determining (CDR)
Residues of V-regions of Light and Heavy Chains**

	V_L	V_H		V_L	V_H
FR1	1–23	1–30	CDR1	24–34	31–35B
FR2	35–49	36–49	CDR2	50–56	50–65
FR3	57–88	66–94	CDR3	89–97	95–102
FR4	98–107	103–113			

curred in V_κII, V_κIII, and V_κIV, and an FR4 segment of eleven residues was seen in two mouse and one human V_HIII.

The genetic units for an immunoglobulin framework are thus defined not as a stretch of DNA coding for the entire V_L or V_H framework,

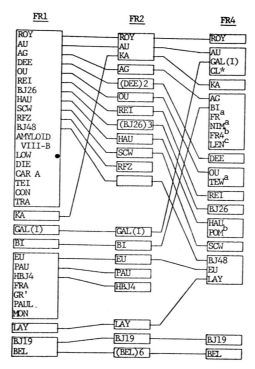

Fig. 1. Assembly of the frameworks of human V_κI chains by assortment of FR sets. ●, Cold agglutinin with anti-blood group I activity; (a) human κ light chain subgroup II; (b) human κ light chain subgroup III; (c) human κ light chain subgroup IV. From Kabat et al. (1).

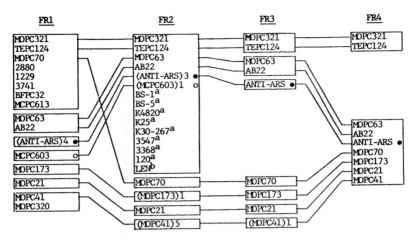

Fig. 2. Assembly of the frameworks of mouse V_κ chains by assortment of FR sets. ●, Anti-p-azophenylarsonate; ○, Anti-phosphocholine; (a) rabbit κ light chain; (b) human κ light chain subgroup IV. From Kabat *et al.* (1).

as has been almost universally accepted, but as smaller stretches coding for the individual FR segments and we have termed these minigenes (1).

These findings resolve many of the earlier difficulties but also require extensive rethinking of the hypotheses for the genetic control of immunoglobulin chains and for the generation of antibody diversity. The following inferences follow directly from the data:

(1) Earlier studies on subgrouping of V_L (4–6) and V_H (7,8) regions of various species were based entirely on FR1 and could never be extended to the rest of the framework. It is clear from Figs. 1–4 that, since the sets for each FR are independent of one another, subgrouping the entire framework sequence is not possible. Moreover, even in the inbred mouse, subgrouping of V_κ chains into isotypes (9) based entirely on FR1 required including chains with three amino acid differences as belonging to a given isotype; these differences were ascribed to somatic mutation. The ability to classify mouse V_κ chains into sets with multiple members of identical sequences in FR1, makes the somatic mutation hypothesis unnecessary.

(2) It has been suggested that if one accepted somatic mutation as occurring and rearranged the data in Figs. 1–4 in order of increasing numbers of amino acid differences from a prototype, the set with the greatest number of members, the assortment of minigene sets would not be random. Figures 5, 6, and 7 show the results of such a

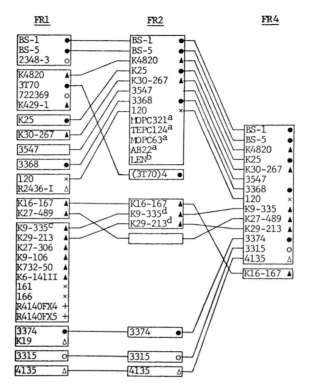

Fig. 3. Assembly of the frameworks of rabbit V_κ chains by assortment of FR sets. ●, Anti-type III pneumococcal polysaccharide; ○, anti-type VIII pneumococcal polysaccharide; ▲, anti-streptococcal group A variant carbohydrate; △, anti-streptococcal group C carbohydrate; +, anti-p-azophenylarsonate; ×, anti-*Micrococcus lysodeikticus;* (a) mouse κ light chain; (b) human κ light chain subgroup IV; (c) K9-335 has the same sequence as K9-338; (d) the residue at position 36 (2) has been changed from Tyr to Phe for K29-213, K9-335, and K9-338 (3). From Kabat *et al.* (1).

rearrangement of Figs. 1–3. The set at the top for each FR segment is the prototype; above it is listed the amino acid for each position at which another set differs from it. The amino acid differences from the prototype set at each position are then given above each of the other sets. Substitutions which involve two or three base changes are given in parentheses alongside the amino acid.

It is evident from Figs. 5–7 that attempting to order the sets has made Figs. 2–4 much more complex and that the number of crossovers has substantially increased. Thus the assortment of the FR sets is totally unrelated to the number of amino acid differences between the

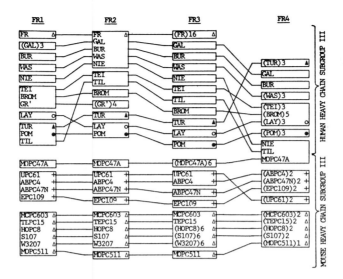

Fig. 4. Assembly of the frameworks of human and of mouse V_HIII chains by assortment of FR sets. ●, Anti-human gamma G1 globulin; ○, anti-human gamma G1 and G3 globulin; ▲, cold agglutinin with anti-blood group I activity; △, anti-phosphocholine; +, anti-β2 → 1-fructosan. From Kabat et al. (1).

prototype set and the other FR sets. These findings and the substantial number of two and three base changes also eliminate somatic mutation as a significant mechanism for the variation in framework sequences.

(3) The generation of V-region frameworks by assortment of the minigene sets increases by several orders of magnitude the numbers of different frameworks over that proposed earlier on the assumption that the structural genes for the entire framework corresponded in number to subgroups or isotypes, each of which was considered to represent a germ-line gene for the entire framework. Thus if these different minigene sets are all present in the germ line already assorted and joined to the three complementarity-determining segments as proposed by Tonegawa et al. (10) and by (P. Seidman et al. (10a) et al. (personal communication)[1] from their cloning studies, one has arrived at a germ-line theory far more complex than had ever been envisioned and which is clearly contrary to the hybridization studies (11) which have uniformly indicated the presence of a small number of V_κ and V_λ genes. This is not so if the DNA coding each complete V domain is assembled by recombining the various germ-line minigenes for the framework with those for the CDR.

(4) Generation of the V-region frameworks from minigene sets

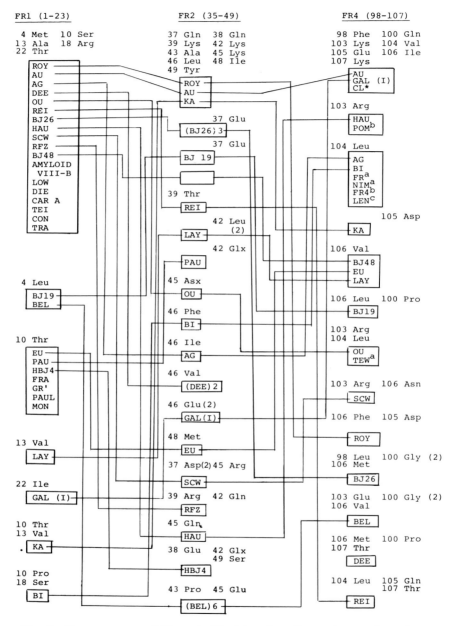

Fig. 5. Rearrangement of FR sets in Fig. 1 in order of increasing numbers of amino acid differences from the prototype. The top set of each FR represents the prototype; the numbers and amino acids given above it indicate the residues present and which residues differ in other sets. The number and amino acid above each of the other sets indicates the position and residue at which the set differs from the prototype. Two and three base changes from the prototype are indicated in parentheses. See Fig. 3 for definition of symbols.

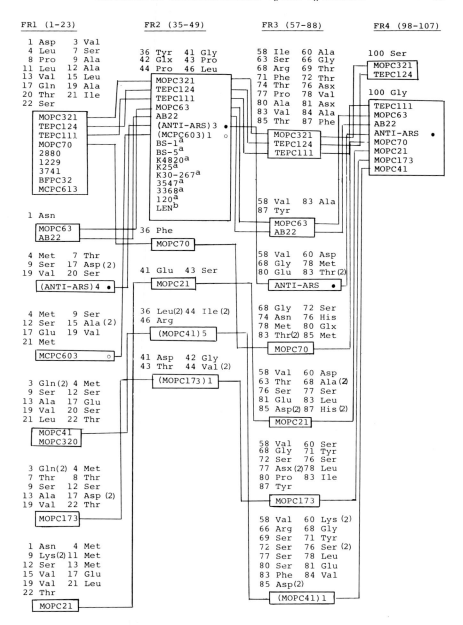

Fig. 6. Rearrangement of FR sets in Fig. 2 in order of increasing numbers of amino acid differences from the prototype. (Sets are ordered as described in **Fig. 5**). See **Fig. 3** for definition of symbols.

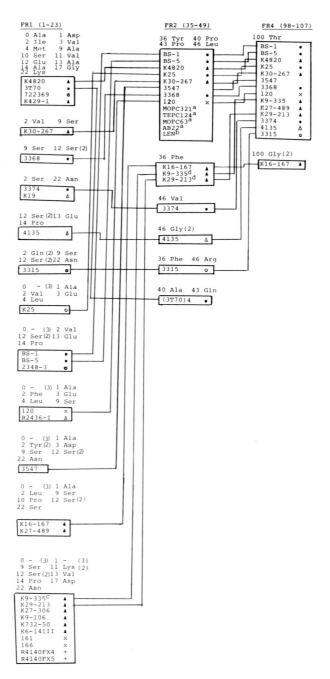

Fig. 7. Rearrangement of FR sets in Fig. 3 in order of increasing numbers of amino acid differences from the prototype. (Sets are ordered as described in Fig. 5). See Fig. 3 for definition of symbols.

increases the number of possible idiotypic determinants by several orders of magnitude and accounts completely for the findings of Oudin and Casenave (12,13) that antibodies of given specificity may have many different idiotypic specificities and that antibodies of different specificities as well as antibodies and immunoglobulins lacking known antibody specificity from the same immunized animal may show cross-reactive idiotypes. Idiotypic determinants could be of several types (14) depending on whether the idiotypic determinant involved: (1) residues making up the CDR; (2) those making up the CDR as well as those making up one or another of the FR segments; and (3) those involving only FR segments. In addition, since many idiotypic specifities may be expressed only when the light and heavy chains are combined (15) and although there is frequently an apparent linkage of idiotype to heavy chain allotypes, such idiotypes may require the presence of both V_H and V_L and thus not be determined solely by the structure of V_H. The a allotypes, however, which appear to involve residues in FR1 and FR3 have been shown to be linked to C-region allotypes (16).

In view of these conclusions it was hypothesized (1) that the minigene sets generating the immunoglobulin framework together with the three CDR were assembled somatically during differentiation and embryonic development by a process of recombination or insertion, perhaps involving intervening sequences. This hypothesis has the advantage of requiring only a limited number of germ-line FR genes from which the entire repertoire of V-region sequences could be generated. The CDR segments represent an additional order of diversity since only a few instances with identical CDR have been found (3,17,18) and one suspects that the germ-line minigenes for the CDR will be found separated in the genome from those for the FR, and that some insertional mechanism of assembly as originally proposed by Wu and Kabat (19) and subsequently by Capra and Kindt (20,21) will be involved.

The findings of Tonegawa et $al.$ (10) that in the 12-day mouse embryo a phage clone containing mouse V_λ DNA sequences had a linear sequence of nucleotides coding for residues 1–96 (numbering as in Kabat et $al.$, 1) and similar findings with phage clones of mouse V_κ chains by P. Seidman et $al.$ (10a) from adult myeloma, has been taken to indicate that the genome contained the DNA coding for this stretch in a linear sequence. However, all of these clones lack FR4. All X-ray crystallographic studies (22–26, cf. 27,28) show FR4 to be an integral part of the V_L and V_H domains and involved in formation of a β-sheet for the V framework. Attachment of the DNA for FR4 to the

DNA for the rest of the V region could thus be crucial for the transcription of the complete V_H and V_L domains and the biosynthesis of the entire chain.

Translation of the nucleotide sequences of the mouse V_λ clone from 12-day-old mouse embryo into amino acids (10) and comparison of these with the reported amino acid sequences showed that the framework portion could just as well be viewed as a double recombinant (1) of FR1 and FR3 from $V_\lambda II$ with an FR2 from $V_\lambda I$ rather than as a somatic mutation. It thus appears possible that the cell of the 12-day-old mouse embryo donating the DNA might already have differentiated to an extent at which all the DNA for all 96 residues was already in a continuous sequence, and it was therefore proposed (1) that the hypothesis that the minigenes were separated in the genome could then be tested only by examining sperm DNA, which would contain a representation of germ-line DNA. In such studies one must be especially careful to separate the sperm from the somatic cells present in semen (29) which could lead to erroneous results. The finding of FR sets of identical sequence in several species makes it possible both to obtain clones and to hybridize sperm DNA from species such as rabbit and man with mouse mRNA or cDNA, to attempt to locate these minigene sequences, to determine the number of copies present, and to see if intervening sequences are present.

Brack *et al.* (30) have now isolated another clone from H2020, a mouse λ myeloma, and have found the genetic information for the V and C domains in the same clone. The nucleotides for the entire V region exist in a continuous sequence with a 1250 base intervening sequence between the V and C regions. Thus the hypothesis (1) of somatic assembly during differentiation to the adult myeloma is already established for FR4.

One could also approach the problem of identifying the minigene sets by obtaining antisera to the various FR segments. FR peptides are now well within the capacity of synthetic methods. With antisera to FR1, FR2, FR3, and FR4 peptides coupled to insoluble absorbents, serum immunoglobulins and antibodies could be fractionated and examined to identify framework recombinants.

One could also carry out breeding studies in various species, immunizing the various generations to obtain monoclonal antibodies to dextrans, pneumococcal type specific and streptococcal group specific antibodies and use the antisera to the FR segments in studying the assortment of the framework segments. A similar study could be attempted by obtaining antibodies to the CDR segments and searching for identical CDR sequences.

Another approach would be to isolate nucleotide sequences of FR sets and to use these as probes to identify sets in DNA of germ line and somatic cells by hybridization and by cloning. It might also be possible to synthesize the oligonucleotide probes for various minigene sets, taking account of the nucleotide sequences found in clones to avoid uncertainties in the third base. In addition one could look for the minigene sets in chromosomes by *in situ* hybridization techniques.

It is evident that the demonstration of the seemingly random assortment of framework segments of immunoglobulin chains is opening a new phase in the search for understanding the generation of antibody diversity.

ACKNOWLEDGMENTS

Work of the laboratories is supported by a grant from the National Science Foundation NSF 76-81029. The data base of variable region sequences is maintained in the PRO-PHET computer system sponsored by the National Cancer Institute, National Institute of Allergy and Infectious Diseases, National Institute of Arthritis, Metabolism and Digestive Diseases, National Institute of General Medical Sciences, and the Division of Research Resources (Contract No. N01-RR-4-2147), of the National Institutes of Health.

REFERENCES

1. Kabat, E. A., Wu, T. T., and Bilofsky, H. (1978) *Proc. Natl. Acad. Sci. U.S.A.* **75,** 2429–2433.
2. Kabat, E. A., Wu, T. T., and Bilofsky, H. (1976) "Variable Regions of Immunoglobulin Chains." Bolt, Beranek & Newman, Cambridge, Massachusetts.
3. Braun, D. G., and Huser, H. (1977) *Prog. Immunol. Proc. 3rd Int. Cong. Immunol. 1977* pp. 255–264.
4. Milstein, C. (1967) *Nature (London)* **216,** 330–332.
5. Niall, H., and Edman, P. (1967). *Nature (London)* **216,** 262–263.
6. Hood, L., Gray, W. R., Sanders, B. G., and Dreyer, W. J. (1967) *Cold Spring Harbor Symp. Quant. Biol.* **32,** 133–145.
7. Barstad, P., Farnsworth, V., Weigert, M., Cohn, M., and Hood, L. (1974) *Proc. Natl. Acad. Sci. U.S.A.* **71,** 4096–4100.
8. Capra, J. D., and Kehoe, J. M. (1975) *Adv. Immunol.* **20,** 1–40.
9. Potter, M. (1978) *Adv. Immunol.* **25,** 141–211.
10. Tonegawa, S., Maxam, A. M., Tizard, R., Bernard, O., and Gilbert, W. (1978) *Proc. Natl. Acad. Sci. U.S.A.* **75,** 1485–1489.
10a. Seidman, J. G. (1978). *Science* **202,** 11–17.
11. Rabbits, T. H. (1977) *Immunol. Rev.* **36,** 29–50.
12. Oudin, J., and Casenave, P.-A. (1971) *Proc. Natl. Acad. Sci. U.S.A.* **68,** 2616–2620.
13. Casenave, P.-A., Ternynck, T., and Avrameas, S. (1974) *Proc. Natl. Acad. Sci. U.S.A.* **71,** 4500–4502.
14. Kabat, E. A. (1976) "Structural Concepts in Immunology and Immunochemistry," 2nd ed., p. 334–345. Holt, New York.

15. Laskin, J. A., Gray, A., Nisonoff, A., Klinman, N., and Gottlieb, P. (1977) *Proc. Natl. Acad. Sci. U.S.A.* **74**, 4600–4604.
16. Mage, R. G. (1977) *Prog. Immunol., Proc. Int. Cong. Immunol., 3rd, 1977* pp. 289–297.
17. Wu, T. T., Kabat, E. A., and Bilofsky, H. (1975) *Proc. Natl. Acad. Sci. U.S.A.* **72**, 5107–5110.
18. Klapper, D. G., and Capra, J. D. (1976) *Ann. Immunol.* (Paris) **127**, 261–271.
19. Wu, T. T., and Kabat, E. A. (1970) *J. Exp. Med.* **132**, 211–250.
20. Capra, J. D., and Kindt, T. J. (1975) *Immunogenetics* **1**, 417–427.
21. Kindt, T. J., and Capra, J. D. (1978) *Immunogenetics* **6**, 309–321.
22. Schiffer, M., Girling, B. L., Ely, K. R., and Edmundson, A. B. (1973) *Biochemistry* **12**, 4620–4631.
23. Poljak, R. J., Amzel, L. M., Avey, H. P., Chen, B. L., Phizackerley, R. P., and Saul, F. (1973) *Proc. Natl. Acad. Sci. U.S.A.* **70**, 3305–3310.
24. Segal, D. M., Padlan, E. A., Cohen, G. H., Rudikoff, S., Potter, M., and Davies, D. R. (1974) *Proc. Natl. Acad. Sci. U.S.A.* **71**, 4298–4302.
25. Epp, O., Colman, P., Fehlhammer, H., Bode, W., Schiffer, M., and Huber, R. (1974) *Eur. J. Biochem.* **45**, 513–524.
26. Saul, F. A., Amzel, M., and Poljak, R. J. (1978) *J. Biol. Chem.* **253**, 585–597.
27. Padlan, E. A. (1977) *Q. Rev. Biophys.* **10**, 35–65.
28. Kabat, E. A. (1978) *Adv. Protein Chem.* **32**, 1–75.
29. Phillips, S. G., Phillips, D. M., Kabat, E. A., and Miller, O. J. (1978) *In Vitro* **14**, 639–650.
30. Brack, C., Hirama, M., Lenhard-Schuller, R., and Tonegawa, S. (1978) *Cell* **15**, 1–14.

Immunoglobulin Genes
and Nuclear RNA Precursors

RANDOLPH WALL, EDMUND CHOI,
MICHAEL KOMAROMY,
MAUREEN GILMORE-HEBERT

Department of Microbiology and Immunology
UCLA School of Medicine
and
The Molecular Biology Institute
University of California
Los Angeles, California

AND

KATHLEEN HERCULES

Department of Biological Chemistry
UCLA School of Medicine
and
The Molecular Biology Institute
University of California
Los Angeles, California

INTRODUCTION

The constant and variable regions in immunologlobulin light and heavy chains are apparently each coded by a distinct gene (reviewed in Hood et al., 1–3). Nucleotide sequence studies now indicate that variable and constant regions are contiguous in immunologlobulin mRNA (4,5). Until recently, it was postulated that variable and constant regions are joined through somatic rearrangements in DNA during the early stages of lymphoid cell development (reviewed in Hozumi et al., 6,7). Brack and Tonegawa have now cloned a DNA fragment containing variable and constant regions from a λ light chain-producing myeloma cell line (8). In this cloned DNA, presumably containing the λ light chain structural gene sequences

45

being expressed in these cells, the λ variable and constant regions are separated by 1.25 kb.* Hybridization studies by Rabbitts (9) suggest that κ light chain variable and constant regions also may not be contiguous in the DNA of κ light chain-producing myeloma cells. These insights into immunoglobulin gene structure are paralleled by similar findings in virtually every eukaryotic gene studied to date. Intervening sequences separating the structural gene or coding sequences in cellular DNA have been found in a variety of eukaryotic cellular genes including: globin (10,11), ovalbumin (12,13), a fraction of *Drosophila* ribosomal RNA genes (14–16), and yeast tRNA's genes (17–19).

Early in the fall of 1977, the convergence of results from independent studies on the structure and on the biogenesis of the late mRNA's transcribed from adenovirus DNA unexpectedly suggested that mRNA in eukaryotic cells could be generated from widely separated sequences in DNA by nuclear RNA splicing (reviewed in Darnell, 20). In this report, we summarize our present results on the transcription and processing of the nuclear RNA precursors to immunoglobulin κ light chain mRNA. These studies indicate that κ light chain variable and constant regions are not contiguous in myeloma cell DNA, but rather are separated by approximately 2.0 kb within the 10 kb transcription unit which comprises the active light chain gene. The separated variable and constant regions appear to be spliced together in the post-transcriptional processing of a 10 kb nuclear RNA precursor (21) to κ light chain mRNA.

RESULTS AND DISCUSSION

SPECIFIC HYBRIDIZATION PROBES FROM THE MOLECULAR CLONING OF IMMUNOGLOBULIN mRNA

Since none of these studies would be feasible without the resolution offered by recombinant DNA probes, we will first describe the clones constructed from immunoglobulin mRNA. We previously established general procedures which allow the construction of recombinant clones from any poly(A)-containing mRNA (22). Other laboratories, using similar experimental approaches, have independently established successful methods for the molecular cloning of poly(A)-

---

* kb, kilobases or kilobase pairs.

containing mRNA (23–27). Such recombinant clones containing specific eukaryotic structural gene sequences (i.e., mRNA sequences) provide pure hybridization probes for studies on the nature and expression of eukaryotic genes. We have now constructed recombinant DNA clones from several different immunoglobulin light chain mRNA and heavy chain mRNA. Basically, in the molecular cloning of these immunoglobulin mRNA, complementary DNA (cDNA) synthesized on purified light or heavy chain mRNA by reverse transcriptase, was made double-stranded, inserted into the plasmid vector pMB9 (28) or pBR322 (29) and transformed into *Escherichia coli* by procedures similar to those we first reported for the recombinant cloning of rabbit globin mRNA (22). Recombinant clones containing specific immunoglobulin mRNA sequences were initially identified among the transformed colonies selected by antibiotic resistence using the Grunstein–Hogness colony hybridization with ^{32}P-cRNA prepared from the cDNA used in constructing the clones (30). Transformed colonies giving a positive hybridization signal in this test were selected and further characterized by restriction enzyme mapping and nucleotide sequencing using the rapid procedures developed by Maxam and Gilbert (31). The studies reported here employ several of the recombinant clones prepared from MOPC 21 κ light chain mRNA which now have been extensively characterized.

Figure 1 shows the detailed restriction maps of three κ light chain mRNA recombinant clones designated (pL21-1, pL21-1V, and pL21-5) in relation to the κ light chain mRNA. The κ light chain mRNA sequences in these clones have been definitely identified by the presence of multiple restriction sites predicted from the published nucleotide sequences for the MOPC 21 κ mRNA constant region (4,32), by the correspondence of nucleotide sequences determined in these clones with the published amino acid sequence (33) for the MOPC 21 κ light chain (submitted for publication elsewhere). The cDNA used in constructing these κ light chain clones was synthesized under reverse transcriptase reaction conditions promoting long transcripts (25). Approximately 50–60% of the light chain cDNA appeared to be full length transcripts of MOPC 21 κ light chain mRNA. In the construction of these clones, no attempt was made to select full length double-stranded molecules following complementary strand synthesis by DNA polymerase I and S_1 nuclease digestion (22,25). Provided that the DNA polymerase I reaction does not always produce full length complementary strands, this approach should be expected to produce clones containing sub-

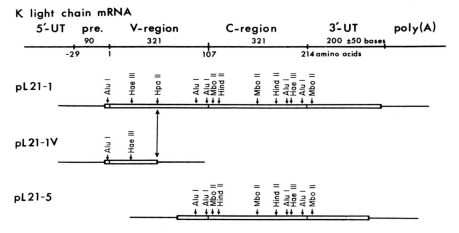

Fig. 1. Recombinant DNA probes containing κ light chain mRNA sequences. Restriction maps of κ light chain plasmids pL21-1, pL21-5, and pL21-1V are presented in relation to their location in κ light chain mRNA. The restriction map of pL21-5 was determined by Pat Clarke. Recombinant plasmids, pL21-1 and pL21-5, were cloned in pMB9. The variable region-specific plasmid pL21-1V was derived from a *Hpa* II fragment of pL21-1 recloned in PBR322. Only the inserted κ light chain mRNA sequences are shown in detail (□). Not all restriction sites mapped in the κ light chain mRNA sequences are shown. Restriction sites which correspond to those established in the nucleotide sequences of the constant region and 3'-untranslated region (3,4) are: *Alu* I at Ser$_{208}$ and Ser$_{191}$, *Hae* III at Ala$_{196}$, *MBO* II recognition site at Lys$_{149}$ (cleavage at Gly$_{152}$), *Hind* II at Leu$_{181}$. A *Hin* f restriction site determined 13 nucleotides from the terminal poly(A) segment is present in pL21-1 (not shown) but not pL21-5. Flanking dA : T insertion sequences and plasmid vector sequences are shown by thin lines (——).

stantial or complete copies of κ mRNA, as well as clones with segments from the 3' and 5' regions of κ light chain mRNA. Our characterization of the κ light chain clones confirms this expectation.

Immunoglobulin κ light chain clone, pL21-1, contains 930 mRNA bases of mRNA sequence extending from the 3'-poly(A) segment through the C and V regions and ending about 30 nucleotides into the precursor or leader coding sequence. A κ light chain variable region-specific recombinant clone (pL21-1V) was constructed by recloning the designated *Hpa* II fragment from pL21-1 which contains the first 150 nucleotides of the variable region (Fig. 1). The nucleotide sequence determined from the internal *Hae* III–*Alu* I fragment from pL21-1V exactly corresponds to the MOPC 21 light chain variable region amino acid sequence through Lys$_{24}$. Recombinant clone, pL21-5, was used as the constant region probe. This recombinant plasmid contains approximately 600 nucleotides of κ light chain mRNA sequences beginning in the 3′-untranslated region and includes the entire constant region with less than 100 nucleotides of κ light chain variable region past the V–C juncture (amino acid 107).

These cloned plasmid DNA's containing C, V, and $V + C$ as well as 3′-terminal MOPC 21 κ light chain mRNA sequences have been used in the studies in the following sections which define nuclear RNA precursors and the processing steps leading to cytoplasmic κ light chain mRNA and establish the nature of the variable and constant regions in the active κ light chain gene (i.e., in the κ light chain transcription unit) being transcribed in P3 myeloma cells.

IMMUNOGLOBULIN κ LIGHT CHAIN mRNA IS MADE FROM A LARGE NUCLEAR RNA PRECURSOR

It is now well established that most mRNA in eukaryotic cells are derived from nuclear RNA through post-transcriptional modifications. These include poly(A) addition, methylation, and the addition of 5′ terminal "caps" which have the general structure, $m^7G(5')pppN'm$-$N'(m)p$. In addition, most mRNA in eukaryotic cells are likely to be generated by the post-transcriptional cleavage of larger nuclear RNA (reviewed in Darnell, 20,34). We have used recombinant DNA probes, produced by the molecular cloning of immunoglobulin κ light chain mRNA to detect rapidly-labeled nuclear RNA containing κ light chain mRNA sequences and to examine their kinetic relationship to cytoplasmic mRNA. Immunoglobulin-producing P3 mouse myeloma cells were pulse-labeled with ^{3}H-uridine, the nuclear RNA was extracted and fractionated by density gradient sedimentation after stringent denaturation which has been shown to eliminate aggregated RNA complexes (35). Individual gradient fractions were then exhaustively hybridized with κ light chain recombinant plasmid DNA bound to nitrocellulose filters. We were able to resolve three discrete classes of nuclear RNA containing κ mRNA sequences (21). Two of these sedimenting at 40 and 24 S, are substantially larger than 13 S κ mRNA (approximately 10 kb and 3–4 kb in size), while the third is similar in size to 13 S κ mRNA (1.2 kb) (Fig. 2A). The kinetics of appearance of these κ specific nuclear RNA and cytoplasmic κ light chain mRNA are shown in Fig. 2B. Beginning with the 40 S nuclear RNA species, the sequential appearance of these three classes of nuclear RNA precedes the first appearance of newly synthesized 13 S κ light chain mRNA in the cytoplasm. The results presented here suggest that immunoglobulin κ light chain mRNA is generated by the stepwise cleavage and processing of the large 40 S nuclear RNA transcript. The

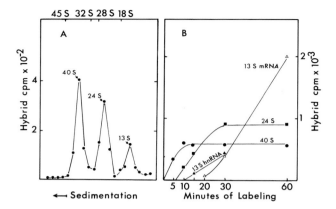

Fig. 2. Kinetic evidence for the biogenesis of κ light chain mRNA from a large nuclear RNA precursor. The pulse-labeling results in this figure have been previously published in detail (21). (A) shows the sedimentation analysis of 15 min labeled nuclear RNA hybridized with κ light chain mRNA clone pL21-1. (B) shows the kinetics of appearance of the 40 S (10 kb) nuclear RNA precursor and the nuclear RNA processing intermediates (24 S, 3–4 kb; 13 S, 1.2 kb) in relation to 13 S cytoplasmic κ light chain mRNA.

ordered appearance of label in these discrete nuclear RNA species containing κ mRNA sequences clearly occurs in a manner consistent with a precursor–product relationship to cytoplasmic κ light chain mRNA suggesting the following pathway for the biogenesis of κ light chain mRNA:

$$40 \text{ S} \longrightarrow 24 \text{ S} \longrightarrow 13 \text{ S} \xrightarrow[\text{the cytoplasm}]{\text{transport to}} 13 \text{ S } \kappa \text{ mRNA}$$
$$(10 \text{ kb}) \quad (3\text{–}4 \text{ kb}) \quad (1.2 \text{ kb}) \qquad\qquad (1.2 \text{ kb})$$

In establishing the precursor–product relationship between a given mRNA and nuclear RNA it is essential to demonstrate that the mRNA is *obligatorily* derived from that nuclear RNA. Pulse-chase experiments using glucosamine treatment which irreversibly depletes the intracellular UTP pools by the production of UDP-*N*-acetyl-glucosamine (36), have now been carried out to establish that κ light chain mRNA is obligatorily derived through this proposed pathway. These studies demonstrate that at least 60–80% of κ sequences in the 40 S nuclear RNA synthesized in 5 min of pulse labeling are "chased" into cytoplasmic 13 S κ light chain mRNA. A more detailed account of these "pulse-chase" experiments will appear elsewhere (36a).

Now to the point of these studies which relates to κ light chain genes. Since the 40 S (10 kb) species is the only reproducible class of κ specific nuclear RNA seen in the shortest pulse labels (i.e., in 5 min,

Fig. 2B), this species could represent the primary transcript (i.e., the direct unprocessed transcription product) of the immunoglobulin κ light chain gene. In this case, isolation and mapping studies on this 40 S species represents a direct means of dissecting the features of the transcription unit in myeloma DNA coding for immunoglobulin κ light chain mRNA (including the arrangement of variable and constant regions). These structural studies are now underway. However, in the next section we present a quite different experimental approach for resolving the nature of immunoglobulin genes.

V AND C REGIONS ARE SEPARATED IN THE TRANSCRIPTION UNIT IN MYELOMA CELL DNA CODING FOR THE LARGE PRECURSOR TO κ LIGHT CHAIN mRNA

We have used the technique of UV transcription mapping with recombinant DNA hybridization probes containing immunoglobulin κ light chain variable or constant region sequences, to determine the size of the transcription unit coding for κ light chain mRNA and to establish the arrangement of variable and constant regions in this transcription unit. This procedure, developed in prokaryotic and phage systems (reviewed in Sanerbier, 37), has recently emerged as an elegant and powerful means for mapping transcription units (i.e., DNA regions transcribed from a single initiation site or promoter) in eukaryotic cells. This procedure involves the random introduction of transcription terminating UV lesions in DNA (presumably pyrimidine dimers). These lesions result in the release of growing nascent RNA chains at the UV damaged site without inhibiting the re-initiation of RNA synthesis at promoter sites in DNA (37). Within a transcription unit, UV irradiation causes an exponential decrease in transcription with increasing distance from the promoter or initiation site. UV transcription mapping has recently been used to define the size of the transcription units for cellular hnRNA* and mRNA (38,39), and rRNA (40,41) as well as for early (39,42) and late adenovirus mRNA (43,44).

We initially determined the effects of UV irradiation on the well characterized transcription unit coding for the 45 S precursor to 18 and 28 S rRNA to provide standards for converting UV survival rate to the distance (in base pairs) from the promoter or transcription initiation site in DNA. The transcription unit coding for the 45 S ribosomal RNA precursor in mouse is 13.9 kb (45). The 32 and 28 S map at 8.9 kb from the initiation site, while the 18 S rRNA maps at 4.4 kb (Table I). These

* hnRNA, heterogeneous nuclear RNA.

TABLE I
Summary UV Transcription Mapping Data

MOPC 21 rRNA

Species	$D_{37}{}^a$	UV target size
45 S	100	13.9 kb
32 S	155	8.9 kb
28 S	155	8.9 kb
18 S	310	4.4 kb

15 min κ specific nuclear RNA

Probe	D_{37}	UV target size
pL21-5	145	9.6 kb[b]
pL21-1V	180	7.6 kb
pL21-4	Complex curve, resolved into 2	6.6 kb
	equal components	0.23 kb

[a] D_{37} = UV dose (in erg/sec/mm²) giving 37% survival of an RNA species or of total plasmid DNA hybridized cpm relative to an unirradiated control.

[b] Calculation of the UV target size of pL21-5 transcription into hnRNA using 45 S pre-rRNA standard.

$$\text{UV target size pL21-5} = \frac{D_{37}\ 45\ \text{S standard}}{D_{37}\ \text{pL21-5 hybrid}}$$
$$\times\ \text{size 45 S standard}$$
$$= \frac{100\ \text{erg/sec/mm}^2}{145\ \text{erg/sec/mm}^2} \times 13.9\,\text{kb}$$
$$= 9.6\ \text{kb}$$

values are in excellent agreement with the reported rRNA transcription units for mouse cells determined by UV transcription mapping and other gene mapping techniques (40,45,46).

Next, we determined the effect of UV irradiation on the transcription of κ light chain variable and constant region sequences into rapidly-labeled nuclear RNA. Samples of P3 cells were exposed to different doses of UV, incubated 20 min to permit previously initiated nascent RNA chains to be completed, and then incubated for 15 min with ³H-uridine to label hnRNA. If the variable and constant regions are contiguous in the κ light chain transcription unit as they are in the mRNA (4,5), then the UV sensitivities of these two κ mRNA domains would be indistinguishable. Instead, we found that the UV sensitivity of variable and constant regions was very different. The UV sensitivity of labeled hnRNA hybridization to the constant region probe (pL21-5) gave a UV target size, relative to 45 S pre-rRNA (13.9 kb), of 9.6 kb (Fig. 3). This value is in excellent agreement with the size of the 40 S (approximately 10 kb) nuclear RNA precursor to κ light chain rRNA previously detected in pulse labeling experiments (21). Nuclear RNA hybridization to the variable region probe (pL21-1V) exhibited a UV target size of 7.6 kb in relation to the 45 S pre-rRNA standard. Both κ light chain variable and constant regions are present in the same 40 S hnRNA precursor molecules (results not shown) and are presumably transcribed from a single transcription unit in DNA. Accordingly, the UV mapping data cited above suggest that κ light variable and constant regions are separated by approximately ~2 kb within a 10 kb transcription unit coding for κ light chain mRNA. This approach represents a novel application of the UV transcription mapping technique, since it is the first time it has been applied to determining the arrangement of specific mRNA sequences within a transcription unit.

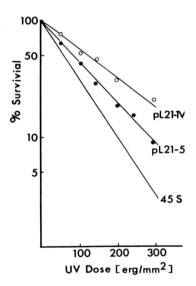

Fig. 3. UV mapping of the light chain transcription unit in P3 cells. The hybridization of 15 min labeled hnRNA to 20 μg constant region DNA filters (pL21-5, ●——●) and 20 μg variable region DNA filters (pL21-1V, O——O) is plotted versus increasing UV dose. Hybridization was scored after T_1 and pancreatic RNAse digestion. The recoveries of hnRNA from each UV dose were normalized to the amount of 32 S in each sample. The accuracy of the target size determined from these hybridizations is ±0.2 kb.

This obviously represents a relatively rapid means for mapping the arrangement of structural gene (i.e., mRNA) coding sequences within the transcription units of other eukaryotic genes.

We also have used UV mapping to independently confirm that cytoplasmic κ light chain mRNA is derived from a 10 kb transcription unit. The κ light chain mRNA in the cytoplasm should exhibit the UV target size of the most promoter-distal sequence in the DNA transcription unit required for the production of the messenger RNA. The UV sensitivities of the constant region (pL21-5) sequences in both nuclear RNA and cytoplasmic RNA have been shown to be identical indicating that κ light chain mRNA is derived from a 10 kb transcription unit. UV mapping provides a static comparison of the transcription units for κ light chain mRNA and hnRNA and establishes that both are coded by a 10 kb transcription unit. However, these findings, in conjunction with the kinetic labeling studies already described, strongly suggest that κ light chain mRNA is derived from the *same* 10 kb transcription unit coding for the 40 S nuclear RNA precursor (21).

CLOSING REMARKS

These studies provide a number of important insights into the nature and expression of the immunoglobulin κ light chain genes undergoing transcription in myeloma cells. The model in Fig. 4 summarizes the features of the κ light chain transcription unit and the

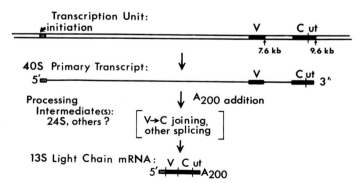

Fig. 4. The production of κ light chain mRNA from a 10 kb transcription unit in which variable and constant regions are separated. The model proposes that the joining of variable and constant regions occurs in the post-transcriptional processing of a 10 kb primary transcript. Further details are presented in the text.

nuclear RNA processing events leading to κ light chain mRNA. Variable and constant regions are separated by ~2 kb in the 10 kb light chain transcription unit and are present in a $5' \to 3'$ orientation colinear with that in κ light chain mRNA. The constant region and 3' untranslated regions are shown as the most promoter-distal sequences, presumably at the termination site of the transcription unit.

As presented, this is a simple transcription unit (i.e., coding for a single mRNA) in which the P3 κ light chain mRNA sequences comprise only about 1.2 kb of the total sequences in the 10 kb transcription unit. This is in contrast to the now well established complex transcription units in adenovirus (47–49) and SV40 (50,51) in which multiple viral mRNA's, coded by the same transcription unit in viral DNA, are generated by different patterns of post-transcription processing and splicing (reviewed in Darnell, 20). Considerable evidence indicates a single κ constant region per haploid genome (reviewed in Hood *et al.*, 2,3). It is now apparent that multiple κ variable regions must be present in germ line DNA (reviewed in Hood *et al.*, 2,3,7,9). It is interesting to speculate whether other κ variable regions besides the P3 variable region might be present in this large transcription unit. If so, then somatic rearrangements in DNA (7,9) or different nuclear RNA splicing patterns might promote the joining of the constant region with such variable regions, thereby generating other κ mRNA's. At present, this speculation is unrestrained by experimental evidence.

It is proposed that the 40 S nuclear RNA species detected in pulse labeling studies (21), comprises the primary transcript in which variable and constant regions are separated by same extent as in the DNA transcription unit (Fig. 4). Of the various mechanisms proposed for joining structural gene sequences separated by intervening sequences (reviewed in Darnell, 20), the most plausible involves splicing of separated RNA sequences transcribed directly into a primary hnRNA transcript. Nuclear RNA splicing in the generation of cytoplasmic mRNA from widely separated sites in viral DNA is now established for adenovirus and SV40 (reviewed in Darnell, 20) and for B-globin nuclear RNA where it has been recently shown that the isolated 15 S B-globin nuclear RNA precursor contains two intervening sequences separating B-globin mRNA coding sequences (52). Accordingly, the model in Fig. 4 predicts that κ light chain variable and constant regions which are contiguous in κ ligh chain mRNA (4,5) are joined by a splicing event in the post-transcriptional processing of the 10 kb nuclear RNA precursor. Since both κ variable and constant region sequences are present in the same 10 kb nuclear RNA precursor molecules, the joining of V and C involves intramolecular splicing mechanisms. Preliminary results (not shown) indicate that sequences apparently derived from the 5′ terminus of κ mRNA map at the promoter (i.e., within approximately 0.2 kb) of the light chain transcription unit. Accordingly, we propose that the processing of κ light chain mRNA from its large nuclear RNA precursor involves at least two nuclear RNA splicing events.

While the nature of splicing/processing intermediates is not specified in the model (Fig. 4), pulse-labeling experiments (21) and other UV transcription results (36a) definitively establish a 24 S nuclear RNA species as a processing intermediate (approximately 3–4 kb long) in the pathway to cytoplasmic 13 S κ light chain mRNA. We are now engaged in electron microscope mapping of both the 40 and 24 S light chain nuclear RNA precursors hybridized with recombinant plasmid clone, pL21-1, (in which V and C are contiguous, Fig. 1), to determine the sequence arrangement of these hnRNA species. The results of these studies are expected to conclusively establish that κ light chain variable and constant regions are spliced together in the post-transcriptional processing of the large precursor to κ mRNA.

It now appears that the joining of immunoglobulin light chain variable and constant regions occurs by a striking and previously unexpected molecular mechanism which likely is not unique to immunoglobulin genes. Nonetheless, the demonstration that nuclear RNA splicing appears to be involved in the expression of immunoglobulin genes (and apparently most other eukaryotic genes as well) raises the possibility that such processes may be involved in the regulation of eukaryotic gene expression. It is especially intriguing to speculate that ordered patterns of gene expression in cell development might be manifested through changes in nuclear RNA splicing. An obvious example in the development of the immune response is the IgM → IgG transition where alternate patterns of nuclear RNA splicing could result in the simultaneous production of μ and γ heavy chains containing identical variable regions.

ACKNOWLEDGMENTS

These studies were supported by National Institutes of Health grant AI 13410 and Program Project CA 12800. Maureen Gilmore-Hebert was the recipient of US Public Health Service postdoctoral fellowship GM 5477. Edmund Choi was supported on US Public Health Service Training Grant GM 7185. The restriction map of recombinant plasmid pL21-5 was determined by Pat Clarke. We wish to thank Jean Mueller for excellent technical and administrative support.

REFERENCES

1. Hood, L. (1972) *Fed. Proc., Fed. Am. Soc. Exp. Biol.* **31**, 177–187.
2. Hood, L., Campbell, J. H., and Elgin, S. C. R. (1975)*Annu. Rev. Genet.* **9**, 305–353.
3. Kuehl (1977) *Curr. Top. Microbiol. Immunol.* **76**, 2–47.
4. Milstein, C., Brownley, G. G., Cartwright, E. M., Jarvis, J. M., and Proudfoot, N. J. (1974) *Nature (London)* **252**, 354–359.
5. Milstein, C., Brownley, G. G., Cheng, C. C., Hamlyn, P. N., Proudfoot, N. J., and Rabbitts, T. H. (1976) *Mosbacher Colloq.* **27**, 75–90.
6. Hozumi, N., and Tonegawa, S. (1976) *Proc. Natl. Acad. Sci. U.S.A.* **73**, 3628–3632.
7. Tonegawa, S., Hozumi, N., Matthyssens, G., and Schuller, R. (1976) *Cold Spring Harbor Symp. Quant. Biol.* **41**, 877–889.
8. Brack, C., and Tonegawa, S. (1977) *Proc. Natl. Acad. Sci. U.S.A.* **74**, 5652–5656.
9. Rabbitts, T. H., and Forster, A. (1978) *Cell* **13**, 319–327.
10. Jeffreys, A. J., and Flavel, R. A., II (1977) *Cell* **12**, 1097–1108.
11. Tilghman, S. M., Tiemeier, D. C., Seidman, J. G., Peterlin, B. M., Sullivan, M., Maizel, J. V., and Leder, P. (1978) *Proc. Natl. Acad. Sci. U.S.A.* **75**, 725–727.
12. Breathnach, R., Mandel, J. L., and Chambon, P. (1977). *Nature (London)* **270**, 314–319.
13. Weinstock, R., Sweet, R., Weiss, M., Cedar, H., and Axel R. (1978). *Proc. Natl. Acad. Sci. (London)* **75**, 1299–1303.
14. White, R., and Hogness, D. (1977) *Cell* **10**, 177–192.
15. Wellauer, P. K., and David, I. B. (1977) *Cell* **10**, 193–212.
16. Pelligrini, M., Manning, J., and Davidson, N. (1977) *Cell* **10**, 213–224.
17. Goodman, H. M., Olsen, M. V., and Hall, B. D. (1977) *Proc. Natl. Acad. Sci. U.S.A.* **74**, 5453–5457.
18. Valenzuela, P., Venegas, A., Weinberg, F., Bishop, R., and Rutter, W. J. (1978) *Proc. Natl. Acad. Sci. U.S.A.* **75**, 190–194.
19. Knapp, G., Beckmann, J. S., Johnson, P. F., Fuhrman, S. A., and Abelson, J. (1978) *Cell* **14**, 221–236.
20. Darnell, J. E. (1978) *Prog. Nucleic Acid Res. Mol. Biol.* (in press).
21. Gilmore-Hebert, M., and Wall, R. (1978) *Proc. Natl. Acad. Sci. U.S.A.* **75**, 342–345.
22. Higuchi, R., Paddock, G. V., Wall, R., and Salser, W. (1976) *Proc. Natl. Acad. Sci. U.S.A.* **73**, 3146–3150.
23. Rougeon, F., Kourilsky, P., and Mach, B. (1975) *Nucleic Acids Res.* **2**, 2365–2378.
24. Rabbitts, T. H. (1976) *Nature (London)* **260**, 221–225.
25. Maniatis, T., Kee, S. G., Efstratiadis, A., and Kafatos, F. C. (1976) *Cell* **8**, 163–182.
26. Rougeon, F., and Mach, B. (1976) *Proc. Natl. Acad. Sci. U.S.A.* **73**, 3418–3422.
27. Ullrich, A., Shine, J., Chirgwin, J., Pictet, R., Tischer, E., Rutter, W., and Goodman, H. (1977) *Science* **196**, 1313–1319.
28. Boliver, F., Rodriquez, R., Greene, P., Betlach, M., Heyneker, H., and Boyer, H. (1977) *Gene* **2**, 95–113.
29. Bolivar, F., Rodriquez, R. L., Betlach, M. C., and Boyer, H. W. (1977) *Gene* **2**, 75–93.
30. Grunstein, M., and Hogness, D. S. (1975) *Proc. Natl. Acad. Sci. U.S.A.* **72**, 3961–3965.
31. Maxam, A. M., and Gilbert, W. (1977) *Proc. Natl. Acad. Sci. U.S.A.* **74**, 560–564.
32. Seidman, J. G., Edgell, M. H., and Leder, P. (1978) *Nature (London)* **271**, 582–585.
33. Svasti, J., and Milstein, C. (1972) *Biochem. J.* **128**, 427–444.
34. Darnell, J. E. (1976) *Proc. Nucleic Acid Res. Mol Biol.* **19**, 493–511.
35. Federoff, N., Wellauer, P. K., and Wall, R. (1977) *Cell* **10**, 597–610.

36. Scholtissek, C. (1971). *Eu. J. Biochem.* **24**, 358–365.
36a. Gilmore-Hebert, M., and Wall, R. (1979). Submitted for publication.
37. Sauerbier, W. (1976) *Adv. Radiat. Biol.* **6**, 60–106.
38. Giorno, R., and Sauerbier, W. (1976) *Cell* **9**, 775–783.
39. Goldberg, S., Schwartz, H., and Darnell, J. E. (1977) *Proc. Natl. Acad. Sci. U.S.A.* **74**, 4520–4523.
40. Hacket, P. B., and Sauerbier, W. (1975) *J. Mol. Biol.* **91**, 235–256.
41. Carlson, J., Ott, G., and Sauerbier, W. (1977) *J. Mol. Biol.* **112**, 353–357.
42. Berk, A. J., and Sharp, P. A. (1977) *Cell* **12**, 45–55.
43. Goldberg, S., Weber, J., and Darnell, J. E. (1977) *Cell* **10**, 617–621.
44. Goldberg, S., Nevins, J., and Darnell, J. E. (1978) *J. Virol.* **25**, 806–810.
45. Wellauer, P. K., David, I. B., Kelley, D. W., and Perry, R. P. (1974) *J. Mol. Biol.* **89**, 397–407.
46. Cory, S., and Adams, J. M. (1977) *Cell* **11**, 795–805.
47. Nevins, J., and Darnell, J. E. (1978) *J. Virol.* **25**, 811–823.
48. McGrohan, M., and Raskas, H. J. (1978) *Proc. Natl. Acad. Sci. U.S.A.* **75**, 625–629.
49. Ziff, E., and Fraser, N. (1978) *J. Virol.* **25**, 897–906.
50. Berk, A. J., and Sharp, P. A. (1978) *Proc. Natl. Acad. Sci. U.S.A.* **75**, 1274–1278.
51. Hsu, M. T., and Ford, J. (1977) *Proc. Natl. Acad. Sci. U.S.A.* **74**, 4982–4985.
52. Tilghman, S. M., Curtis, P. D., Tiemeir, D. C., Leder, P., and Weissman, C. (1978) *Proc. Natl. Acad. Sci. U.S.A.* **75**, 1309–1313.

Studies on mRNA Sequence and Immunoglobulin Gene Organization Using Synthetic Oligonucleotides

P. H. HAMLYN AND C. MILSTEIN

MRC Laboratory of Molecular Biology
Cambridge, England

INTRODUCTION

Until quite recently the genetic origin of antibody diversity could only be studied at a molecular level by an examination of the final gene products—the immunoglobulin molecules themselves. This indicated that the constant (C) region genes of the light and heavy chains must be shared by multiple variable (V) region genes for the corresponding chains and that therefore a mechanism for V and C gene integration was required at the somatic level. Protein structure studies alone could not hope to elucidate the mechanism of integration of the V and C genes, nor could they be used to determine if or how differentiation, i.e., changes in the genetic material coding for immunoglobulins, takes place in the development of lymphocytes. The isolation of partially purified IgG light chain mRNA as a probe of gene organization marked the beginning of a more direct approach to the understanding of the genetic basis of antibody production. Such mRNA was isolated from myeloma cells, which grow in tissue culture either in mass quantities or after incorporation of ^{32}P to yield ^{32}P-mRNA of relatively high specific activity. Studies in this laboratory have been concentrated in the myeloma line P3 derived from the mouse tumour MOPC 21 (1,2).

STUDIES WITH ^{32}P-mRNA AND cDNA PRIMED WITH OLIGO(dT)

Initially light chain ^{32}P-mRNA was used for direct nucleotide sequence analysis (1,2) and as such was one of the first eukaryotic mRNA's to be described at this level. The usefulness of the chemical characterization which this approach afforded was evident, for example, in the demonstration that the molecular species which hybridize to nonrepetitive DNA contain light chain mRNA sequences for both C and V regions (3).

The discovery that reverse transcriptase could be used to copy mRNA into complementary (c) DNA using the poly(A) tail as a binding site for the primer oligo(dT) was quickly adapted for the production of light chain cDNA (4). For hybridization studies cDNA has the advantage over ^{32}P-mRNA of greater stability (being DNA rather than RNA) and the possibility of being labeled to a much higher specific activity. Oligo(dT) in theory can initiate transcription on all mRNA's with poly(A) tails but it is uncertain to what extent there is preferential transcription of some mRNA's. In fact some results based on the presence and absence of repetitive components suggested that short copies were enriched while long copies were depleted of L-chain mRNA (5,6). At any rate the cDNA was not substantially purer than the template mRNA, which is in general about 50% pure, and chemical studies were again required to characterize it. To achieve greater purity primers have to be selective, being complementary only (or mainly) to a sequence in the light chain mRNA.

STUDIES WITH SPECIFIC PRIMERS

Three oligonucleotides prepared either chemically (7) or chemically and enzymatically (5,8) have been found to initiate preferential transcription on light chain mRNA. The resultant cDNA's are thus purer light chain sequences than the mRNA used to prepare them. The priming sites of these three oligonucleotides are illustrated in Fig. 1. This advantage was used both to analyze the arrangement of IgG genes and for further sequence analysis. The greater purity of the cDNA prepared using the specific hexanucleotide primer $d(T_2\text{-}G_3\text{-}T)$ (see Fig. 1), eliminated the repetitive component which had been observed in ^{32}P light chain mRNA and cDNA prepared using oligo(dT) (6) and thus substantiated the earlier conclusion that the number of V genes similar to MOPC 21 was small in number. It also allowed a more

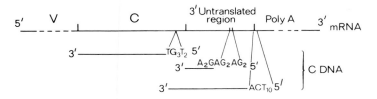

Fig. 1. The priming sites of $d(T_2\text{-}G_3\text{-}T)$, $d(pG_2\text{-}A\text{-}G_2\text{-}A\text{-}G\text{-}A_2)$, and $d(pT_{10}\text{-}C\text{-}A)$. The diagram illustrates (approximately to scale) the priming sites of the three oligonucleotide primers used in these experiments. The length of the cDNA's approximates to the region each was used to sequence.

accurate estimation of the number of cross-hybridizing germ line genes by saturation analysis (5).

The use of specific primers for the production of cDNA had even greater consequences for nucleotide sequence analysis. It meant that the laborious traditional methods involving degradation into oligo-nucleotides and sequence analysis of these smaller fragments (with the problem of "overlapping" the small fragments to obtain a continuous sequence) could be abandoned in favor of the rapid gel electrophoresis methods which had revolutionized DNA sequencing (9) and had been adapted for cDNA copies of RNA by Brownlee and Cartwright (10). These rapid methods are dependent on the popula-tion of cDNA's having the same 5′ ends but different 3′ ends, a requirement easily met using specific primers to produce the cDNA.

Recent further improvements in DNA sequencing technology (11) involving the use of 2′,3′-dideoxyribonucleotide triphosphates in conditions which partially and base specifically inhibit transcription have now been adapted for mRNA sequencing. These substrate analogues are recognized by the enzyme and incorporated into the growing cDNA. They do not possess a 3′-OH group and therefore act as chain terminators. By arranging that transcription takes place in an incubation containing all deoxyribonucleotides and, for example, dideoxy C the termination is partial, and being random a population of cDNA's is produced which is terminated in all positions at which dCTP is incorporated into the cDNA. Other separate reactions pro-duce cDNA's terminating in A,G, and T. Parallel gel electrophoresis of the four populations of cDNA allows the nucleotide sequence of the cDNA to be read off the gels directly. When this method of generating sequence data is used with polyacrylamide gels of increased resolu-tion (12) stretches of up to 300 nucleotides can be deduced from one priming site. Using this method the nucleotide sequence has been deduced of the mRNA coding for the constant region and also that for the 3′ noncoding region of IgG light chain (12a). The complete sequence is shown in Fig. 2.

Primed synthesis of cDNA has proved useful for sequence analysis of mRNA's other than IgG light chain. For example, the 3′ noncoding regions (13) and the 5′ noncoding regions (14,15) of various globin mRNA's have been elucidated by this method. A severe limitation to the general application of the method is the requirement for some prior knowledge of the RNA sequence before a complementary oligonucleotide can be constructed. Even with this information very few of the complementary primers (up to a length of nine nucleotides) we have tested have initiated transcription, or when they have, it has not always been exclusively at the desired site. This latter problem can be overcome by manipulating the conditions of transcription, usually by reducing one of the nucleotide triphosphate concentrations, so that one site is greatly preferred to the other, or by enzymatic addition of another base to the oligonucleotide, thus increasing its specificity.

An example of manipulation of the conditions of transcription is illustrated below with the primer d(p T-T-C-T-G-T-T-G-A). This oligonucleotide was found to initiate transcription in two places as illustrated.

V region site

34						
Ser	Trp	Tyr	Gln	Gln	Lys	Amino acid
AGX	UGG	UAU	CAA	CAG	AAA	RNA
		1	111	111	11	
		A	GTT	GTC	TT	DNA

     ↑

C region site

207						
Lys	Ser	Phe	Asn	Arg	Asn	Amino acid
AAG	AGC	UUC	AAC	AGG	AAU	RNA
		11	111	11	1	
		AG	TTG	TCT	T	DNA

     ↑

By allowing transcription to take place in the absence of dGTP, only short cDNA was made. Examination of the two priming sites shows that the cDNA made at the V region site can be transcribed for longer without insertion of a dGTP than the cDNA at the C region site. The position of insertion of dGTP is marked with arrows. Using these special conditions (i.e., no dGTP in the transcription mixture) short cDNA of different lengths corresponding to different priming sites can

```
        110                                                  120
ARG ALA ASP ALA ALA PRO THR VAL SER ILE PHE PRO PRO SER SER GLU GLN LEU THR SER
CGG GCT GAT GCT GCA CCA ACT GTA TCC ATC TTC CCA CCA TCC AGT GAG CAG TTA ACA TCT
                                                            HindII
                                                            HpaI
                                          MboII


        130                                                  140
GLY GLY ALA SER VAL VAL CYS PHE LEU ASN ASN PHE TYR PRO LYS ASP ILE ASN VAL LYS
GGA GGT GCC TCA GTC GTG TGC TTC TTG AAC AAC TTC TAC CCC AAA GAC ATC AAT GTC AAG
Mn'I    Mn'I


        150                                                  160
TRP LYS ILE ASP GLY SER GLU ARG GLN ASN GLY VAL LEU ASN SER TRP THR ASP GLN ASP
TGG AAG ATT GAT GGC AGT GAA CGA CAA AAT GGC GTC CTG AAC AGT TGG ACT GAT CAG GAC
MboII                                                            MboI


        170                                                  180
SER LYS ASP SER THR TYR SER MET SER SER THR LEU THR LEU THR LYS ASP GLU TYR GLU
AGC AAA GAC AGC ACC TAC AGC ATG AGC AGC ACC CTC ACG TTG ACC AAG GAC GAG TAT GAA
                                                        MnII    HindII


        190                                                  200
ARG HIS ASN SER TYR THR CYS GLU ALA THR HIS LYS THR SER THR SER PRO ILE VAL LYS
CGA CAT AAC AGC TAT ACC TGT GAG GCC ACT CAC AAG ACA TCA ACT TCA CCC ATT GTC AAG
        HaeIII                                                   HphI
        Alu


        210
SER PHE ASN ARG ASN GLU CYS  term
AGC TTC AAC AGG AAT GAG TGT TAG AGA CAA AGG TCC TGA GAC GCC ACC ACC AGC TCC CCA
Alu                                                              Hga I
                                                                 Alu

GCT CCA TCC TAT CTT CCC TTC TAA GGT CTT GGA GGC TTC CCC ACA AGC GAC CTA CCA CTG
Alu
MboII

TTG CGG TGC TCC AAA CCT CCT CCC CAC CTC CTC CTC CTC CTC CCT TTC CTT GGC TTT

TAT CAT GCT AAT ATT TGC AGA AAA TAT TCA ATA AAG TGA GTC TTT GCA CTT G Poly(A)
                                                                  Hinf
```

Fig. 2. The nucleotide sequence of MOPC 21 C and 3'-untranslated regions. The mRNA sequence is written with the U's as T's to identify the restriction sites that are shown in the figure. Restriction sites tested for but not found in the sequences were *Hae* II, *Hind* III, *Hpa* II, *Eco* RI and II, *Ava* I, *Bam* I, *Bgl* I and *Pst*. The amino acids are numbered conventionally.

be prepared and isolated. An isolated "extended cDNA" can in turn be used as a primer although its low yield and contamination during isolation make it much less effective (although much more specific) than the original oligonucleotide.

An alternative to preparing an "extended primer" in a transcription reaction is to permanently modify the oligonucleotide. The oligo-nucleotide $d(T_2-G_3)$ was found to initiate transcription in two places on the light chain mRNA (16). Enzymatic conversion of the sequence to $d(T_2-G_3-T)$ resulted in complete specificity. Presumably there exists a minimum size of primer (larger than nine nucleotides) which would ensure completely specific hybridization to a messenger RNA of a given length.

The need to use primers for nucleotide sequence analysis of mRNA's can be circumvented if cDNA prepared from mRNA is made double-stranded and then inserted into a plasmid or λ phage and the recombinant cloned. The inserted DNA can then be sequenced by rapid methods for sequence analysis of double-stranded DNA (17). However, this procedure has the disadvantage that each mRNA for which nucleotide sequence data is required must be separately cloned, whereas a primer made for a region common to several IgG mRNA's could be used to sequence all of them. Of course the primer does not have to be chemically synthesized, a restriction fragment from .cloned DNA could be used which corresponds to a sequence common to several IgG mRNA's, as short as possible, but long enough to ensure that it primes in one position only on each mRNA. The advantage of chemically synthesized primers is that they can be prepared in bulk.

THE USES OF mRNA NUCLEOTIDE SEQUENCE DATA

It has been an important aspect of the approach of this laboratory that nucleotide sequence studies have always been made on the mate-rial used for hybridization analysis to test its authenticity and its purity. Establishing the nucleotide sequence of the C region has pro-vided a check on the determination of the amino acid sequence and corrected an error made in the previously published sequence (18). This error arose in a region of the amino acid sequence which had proved difficult to elucidate because of extensive deamination and the occurrence of a tryptophan. Several alternative sequences were purposed; see Table I. A revision of the amino acid sequence at posi-

TABLE I

Comparison of Different Sequences Obtained for Amino Acids
161–165 in Mouse IgG$_K$ Light Chain

Protein	Sequence	Reference
	161 165	
MOPC 21	Asx-Ser-Asx-Thr-Glx-Trp	(18)
MOPC 321	Glx-Ser-Asx-Thr-Asx-Trp	(19)
MOPC 173	Asx-Ser-Asn-Thr-Glu-Trp	(20)
SP3/HL	Asn-Ser-Trp-Thr-Asp-Gln	(12a)
MOPC 21 mRNA	Asn-Ser-Trp-Thr-Asp-Gln	

tions 163 to 166 using improved automatic techniques now agrees
with the nucleotide sequence data, the new sequence being 163–166,
Trp-Thr-Asp-Gln.

Nucleotide sequence data is also useful in determining the position
at which restriction enzymes will cut the double-stranded cDNA
incorporated into a plasmid, or the genomic DNA. In recent
experiments in which embryonic and myeloma DNA was digested
with Bam HI it was shown that the V and C genes were on separate
restriction fragments in the embryonic DNA but on the same one in
the myeloma DNA (21). A similar situation has been shown for a κ
producing myeloma by Rabbitts and Forster (22). This observation is
taken to indicate movement of the genes during differentiation.
However, a trivial explanation could be that a Bam HI site present
near the V–C junction in the embryonic DNA resulting in separate
restriction fragments for V and C regions, could have been altered by
mutation (or modified) during differentiation so that it is no longer a
site for Bam HI digestion. As a consequence the myeloma DNA could
contain both V and C sequences in a single fragment bigger than either
of them. Examination of the nucleotide sequence of MOPC 21 mRNA
in the region of the V–C join indicates a sequence G-T-A-T-C-C (amino
acids 115–116) which is only one base different from the sequence
recognized by Bam HI, i.e., G-G-A-T-C-C. However, to invoke this as
an explanation for the changes in pattern of restriction cuts between
embryonic and myeloma DNA requires that other Bam HI sites should
be regenerated in order to make the size of the fragments add up. A
trivial mutation or a modification, therefore, does not constitute a satis-
factory explanation for the pattern change from embryonic to
committed cells, but serves to illustrate how knowledge of the se-

quence can be useful in supporting speculations on the behavior of V and C genes. It may further provide essential clues as to the process of final expression of an integrated $V–C$ mRNA. In this connection it is relevant to reiterate the fact that even myeloma cells, which already have had their DNA altered with respect to the embryonic DNA, do not contain a contiguous sequence, including the V and C regions (21,22). The mRNA sequence analysis discussed here further extended the previous sequence evidence (2) demonstrating that the V and C sequences are uninterrupted and that the protein is therefore translated from a simple continuous mRNA, indicating that a final rearrangement or splicing takes place somewhere between the transcription of a discontinuous V and C myeloma DNA and the expression of a continuous mRNA.

HYBRID MYELOMA CELLS AND THE SPECIFICITY OF $V–C$ INTEGRATION

This splicing seems to be cis in the sense that V and C regions from the nonhomologous chromosomes do not integrate. This evidence is derived from the studies on hybrid cells expressing two different sets of V and C region kappa light chains performed by Cotton and Milstein in 1973 (23). The C region difference required the use of mouse and not cells since in the mouse, the $C\kappa$ region does not carry genetic markers. The experiment has been extended to the H chain where the V_H region is shared by all classes and subclasses of heavy chains. Studies within an inbred strain are therefore possible. Cis expression has been obtained in all the cases tested (24). In some experiments efforts to induce trans integration have not met with success. Hybrid cells expressing two antibodies, one of the μ class capable of lysis of sheep red blood cells and the other an IgG_1 myeloma protein with no such activity, retain their separate expression. Out of over 10^5 cells, none was found capable of anti-SRBC activity expressed on the IgG_1 molecule, even after a passage of the hybrid cells in vivo (25).

SUMMARY

V and C genes occur separately in the germ line and during differentiation a rearrangement of the DNA takes place involving a single V and a single C gene for each light and heavy chain. However, even in cells committed to the production of a single Ig, V and C genes remain separated in their genomic DNA. Since the mRNA is found as a continuous sequence with no interruption in the V–C boundary, an additional rearrangement takes place between the transcription of a discontinuous V and C myeloma DNA and the production of mRNA. Cell fusion between two myeloma producing cells indicate that the rearrangement is cis and therefore likely to involve an intra-molecular splicing.

The understanding of the arrangement of genes coding for antibody molecules and the elucidation of the nucleotide sequence of mRNA— the intermediate between the genes and the protein—have been parallel activities. Both studies have recently been based on the use of specific primers for the production of cDNA of a high purity. As sequence studies on the genes coding for V and C regions become available it will be extremely useful to know which of these sequences appears in the final translatable product, and for this the nucleotide sequence of that molecule is required.

REFERENCES

1. Brownlee, G. G., Cartwright, E. M., Cowan, N. J., Jarvis, J. M., and Milstein, C. (1973) *Nature (London)* **244**, 236.
2. Milstein, C., Brownlee, G. G., Cartwright, E. M., Jarvis, J. M., and Proudfoot, N. J. (1974) *Nature (London)* **252**, 354.
3. Rabbitts, T. H., Jarvis, J. M., and Milstein, C. (1975) *Cell* **6**, 5.
4. Aviv, H., Packman, S., Swan, D., Ross, J., and Leder, P. (1973) *Nature (London), New Biol.* **241**, 174.
5. Rabbitts, T. H. (1977) *Immunol. Rev.* **36**, 29.
6. Rabbitts, T. H., and Milstein, C. (1975) *Eur. J. Biochem.* **52**, 125.
7. Gait, M. J., and Sheppard, R. C. (1977) *Nucleic Acids Res.* **4**, 4391.
8. Hamlyn, P. H., Gillam, S., Smith, M., and Milstein, C. (1977) *Nucleic Acids Res.* **4**, 1123.
9. Sanger, F., and Coulson, A. R. (1975) *J. Mol. Biol.* **94**, 441.
10. Brownlee, G. G., and Cartwright, E. M. (1977) *J. Mol. Biol.* **114**, 93.
11. Sanger, F., Nicklen, S., and Coulson, A. R. (1977) *Proc. Natl. Acad. Sci. U.S.A.* **74**, 5463.
12. Sanger, F., and Coulson, A. R. (1978) *FEBS Lett.* **87**, 107.
12a. Hamlyn, P. H., Brownlee, G. G., Cheng, C. C., Gait, M. J., and Milstein, C. (1978) *Cell* **15**, 1075.
13. Proudfoot, N. J., Gillam, S., Smith, M., and Longley, J. I. (1977) *Cell* **11**, 807.
14. Baralle, F. E. (1977) *Cell* **12**, 1097.
15. Baralle, F. E., and Brownlee, G. G. (1978) *Nature (London)* **274**, 84.
16. Milstein, C., Brownlee, G. G., Cheng, C. C., Hamlyn, P. H., Proudfoot, N. J., and Rabbitts, T. H. (1976) *Mosbacher Colloq.* p. 75.
17. Maxam, A., and Gilbert, A. W. (1977) *Proc. Natl. Acad. Sci. U.S.A.* **74**, 560.

18. Svasti, J., and Milstein, C. (1972) *Biochem. J.* **128,** 427.
19. McKean, D., Potter, M., and Hood, L. (1973) *Biochemistry* **12,** 760.
20. Schiff, C., and Fougereau, M. (1975) *Eur. J. Biochem.* **59,** 525.
21. Hozumi, N., and Tonegawa, S. (1976) *Proc. Natl. Acad. Sci. U.S.A.* **73,** 3628.
22. Rabbitts, T. H., and Forster, A. (1978) *Cell* **13,** 319.
23. Cotton, R. G. H., and Milstein, C. (1973) *Nature (London)* **244,** 42.
24. Milstein, C., Adetugho, K., Cowan, N. J., Köhler, G., Secher, D. S., and Wilde, C. D. (1976) *Cold Spring Harbor Symp. Quant. Biol.* **51,** 793.
25. Milstein, C., Galfre, G., Secher, D. S., and Springer, T. (1979) *Cell Biology International Reports* **3,** 1.

Comparative Aspects of *in Vitro* and Cellular Assembly of Immunoglobulins

SHERMAN BEYCHOK

Departments of Biological Sciences and Chemistry
Columbia University
New York, New York

The five classes of vertebrate immunoglobulins share a common underlying tetrameric structure, in which two heavy (H) and two light (L) chains are joined together by interchain disulfide bonds and by strong noncovalent interactions (1–4; see also reviews 5–11). Figure 1 is a schematic representation of this general structure with varying numbers and locations of interchain disulfides shown as dashed lines. In most cases, a single disulfide bond links heavy to light chains, and anywhere from one to five disulfides in the hinge region form inter-heavy chain bonds, the actual number depending on heavy chain class and subclass in each species of animal.

The figure also suggests the predominant sites of noncovalent interactions between the domains, drawn as contacting loops, each closed by an intrachain disulfide bond.

The presence of both noncovalent and covalent interactions in a multisubunit structure allows one to consider three distinctive (although not necessarily independent) phases of assembly: (a) folding of the individual chains during and/or after synthesis, which may include closure of the intrachain disulfide bonds; (b) noncovalent association of the folded chains into a tetrameric structure, and (c) covalent assembly through oxidation of the pairs of reduced half-cystine residue that form the correct interchain disulfide bonds. In the synthesis of all classes of immunoglobulins, post-transcriptional modifications such as car-bohydrate addition or proteolytic cleavage may occur, and in two of

69

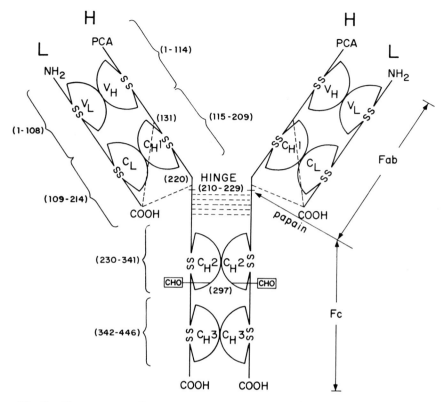

Fig. 1. The structure of immunoglobulin G proteins. The H and L chains are represented by lines showing their N-terminal and C-terminal ends. (PCA is pyrrolidone carboxylic acid, which is the N-terminal residue of most H chains.) The Fab and Fc fragments resulting from papain cleavage are shown on the right. The 12 intrachain disulfides are shown at their relative positions along the chains. The domains of the chains are represented by semicircles which touch at regions of noncovalent interaction. Since the number and location of the interchain disulfides are variable depending on the IgG subclass, only their possible locations are indicated by dashed lines. The residue numbers refer to the human IgG₁ protein (*Eu*) (11a). The sites of carbohydrate attachment to the H chain of *Eu* are indicated by the symbol CHO. Adapted from figures published by Edelman and Gall (5), Dorrington and Tanford (8), and Milstein and Pink (7); taken from Sears (12).

the classes (IgA and IgM), polymerization of the fundamental four-chain unit into larger structures with additional disulfide bonds and peptide components represents a final assembly process (13–16).

Phase (a), that is the rates and pathways of individual domain and chain folding, is under investigation in our laboratory at present, and will not concern us in this paper except for a few brief remarks at the conclusion. Phases (b) and (c), which describe the self-assembly steps, are the subjects of this talk.

In an early one of the long and important series of papers by Scharff and his associates on intracellular assembly of immunoglobulins, it was noted that assembly of the four-chain structure could occur by three pathways (17):

$$\text{I. } H + L \rightarrow HL \xrightarrow{HL} H_2L_2$$
$$\text{I. } H + H \rightarrow H_2 \xrightarrow{L} H_2L \xrightarrow{L} H_2L_2$$
$$\text{III. } H + L \rightarrow HL \xrightarrow{H} H_2L \xrightarrow{L} H_2L_2$$

Although these pathways can represent either noncovalent or covalent assembly (18, and see below) the experimental procedures in both intracellular and *in vitro* studies more often identify the covalent intermediate states, and we shall therefore first direct our attention to the covalent process. In each of these pathways, at least one of the three possible covalent intermediates—HL, H_2, H_2L—does not occur. Consequently if only one of the covalent routes were used in the assembly of a particular protein, the pathway is established by analysis of intermediates. Studies on many mouse myeloma proteins, using both tumor and cultured cells, on several human meylomas as well as on normal mouse and rabbit lymph node cells (reviewed by Scharff, 18) have revealed that there are preferred pathways of assembly, intracellularly, but that minor pathways invariably occur. In general, the major pathway depends on the structure of the heavy chain, but the relative amounts of the covalent intermediates and the kinetics of assembly vary from tumor to tumor, with average half-times about 7 min for complete covalent assembly of the chains (19,20). By way of summary, mouse IgG_1, IgG_{2a} and IgA assemble predominantly via pathway (II); IgM assembles mainly through (I), and IgG_{2b} assembles through (I) and (III). An especially interesting case is that of the MPC-11 myeloma protein, whose assembly has been studied in both tumor and cultured cells (21). In both instances, HL half-molecules are formed in significant quantities, but in the tumor cells HL intermediates are blocked toward further assembly and secreted as covalent half-molecules. We shall return to this case later.

Our own efforts have been concentrated entirely on developing an *in vitro* system to serve as a counterpart to these cellular investigations (22–28). Two facts, applying equally to the *in vivo* and *in vitro* situations, make these studies possible. The first is that the assembly process is relatively slow, so that the time dependence of the growth and decay of intermediates can be followed. The second is that owing to the molecular weight difference between heavy and light chains, and to the composition of intermediates, the progress of the reassembly reaction is readily followed by SDS gel analysis. Thus the observable species L, H, HL, H_2, H_2L, and H_2L_2 form a series of increasing molecular weight, the difference being approximately 25,000 daltons between succeeding members.

The protein we have studied most extensively, IgG^{Fro}, is a human $IgG_{1\kappa}$ generously provided over a period of several years by Dr. E. F. Osserman, and isolated from the plasma of a patient with the clinical symptoms of a plasma cell dyscrasia (29). In early experiments (22,23), we sought to establish an analytical approach to the complex reoxidation kinetics and, at the same time, find a basis for comparison with studies of intracellular covalent assembly carried out by other investigators. To do this, we isolated the covalent component of assembly by selective reduction of the interchain disulfides and then studied the reoxidative behavior of the molecule under nondissociating conditions, in which the pre-existing state of noncovalent chain association is maintained even after reduction of the interchain cystine bonds.

Figure 2 shows a representative experiment of this kind. At various times during reoxidation, samples are removed and either alkylated for gel analysis or immediately reacted with Ellmann's reagent (30) for analysis of residual free sulfhydryl titer. Together with the use of methods for the quantitative determination of the concentration of each of the molecular components directly from spectroscopic scans of the gels (23), these experimental procedures enable us to present the kinetics of reoxidation in two different ways, as depicted in Fig. 3. The right side panel simultaneously shows the time-dependent variation in concentration of all observable molecular species and the variation with time of sulfhydryl titer. This is the customary way to display kinetic data and it provides half-times for sulfhydryl disappearance and appearance of the completely reassembled H_2L_2. Moreover, the levels achieved by the intermediates is readily discerned, suggesting in the present case that reoxidation is clearly not restricted to only one of the three pathways (I), (II), or (III). Beyond this information, however, this method of presenting the data is far too complicated for mechanistic analysis. Accordingly, we have chosen to utilize a plot of concentration versus average sulfhydryl titer (left panel of Fig. 3), making time an implicit variable. This method has two important advantages over the conventional function. The first is that it minimizes a major problem inherent in kinetics of air oxidation of thiols, the oxidation kinetics of which are notoriously sensitive to certain trace metals in the buffers, to stirring rates, and other variables that are difficult to

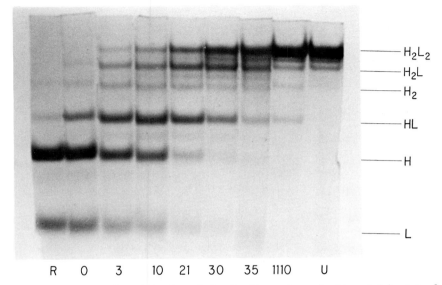

Fig. 2. Strips cut from 5% sodium dodecyl sulfate-polyacrylamide gel slabs stained with Coomassie brilliant blue. Each well (top) was loaded with 24 μg of protein. The various components are identified at the right. The wells labeled U and R represent an unreduced sample and a reduced and alkylated sample taken prior to reoxidation. The remaining strips contain samples alkylated at various times (indicated in minutes at the bottom) in a pH 3.2 → 7.5 reoxidation of reduced *Fro* at a concentration of 4.6 μM. The zero time sample was taken immediately after the protein emerged from the Bio-Gel P2 column. [Taken from Sears *et al.* (22).]

control. The second advantage is that this method makes the experimental results amenable to theoretical analysis of a number of important fundamental questions: What is a random reoxidation and does the system depart from random behavior? Is it possible to discern cooperativity in the covalent assembly, in the sense that the formation of a particular bond alters the rate of formation of another? Is the formation of any one bond favored over any other and, if so, by how much?

Figure 4 shows what random reoxidation would look like for molecules possessing different numbers of inter-heavy chain disulfide bonds. Panel B, for example, corresponds to human IgG$_1$ and IgG$_4$; Panel D to mouse IgG$_{2b}$ and so forth. By random reoxidation, we mean that no one bond is favored over any other throughout the course of the covalent assembly. The only restriction is that the half-cystines are correctly paired.

In the upper part of this figure the components are given in molar

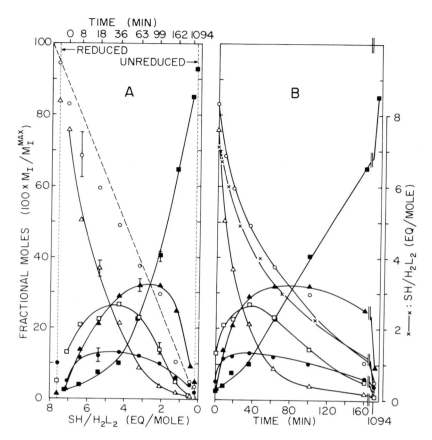

Fig. 3. Analysis of a pH $5.5 \rightarrow 7.5$ reoxidation (protein concentration, 3.3 μM. [Taken from Sears *et al.* (22).]

quantities, as would be measured in an *in vitro* experiment such as that of Fig. 3. In the lower half, components are given in intensities, such as counts of radioactivity, as might be measured in a cellular pulse-chase experiment. For the latter plots, it is assumed that H and L are synthesized in equimolar ratios. Deviation from the curves in Fig. 4 serves to define a preferred pathway for the disulfide bonding arrangements drawn. Comparison of Fig. 3 with the upper part of Panel B shows that the reoxidation of IgG*Fro* is not random.

With the analytical experience gained from these "nondissociated" conditions, we proceeded to examine re-assembly after complete dissociation and separation of component heavy and light chains, fol-

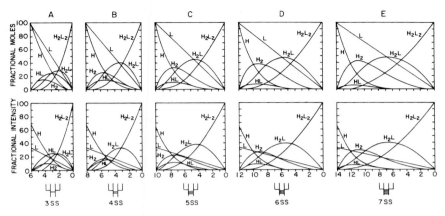

Fig. 4. The hypothetical restricted random reoxidation curves for various patterns of interchain bonding schematically illustrated at the bottom. Each HL and HH bond is assumed to form independently and with the same probability. In the upper panels the components are represented in terms of fractional moles. In the lower panels they are represented in terms of fractional intensities, where intensity here means any conserved property of the H and L chains such as staining intensity or radioactive label. In converting the upper curves to the lower ones, it was assumed that, whatever the property is, it manifests itself in exactly a 2 : 1 ratio for H and L chains. [Taken from Sears *et al.* (22).]

lowed by recombination at various ratios (23,24,31). In particular, it is of interest to know whether actual disruption of the noncovalent bonds leads to any alteration in kinetics and pathway, and whether reoxidation under conditions of light chain excess differs from that at equimolar ratios.

Reoxidation at equimolar levels of H and L chains after chain separation in 1 *M* propionic acid is similar in rate and in assembly pattern to experiments without prior chain separation. Figure 5 shows a reoxidation experiment in which light chains exceed heavy chains in a ratio of greater than 2 to 1. The main additional feature to note is the appearance of a low and almost constant level of covalent L_2 dimer while H_2L_2 is being formed, followed by an increase that begins only after the main assembly reaction is virtually complete. At long times, virtually all of the excess light chain hs been converted into L_2 dimer.

Table I summarizes a number of parameters in the unseparated and separated chain experiments. The main points to be noted are that the average initial rates of sulfhydryl disappearance are the same for both kinds of experiments when the H : L ratio is one, and that the rates of covalent assembly are slowed when L chain is present in excess.

Several other kinds of experiments are possible when partially re-

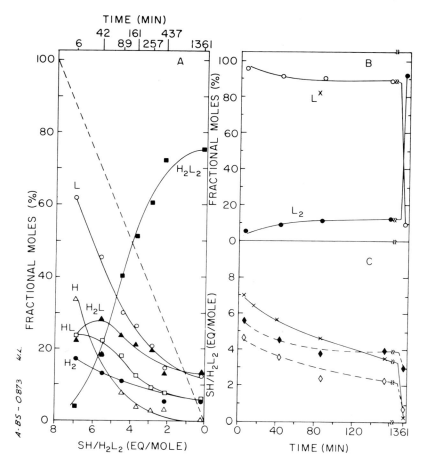

Fig. 5. Recombined chain reoxidation; $R_{L/H} = 2.28$. After reduction of IgG(*Fro*) by DTT, the H and L chains were separated by chromatography on Sephadex G100 in N_2 aerated, 1 *M* propionic acid–1 m*M* EDTA (pH 2.3). The L and H pools were separately chromatographed on Bio-Gel P2 in N_2 aerated 10 m*M* HOAc (pH 3.2), and mixed in a molar ratio of 2.28:1 just prior to raising the pH and ionic strength for reoxidation. In the final reoxidation mixture $(L)_T = 10.5 \, \mu M$, $(H)_T = 4.6 \, \mu M$, and $(H_2L_2)_T = 2.3 \, \mu M$. (A) The L line and the measured SH titer (abscissa) are corrected here for the L excess over H. (B) Fractional moles of the excess L versus time. On the sodium dodecyl sulfate gels, the excess L appears in two forms: either as a monomer, L (○), or as a covalent dimer, L_2 (●). The ordinate has been normalized relative to the total concentration of excess L chains $(L^x + 2L_2)$ which was 0.75 μM in this case. (C)The measured and calculated SH titers versus time as in Fig. 1B. The SH titers are corrected for the SH contribution of L^x and are determined relative to $(H_2L_2)_L$. [Taken from Sears *et al.* (23).]

TABLE I
Comparisons between Unseparated Chain and Recombined Chain Reoxidations[a]

$(H_2L_2)_T$[b]	$R_{L/H}$[c]	$fM_{H_2}max(r)$[d]	$fM_{HL}max(r)$[d]	$fM_{H_2L}max(r)$[d]	t_{av}[e]/SH
		Unseparated chain reoxidations			
3.4	1	25[f]	33(4.8)	28(3.1)	16
3.5	1	18(3.4)	26(4.9)	27(3.4)	18
		Separated-recombined chain reoxidations			
2.9	1.13	24(7.4)	29(6.7)	34(5.0)	15
4.7	1.0	27(6.4)	27(7.1)	43(3.9)	17
2.1	2.19	12[f]	31[f]	26(3.6)	[f]
2.0	2.10	27(7.5)	20(5.9)	33(3.8)	33
1.8	2.28	17(7.0)	24(7.0)	28(5.6)	43
2.2	2.03	26[f]	30(4.2)	22(3.4)	42
1.7	3.46	17(3.9)	30(4.5)	36(3.6)	>50
1.7	3.26	32(7.6)	20(4.9)	39(3.2)	19
1.4	2.80	33(3.9)	25(5.3)	15(3.9)	>50
1.7	3.21	25[f]	16(7.0)	26(4.1)	>50

[a] All experiments are $3.2 \rightarrow 7.5$ reoxidations.
[b] Total possible concentration of H_2L_2 in units of μM.
[c] Molar ratio of L to H.
[d] Fractional moles, in percent; r in parentheses is the corresponding number of SH equivalents per H_2L_2 at the maximum.
[e] Average time in minutes per unit change in the measured SH titer from time zero to the time r = 4.
[f] Insufficient data. [Adapted from Sears *et al.* (23).]

duced, separated H and L chain fractions are prepared. For example, H chain oxidation to H_2 dimers can be studied without the competing and complicating formation of HL bonds (12,23,24). Ordinarily, H chains are not well behaved when alone in the reoxidizing buffer. In addition to the expected formation of the H_2 dimers, higher molecular weight covalent aggregates also readily form, as anticipated from early studies on the behavior of alkylated γ chains in acid and at neutral pH (32,33). In such experiments, the formation of aggregates is too rapid to allow any conclusion about the reoxidation kinetics of inter-heavy chain disulfide bond formation in the absence of L chains.

Three kinds of experiments using partially reduced H chains in combination with modified L chain species are shown in Figs. 6–8. In Fig 6, H chains are oxidized to H_2 dimers in the presence of alkylated light chains, which serve to solubilize the H chains but are blocked from forming HL bonds (12,23). In Fig. 7, solubilization is effected by

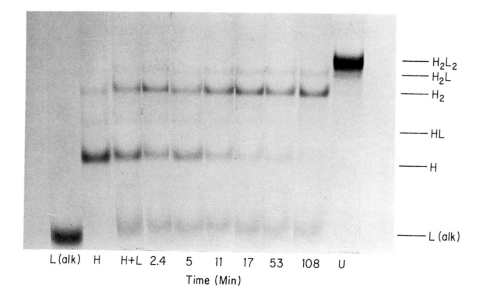

L(alk)　H　　H+L　2.4　　5　　11　　17　　53　　108　　U

Time (Min)

Fig. 6. Sodium dodecyl sulfate-polyacrylamide gels of the reoxidation of H chains mixed with prealkylated L chains, L(alk); $R_{L/H} = 1.5$. The samples in the gels designated L(alk) and H were taken from the respective pools just prior to their being mixed for reoxidation. The gel designated by U is that of an unreduced sample of $IgG^{(Fro)}$, included for reference. In the final reoxidation mixture $(L)_T = 5.5\ \mu M$, $(H)_T = 3.7\ \mu M$, and $(H_2L_2)_T = 1.85\ \mu M$. [Taken from Sears *et al.* (23).]

utilizing V_L fragments [from a 37°C pepsin digestion of Bence-Jones *(Fro)* protein (31)]. V_L does not inhibit covalent polymerization of H chain as well as whole, alkylated L chain, but the reaction is sufficiently orderly that the kinetics of H_2 formation can be studied in the absence of the C_L–C_{H1} domain interaction.

Finally, Fig. 8 shows the reoxidation of H chains in the presence of the L_2 covalent dimer (27). This is a striking experiment which shows that L_2 is rapidly incorporated into the normal pathway of covalent assembly through either of two interchange reactions:

$$IV.\quad H + L_2 \rightarrow HL + L$$
$$IV'.\quad H_2 + L_2 \rightarrow H_2L + L$$

Thus, when excess L chain is present, an additional pathway for assembly is provided. Any excess L that has been converted into L_2 may react with either H or H_2 through a disulfide interchange reaction.

To summarize thus far, the overall reoxidative assembly patterns in experiments with H and L separated prior to recombination are similar

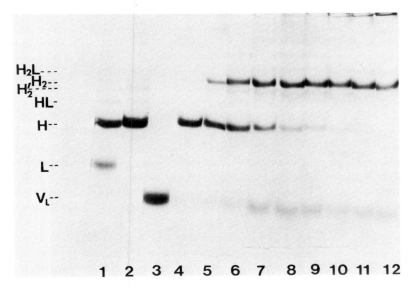

Fig. 7. SDS polyacrylamide gels of $H_{SH} + V_L$ reoxidation. Wells 1 and 2 represent the partially-reduced myeloma protein and the purified H chain fraction, respectively. Well 3 is the V_L fragment isolated from a 37°C partial pepsin digest of B J protein. Well 4 is the $H + V_L$ mixture (1 : 1) that was alkylated before raising the pH. Wells 5–12 represent aliquots from the reoxidation mixture alkylated at various times. Well 5: 3.5 min; well 6: 18.0 min; well 7: 39.5 min; well 8: 73.0 min; well 9: 102.0 min; well 10: 145.5 min; well 11: 192.0 min; well 12: 1080.0 min. [Taken from Kazin (31).]

to those observed when the chains remain noncovalently associated throughout. With equimolar mixtures of H and L, the reoxidation rates also are similar to those of unseparated chains. However, when L chains are present in excess, the overall *in vitro* rates of covalent assembly are generally diminished, probably indicating transient non-productive interactions. At the highest molar excesses of L (3 : 1), the assembly pahtways may also be modified. In all experiments with excess L chains, covalent L_2 dimers form at rates which are comparatively slow relative to the H_2L_2 assembly rates. Three kinds of reoxidation experiments with modified L chains are also described. In the first, the free half-cystine of L is irreversibly blocked by reaction with iodoacetamide, and the alkylated L chains are recombined with reduced H chains. This experiment isolates the reactions in which H_2 disulfides are formed without the accompanying formation of HL bonds. Although the alkylated L chains do not play a direct role in the reoxidation, their presence is required to inhibit aggregation and pre-

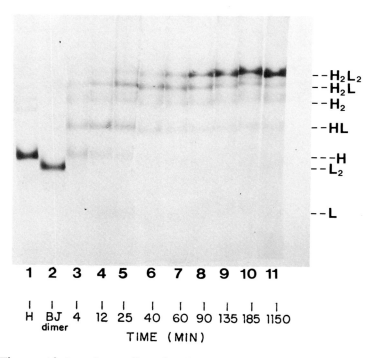

Fig. 8. The reoxidation of partially reduced heavy (H) chain with light chain covalent dimer (L_2) shown on SDS polyacrylamide gel. Wells 1 and 2 represent the purified H chain and Bence-Jones (BJ) covalent L chain dimer, respectively, after Bio-Gel P2 chromatography. The H and L_2 fractions were combined under N_2 at an equimolar ratio in 10 mM acetic acid (final ratio of total L chain of H chain, 1 : 36). The pH of the mixture was then raised to 7.5 and the mixture was exposed to air. The final concentration of H_2L_2 was 1.6 μM. Wells 3–11 represent portions from the reoxidation mixture that were immediately alkylated with 1.0 M iodoacetamide at the times indicated. All gel samples contained 1% SDS and iodoacetamide. [Taken from Kazin and Beychok (27).]

cipitation of high molecular weight products which otherwise ensue; this suggests a possible biological role for excess L *in vivo*. In the second kind of experiment, H chain is oxidized in the presence of the isolated V_L domain. In the third kind of experiment, covalent L_2 dimers are mixed with reduced H chains. L_2 rapidly disappears with the concurrent appearance of HL, H_2L, and fully assembled H_2L_2. H_2 dimers are also reactive in this process.

With respect to the question of random versus nonrandom behavior in the covalent assembly process, Sears and Beychok (24) have carried out a theoretical analysis in which the experimental results are examined in terms of the relative probabilities of H–H and H–L bond formation throughout the course of the reoxidation experiment.

Figure 9 compares the observed probabilities of formation of HH and HL bonds, and their ratio, during an unseparated chain reoxidation, compared to expected theoretical random probabilities. At the outset of the reaction, all bonds can form, but the probability that an HL bond is formed initially is about twice as great as that of an HH

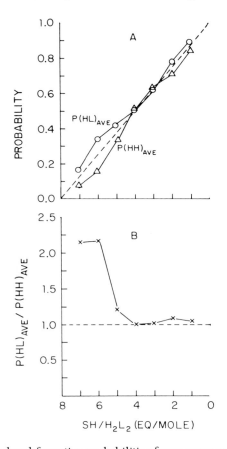

Fig. 9. Disulfide bond formation probabilities for an unseparated chain, 3.2 → 7.5 reoxidation. (A) The average probabilities for forming either an inter-HL bond (O——O) or an inter-HH bond (△——△) were determined from the experimental reoxidation profiles for L, H, etc. and the corresponding SH titers. The diagonal dashed line is the corresponding probability expected for both of these bonds if the reoxidation were random. (B) The ratio (×——×) of the average probabilities shown in (A). The horizontal dashed lines again refer to the random case. [Taken from Sears and Beychok (24).]

bond. As the reaction proceeds, this preference diminishes until about midway in covalent bond formation when the two probabilities become equal.

The essential features of the foregoing studies, then, are: (1) The rate and pattern of covalent chain assembly are qualitatively the same whether the reduced H and L chains remain associated or are separated by propionic acid and recombined prior to establishing reoxidation conditions. (2) Molar excess of L over H chains—up to threefold—do not have a marked effect on the pattern of covalent H_2L_2 assembly, although at molar ratios of greater than $3:1$, the values of fM_{H2}^{max} are increased (in three of four experiments) and the overall rates of sulfhydryl disappearance are diminished, suggesting the possible occurrence of nonproductive transient intermediates. (3) The basic pattern of covalent assembly appears to be characteristic of human IgG_1 proteins in general since Petersen and Dorrington (34) and, very recently, Kishida *et al.* (35) found qualitatively similar reoxidation patterns in studies of other myeloma proteins. (4) Reduced H chains readily reoxidize to H_2 dimers in the presence of alkylated L chains, which have irreversibly lost their capacity to form inter-HL disulfide bonds. (5) A disulfide bond between L chains in the form of L_2 dimers does not prevent the formation of inter-HL disulfide bonds; on the contrary, mixtures of reduced H chains and covalent L_2 dimers readily reoxidize to fully assembled H_2L_2 molecules with concurrent disappearance of L_2 through disulfide exchange.

From the first two observations above, one can draw the broad conclusion that the covalent chain assembly of IgG^{Fro} *in vitro* proceeds in a characteristic fashion which, under the conditions of these experiments, at least, is qualitatively independent of whether the chains are physically separated prior to reoxidation and whether L exceeds H in concentration. The basic similarity between the unseparated chain and recombined chain reoxidations is probably accounted for by the very strong, essentially irreversible, noncovalent affinities between chains which maintain H and L in the assembled H_2L_2 form in both types of experiment. This is the essential concept underlying our analysis of the *in vitro* assembly of IgG molecules.

To prove that the *in vitro* reoxidation conditions establish a stable noncovalently associated tetramer structure very rapidly, we undertook a series of stopped-flow experiments on the kinetics of noncovalent interaction of heavy and light chains in IgG^{Fro} (28). A fluorescent probe, N-(iodoacetylaminoethyl)-8-naphthylamine-1-sulfonic acid (1,8-I-AEDANS) reacts stoichiometrically with the COOH-terminal cysteine residue of the partially reduced L^{Fro} chain. The fluorescence spectra of the modified chain and of the mixture of this chain with an equimolar amount of H chain are shown in Fig. 10, and Fig. 11 shows the fluorimetric titration of L-AEDANS with H chain. The rate of association of these chains is displayed as a second order plot in Fig. 12. The rate constant for this reaction is 6×10^6 liters mol^{-1}sec^{-1} at 20°C, probe, N-(iodoacetylaminoethyl)-8-naphthlamine-1-sulfonic acid (1,8-I-AEDANS) reacts stoichiometrically with the COOH-terminal (36–40).

Since the reaction is second order, the half time is inversely proportional to initial reactant concentration. For the case shown, with a light

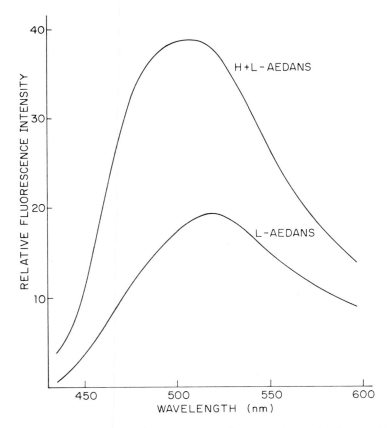

Fig. 10. Emission spectra of L-AEDANS and H + L-AEDANS. The L-AEDANS concentration was 0.20 μM in TE buffer. A small volume of H chain solution was added to a final concentration of 0.22 μM. Temperature was 20°C. Excitation λ, 343 nm; band width was 5 nm for both excitation and emission. [Taken from Friedman *et al.* (28).]

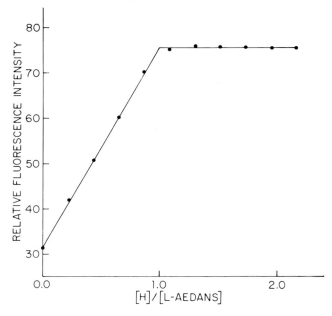

Fig. 11. Fluorometric titration of L-AEDANS with H chain. Small volumes of 2.8 μM H chain were added to a 0.13 μM solution of L-AEDANS in TE buffer and the fluorescent intensities determined after equilibration. Temperature was 20°C. Excitation λ, 343 nm, band width 5 nm; emission λ, 488 nm, band width 10 nm. [Taken from Friedman *et al.* (28).]

chain concentration of $3.3 \times 10^{-8} M$ and heavy chain $5.4 \times 10^{-8} M$, the half time is 2.5 sec, which may be compared with the average of about 15 min for covalent bond formation at still higher concentrations.

We turn now to a comparison of the *in vitro* and cellular assembly. To begin with, it is important to note that the main qualitative results of our *in vitro* work with IgG^{Fro} are not special in kind, or specific for a single protein. As noted above, Petersen and Dorrington (34) and Kishida *et al.* (35) working with different proteins find qualitatively similar patterns of *in vitro* assembly, although their methods of analysis differ considerably from ours. Furthermore other investigations, including work with mouse proteins (41,42), all suggest that there is a fundamental similarity between *in vitro* and cellular processes with respect to the dominant influence of H chain structure on the profile of assembly intermediates (pathway of assembly), as was suggested in the very earliest *in vivo* studies of Scharff's group. This establishes a

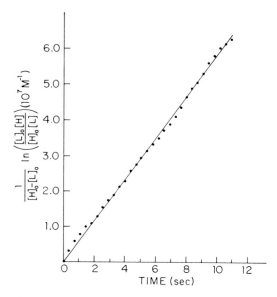

Fig. 12. Second order plot of the association of H with L-AEDANS. Final concentrations were 33 nm L-AEDANS and 54 nm H chain in 25 mM Tris-HCl, 21 mM NaCl, 1 mM sodium acetate, 0.5 mM EDTA, pH 7.5. Temperature, 20°C. [Taken from Friedman *et al.* (28).]

structural basis for control of assembly that is common to cellular and *in vitro* studies and is largely uninfluenced by the specific environmental features of the intracellular assembly sites.

Second, there is at least a rough correspondence, which must have a structural basis, in terms of the rates of assembly. For example, the mouse protein MOPC-31C assembles very slowly intracellularly with less than 40% completion in 18 min compared to an average of about 70% completion (18). Percy *et al.* (41,42) and our laboratory (31) have examined the *in vitro* assembly. We have found low levels of completion (<40% at greater than 100 hr), and a half-time for sulfhydryl disappearance of more than 200 min.

Third, there may be related effects caused by L chain excess in both kinds of experiments. *In vitro*, excess L chain experiments have certain unique features (31): (1) a diminished rate of sulfhydryl disappearance, (2) an inhibition of the usual H chain aggregation and precipitation observed at later times in other reoxidations, (3) a decreased rate of L chain dimerization compared to L chains in solution alone.

Obviously, the L chains are not free to interact because they are complexed with H chains. L chain dimerization does not take place until the H chain sulfhydryls have oxidized. Formation of transient nonproductive intermediates such as HL_2 could account for these effects.

As noted above, the assembly of H and L chains differs in MPC-11 tumors and cultured cell lines, although there appear to be no structural differences in the chains. However, the tumor cells synthesize 3.6 to 4-fold excess of L chains, whereas the cells in culture synthesize about 1.7-fold excess L chain. In the case of the tumor cells, HL is made but does not assemble further into H_2L_2. Baumal and Scharff (20) found these half-molecules in noncovalent association with L chains, and suggested the occurrence of nonproductive complexes such as (LH)L(HL). This may be similar to the situation in our excess L chain experiments, where the diminished rate of assembly has been attributed to transient nonproductive complexes, such as HL_2.

These qualitative similarities certainly indicate that cellular self-assembly requires no special mechanism. However, in detail the *in vitro* and *in vivo* assembly processes may differ considerably. For example, the *in vivo* rates are faster where comparable proteins have been studied. Moreover, the instances of assembly blocks and of high levels of kinetic cooperativity are much more securely established in the cellular studies than in the *in vitro* studies reported to date, with the possible exception of the block in a human IgG_4 reported by Petersen and Dorrington (34).

The final difference to be noted is by far the most serious. In the *in vitro* assembly studies, noncovalent association prior to disulfide bond formation is established beyond reasonable doubt. Indeed, the experiment with L_2 covalent dimer (Fig. 8) demonstrates the thermodynamic control over the assembly process exercised by the correct positioning of L and H chains through noncovalent domain associations. In this view, the kinetic cooperativity observed in covalent assembly of IgG^{Fro} represents a fine-tuning of the tetramer structure initially established by rapid noncovalent interactions. In contrast, few if any H and L chains appear to be noncovalently assembled for any measurable length of time prior to interchain disulfide bond formation intracellularly (43; M. D. Scharff, personal communication). If this is not one of the most important differences thus far observed between *in vitro* and *in vivo* assembly, it is surely one of the most interesting and puzzling, and provides an excellent avenue for future investigations of immunoglobulin assembly.

ACKNOWLEDGMENTS

The author is grateful to former and present collaborators and students who participated in the studies reported herein. In particular he wishes to acknowledge the excellent work and dedication of Prof. Duane Sears, Drs. A. Kazin and M. Pflumm, F. Friedman, M-D. Yang-Chang, J. Mohrer, M. Goldberger, H. Hertan, and C. Beychok.

Many of the concepts and directions of these investigations grew out of discussions with Professors E. A. Kabat, E. Osserman, and M. D. Scharff, to all of whom the author is greatly indebted.

Finally, he thanks Professors Osserman and Scharff for their generosity in providing the proteins studied in these investigations.

This work was supported in part by Grant CA13014 from the National Cancer Institute and Grant PCM77-08537 from the National Science Foundation.

REFERENCES

1. Edelman, G. M. (1959) *J. Am. Chem. Soc.* **81**, 3155.
2. Edelman, G. M., and Poulik, M. D. (1961) *J. Exp. Med.* **113**, 861.
3. Fleischman, J. B., Pain, R. H., and Porter, R. R. (1962) *Arch. Biochem. Biophys.*, *Suppl.* **1**, 174.
4. Fleischman, J. B., Porter, R. R., and Press, E. M. (1963) *Biochem. J.* **88**, 220.
5. Edelman, G. M., and Gall, W. E. (1969) *Annu. Rev. Biochem.* **38**, 415.
6. Metzger, H. (1970) *Annu. Rev. Biochem.* **39**, 889.
7. Milstein, C., and Pink, J. R. L. (1970) *Prog. Biophys. Mol. Biol.* **21**, 211.
8. Dorrington, K. J., and Tanford, C. (1970) *Adv. Immunol.* **12**, 333.
9. Gally, J. A., and Edelman, G. M. (1972) *Annu. Rev. Genet.* **6**, 1.
10. Cathou, R. E., and Dorrington, K. J. (1975) *Biol. Macromol.* **7**, Part C, 91.
11. Nisonoff, A., Hopper, J. E., and Spring, S. B. (1975) "The Antibody Molecule." Academic Press, New York.
11a. Edelman, G. M., Cunningham, B. A., Gall, W. A., Gottlieb, P. D., Rutishauser, U., and Waxdal, M. J. (1969) *Proc. Natl. Acad. Sci. U.S.A.* **63**, 78.
12. Sears, D. W. (1974) Ph.D. Thesis, Columbia University, New York.
13. Parkhouse, R. M. E. (1971) *Biochem. J.* **123**, 635.
14. Parkhouse, R. M. E. (1973) *Transplant. Rev.* **14**, 131.
15. Bevan, M. J. (1971) *Eur. J. Immunol.* **1**, 133.
16. Buxbaum, J., and Scharff, M. D. (1973) *J. Exp. Med.* **138**, 278.
17. Scharff, M. D., and Laskov, R. (1970) *Prog. Allergy* **14**, 37.
18. Scharff, M. D. (1974) *Harvey Lect.* **69**, 125.
19. Baumal, R., Coffino, P., Bargellesi, A., Buxbaum, J., Laskov, R., and Scharff, M. D. (1971) *Ann. N.Y. Acad. Sci.* **190**, 235.
20. Baumal, R., and Scharff, M. D. (1973) *Transplant. Rev.* **14**, 163.
21. Laskov, R., Lanzerotti, R., and Scharff, M. D. (1971) *J. Mol. Biol.* **56**, 327.
22. Sears, D. W., Mohrer, J., and Beychok, S. (1975) *Proc. Natl. Acad. Sci. U.S.A.* **72**, 353–357.
23. Sears, D. W., Kazin, A. R., Mohrer, J., Friedman, F., and Beychok, S. (1977) *Biochemistry* **16**, 2016–2025.
24. Sears, D. W., and Beychok, S. (1977) *Biochemistry* **16**, 2026–2031.

25. Sears, D. W., Mohrer, J., and Beychok, S. (1977) *Biochemistry* **16**, 2031–2035.
26. Beychok, S. (1977) *Proceedings of a Symposium, De La Physique Théorique à la Biologie.* Pergamon, Oxford.
27. Kazin, A. R., and Beychok, S. (1978) *Science* **199**, 688–690.
28. Friedman, F., Yang-Chang, M.-D., and Beychok, S. (1978) *J. Biol. Chem.* **253**, 2368–2372.
29. Osserman, E. (1971) *In* "Cecil-Loeb: Textbook of Medicine" (P. B. Beeson and W. McDermott, eds.), 13th ed., p. 579. Saunders, Philadelphia, Pennsylvania.
30. Ellman, G. L. (1959) *Arch. Biochem. Biophys.* **82**, 70.
31. Kazin, A. R. (1977) Ph.D. Thesis, Columbia University, New York.
32. Stevenson, G. T., and Dorrington, K. J. (1970) *Biochem. J.* **118**, 703.
33. Björk, I., and Tanford, C. (1971) *Biochemistry* **10**, 1271.
34. Petersen, J. G. L., and Dorrington, K. J. (1974) *J. Biol. Chem.* **249**, 5633.
35. Kishida, F., Azuma, T., and Hamaguchi, K. (1976) *J. Biochem. (Tokyo)* **79**, 91.
36. Bigelow, C. C., Smith, B. R., and Dorrington, K. J. (1974) *Biochemistry* **13**, 4602–4608.
37. Azuma, T., Isobe, T., and Hamaguchi, K. (1975) *J. Biochem. (Tokyo)* **77**, 473–379.
38. Azuma, T., Isobe, T., and Hamaguchi, K. (1975) *J. Biochem. (Tokyo)* **78**, 335–340.
39. Azuma, T., and Hamaguchi, K. (1975) *J. Biochem. (Tokyo)* **78**, 341–347.
40. Azuma, T., and Hamaguchi, K. (1976) *J. Biochem. (Tokyo)* **80**, 1023–1038.
41. Percy, M. E., Baumal, R., Dorrington, K. J., and Percy, J. R. (1976) *Can. J. Biochem.* **54**, 675.
42. Percy, J. R., Percy, M. E., and Baumal, R. (1976) *Can. J. Biochem.* **54**, 688.
43. Baumal, R., Potter, M., and Scharff, M. D. (1971) *J. Exp. Med.* **134**, 1316.

Human Immunoglobulin Mutants

EDWARD C. FRANKLIN, BLAS FRANGIONE
Departments of Medicine and Pathology
New York University College of Medicine
New York, New York

AND

JOEL BUXBAUM
Research Service
Veterans Administration Hospital
New York, New York

Structurally altered immunoglobulins in man have been recognized with ever increasing frequency during the last 15 years (1,2). For reasons that remain to be explained, they involve the heavy chains with much greater frequency than light chains. We have studied these variants in the hope that their analysis will complement more classical studies designed to investigate the genetic control of immunoglobulins. This approach has been based on the fact that the deletions encountered do not appear to be random but to involve defined regions of the molecule, most often single intact domains or the hinge (2). While the murine system obviously provides many advantages due to its greater manipulability, the chemical studies of the human variants at this time are far ahead of those of the murine proteins and provide some clues that are not yet available from studies of the mouse (3,4).

If we consider only mutants of the γ heavy chain, it is now well recognized that most commonly they consist of internal deletions which begin or end at the hinge. Figure 1 shows a schematic diagram of eight heavy chain disease proteins belonging to the γ1, 2, and 3 subclasses. All have a part of the V_H sequence which may be normal or abnormal (5) followed by a deletion of the rest of V_H and C_H1 domains and resume normal sequence at the hinge. There is an unexpectedly high frequency of γ3 heavy chain disease proteins and in most of them, the entire quadruplicated hinge is present. However, in at least one, normal sequence appears to resume at one of the quadruplicated units of the hinge rather than the beginning of the hinge (6,7). Also in Fig. 1

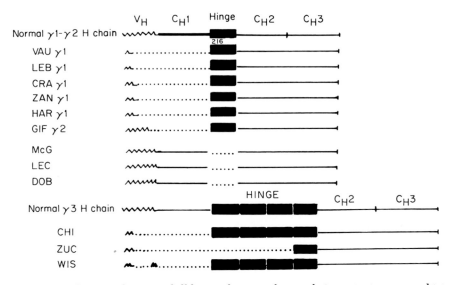

Fig. 1. Schematic diagram of all known human γ heavy chain mutants compared to the normal γ1, γ2, and γ3 heavy chains. Structure of most proteins is summarized in Franklin and Frangione (2). VAU, LEB, ZAN are unpublished. LEC (8), McG (9), DOB (10), CHI (11), WIS (12), ZUC (6). *Top group:* γ1 and γ2 HCD proteins with deletions of part of V_H and C_H1 with resumption of normal sequence at the start of the hinge. *Middle group,* Three myeloma proteins with a deletion of the hinge only. *Bottom group:* Three γ3 HCD proteins. One (CHI) resembles γ1 HCD proteins in having an internal deletion which ends at the start of the quadruplicated hinge, whereas one (ZUC) ends at one of the duplications of the hinge. The third (WIS) is unique in having an internal deletion of the hinge ending at an 8 residue segment corresponding with the VC joining region followed by another deletion ending at the hinge.

are three deleted γ1 myeloma proteins which lack the 15 residues from 216 to 230 which constitute the hinge. Since these molecules are not disulfide linked, they dissociate without reduction (9). These two groups of molecules and one of the murine mutants (3) point to the hinge as a recognition site for some event in RNA processing.

Of great interest is a molecule we have recently encountered which suggests that another recognition site exists at the VC joining region (12). As shown schematically in Fig. 1, in this molecule a small stretch of the amino terminus is followed by a deletion of over 100 residues which ends at the VC joining region where a stretch of 8 residues having striking homology to the carboxyl end of V_H is followed by another deletion which ends at the beginning of the quadruplicated hinge.

Figure 2 shows the amino terminal sequence of this molecule

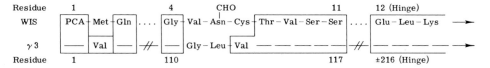

Fig. 2. Amino terminal sequence of WIS aligned for maximal homology. The 3 first residues correspond to the normal amino terminus. The next 8 residues have homology with the VC joining region and from residue 12 on the sequence, corresponds to the hinge of γ3.

aligned for maximal homology with a normal H chain. The first 3 residues PCA–Met–Gln are unusual only in that Met replaces the usual Val at position 2 (13). This can be the result of a single base substitution. The next 8 residues have no homology with the beginning of the V_H domain or the region preceding the hinge but correspond in 5 of 6 invariant residues including Gly (110)* and Thr–Val–Ser–Ser (114–117) to the carboxy terminus of V_H immediately preceding what is regarded as the VC joining region. The substitution of Val (113) by Cys and the finding of carbohydrate at Asn (112) are unique. The next 8 residues starting with Glu–Leu–Lys correspond exactly to the γ3 hinge (Fig. 3). Detailed studies to be published elsewhere (12) have shown the entire quadruplicated hinge to be present and less careful analyses suggest that the remainder of the Fc fragment is intact. Thus, in this protein, it would appear that a mutation–deletion event occurred with splicing to the VC joining region, followed by a second deletion and splicing to the next recognition site of the hinge. Attempts to align the observed sequence either with other regions in V_H or C_H1 or the propeptides of L or H chains proved to no avail.

Before discussing possible mechanisms for these events in light of the discontinuous transcription of DNA and RNA splicing, which has been shown for many proteins recently, I would like to discuss two light chain mutants (SAC and SM) which have been studied by others (15,16) and which are more easy to interpret in light of the elegant studies by Dr. Tonegawa and his colleagues (17). Figure 4 shows that in Tonegawa's studies of a murine λ_{II} chain, there is a large untranslated region of DNA at the end of the propeptide and another one at residue 98 (14) in the embryo and at residue 110 in the adult DNA. When comparing the structure of DNA to the deletions in the two L chain mutants, it is apparent that the deletion in SM ends at residue 110 corresponding to the adult untranslated region and close to the chemically-defined VC joining region of the L chain, while SAC ends

* Numbering corresponds to protein Eu (14).

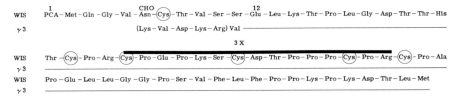

Fig. 3. The amino terminal 95 residues of WIS compared to the hinge of γ3 to show that the entire quadruplicated hinge is present and that the sequence before the hinge of the normal γ3 H chain is different.

at residue 99 which corresponds exactly to the position of the second intron in embryonal λ_{II} defined by Tonegawa. It is of interest that SM resembles the HCD proteins in the first 3 residues following the deletion. Thus, at this early stage it may not be unfounded to postulate that in these deletion mutants, an event occurred which has resulted in splicing at the next available recognition site (i.e., the VC joining region). Depending on the L chain class or subclass, this appears to be somewhere in the vicinity of but not always exactly at the chemically-defined VC joining region.

It seems not unreasonable to attempt to extrapolate these findings correlating the structure of mutant proteins with DNA from the light chain to the heavy chain which is more difficult to study. On the basis of the characterized heavy chain disease mutants, it seems likely that recognition sites or introns may exist not only at the VC joining region but also at the beginning and end of the hinge (Fig. 5). In addition, results with other rarer and less well characterized variants suggest

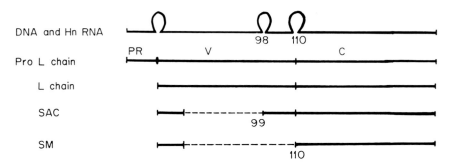

Fig. 4. Schematic diagram showing that the position of untranslated regions in embryonic and adult DNA correspond exactly to the sites of termination of the internal deletions of two light chain mutants.

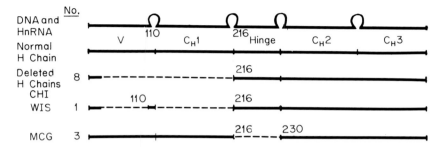

Fig. 5. Schematic diagram predicting the location of untranslated regions of DNA based on structural mutants of heavy chains. Those between the C_H2 and C_H3 domains are based on mutants not shown here.

that each of the domains may correspond to a separate transcriptional unit defined in terms of excision and splicing of HnRNA (2).

There exists in addition another group of heavy chain disease proteins which have been of less interest because they appear to be the result of proteolytic degradation. Figure 6 summarizes the N-terminal sequences of nine of these (six studied by us) and indicates that the amino termini vary and tend to correspond to sites of proteolytic cleavage by a variety of enzymes (18). Studies carried out on one of these (OMM) whose cells are in long-term culture have provided two sorts of evidence that they are indeed breakdown products of true

PROTEIN   RESIDUE

```
          211      215        220          225         230        235         240
γ1         V D K R V E P K S C D K T H T C P P C P A P E L L G G P S V ....
YOK a               S ─────────────────────────────────────────────── ....
    b                              ├───────────────────────────────── ....
DOR a                       ├───────────────────────────────────────── ....
    b                         ├─────────────────────────────────────── ....
AH                                 ├───────────────────────────────── ....
MO                                 ├───────────────────────────────── ....
OA                                 ├───────────────────────────────── ....
VAL                                     ├──────────────────────────── ....
RIP a                                   ├──────────────────────────── ....
    b                                     ├────────────────────────── ....
MAT                                                  ├──( )──────── ....

γ3         ELKTPLGDTTHTCPR(CPEPKSCDTPPPCPR)₃ C P A P E L L G G P S V ....
OMM                 ├───────────────────────────────────────── ....
WIS                                                  ├────────── ....
```

Fig. 6. Sequence of degraded HCD molecules compared to the γ1 and γ3 heavy chains. Structural studies of these proteins are summarized in Franklin (18).

heavy chain disease proteins and not of IgG or intact heavy chains. First, when the heavy chain disease protein was isolated from 10 liters of culture supernatants from OMM cells, it had the same molecular weight as the serum protein but instead of Gly (19), the amino terminus obtained by pronase digestion was PCA-Val (20). We have not obtained the overlapping sequence, but the extra stretch must be small since the molecular weight by SDS-PAGE was indistinguishable from that of the serum protein. Second, when mRNA was isolated from the cells, it was smaller than that of a mouse myeloma tumor (21). The translation product of the mRNA in the wheat germ system was about 2000 daltons larger than the protein synthesized by the cells under conditions where incorporation of carbohydrate was prevented, and much smaller than a normal H chain. Preliminary structural analyses of the radioactive precursor synthesized indicate that the true amino-terminal residue is methionine and that there are 4 to 5 leucines in the first 20 residues. Three of the leucines are consecutive around position 10, a pattern similar to that noted in murine light chain precursors, and consistent with those hydrophobic amino acid sequences found in many other proteins synthesized on membrane-bound polysomes (22). Studies are currently in progress to obtain the sequence of this signal peptide. It appears likely that these apparently degraded proteins are also derived from deleted molecules and that cells from these patients can be used to study biosynthetic events. Hopefully, the discovery and study of additional naturally-occurring variants will correlate with studies of the structure of DNA. In certain instances, they may even predict the nature of unusual events that may be involved in the genetic regulation of antibody structure before biochemical analyses of the DNA can be carried out.

ACKNOWLEDGMENTS

This work was supported in part by U.S. Public Health Service Research Grants no. AM 01431, AM 02594 and CAA12152; The Irvington House Institute.

REFERENCES

1. Franklin, E. C., Lowenstein, J., Bigelow, B., and Meltzer, M. (1964) *Am. J. Med.* **37**, 332.
2. Franklin, E. C., and Frangione, B. (1976) *Contemp. Top. Mol. Immunol.* **4**, 89.
3. Milstein, C., Secher, D. S., Cowan, N. J., Harrison, T. M., Cotton, R. G. H., and

Brownlee, G. G. (1974) *In* "Cellular Selection and Regulation in the Immune Response" (G. M. Edelman, ed.), pp. 245–264. Raven, New York.
4. Scharff, M. (1974) *Harvey Lect.* **69**, 125.
5. Frangione, B., Franklin, E. C., and Smithies, O. (1978) *Nature (London)* **273**, 400.
6. Frangione, B., and Milstein, C. (1969) *Nature (London)* **224**, 597.
7. Michaelsen, T. E., Frangione, B., and Franklin, E. C. (1977) *J. Biol. Chem.* **252**, 883.
8. Rivat, C. *et al.* (1976) *Eur. J. Immunol.* **6**, 550.
9. Fett, J. W., Deutsch, H. F., and Smithies, O. (1973) *Immunochemistry* **10**, 115.
10. Steiner, L., personal communication.
11. Frangione, B. (1976). *Proc. Natl. Acad. Sci. U.S.A.* **73**, 1552.
12. Franklin, E. C., Prelli, F., and Frangione, B. (1979) *Proc. Nat. Acad. Sci., U.S.A.* **76**, 452.
13. Kabat, E. A., Wu, T. T., and Bilofsky, H. (1976) "Variable Regions of Immunoglobulin Chains—Tabulations and Analyses of Amino Acid Sequences." N.I.H., Bethesda, Maryland.
14. Edelman, G. M., Cunningham, W. E., Gall, P. D., Gottlieb, H., Rutishauser, H., and Waxdal, M. J. (1969) *Proc. Natl. Acad. Sci. U.S.A.* **63**, 78.
15. Smithies, O., Gibson, D., Fanning, E. M., Goodfliesh, R. M., Gilman, J. G., and Ballantyne, D. L. (1971) *Biochemistry* **10**, 4912.
16. Garver, F. A., Chang, L., Mendicino, J., Isobe, T., and Osserman, E. F. (1975) *Proc. Natl. Acad. Sci. U.S.A.* **72**, 4559.
17. Tonegawa, S., Maxam, A. M., Tizard, R., Bernard, O., and Gilbert, W. (1978) *Proc. Natl. Acad. Sci. U.S.A.* **75**, 1485.
18. Franklin, E. C. (1978) *J. Immunol.* **121**, 2582.
19. Adlersberg, J., Frangione, B., and Franklin, E. C. (1975) *Proc. Natl. Acad. Sci. U.S.A.* **72**, 723.
20. Franklin, E. C., Frangione, B., and Buxbaum, J. (1978) In preparation.
21. Alexander, A., Barritault, D., and Buxbaum, J. (1978) *Proc. Nat. Acad. Sci., U.S.A.* **75**, 4774.
22. Burstein, Y., and Schechter, I. (1977) *Proc. Natl. Acad. Sci. U.S.A.* **74**, 716.

PART II

CELLULAR
IMMUNOGLOBULIN PRODUCTION

Variable and Constant Region Variants of Mouse Myeloma Cells

WENDY D. COOK, BEN DHARMGRONGARTAMA,
AND MATTHEW D. SCHARFF

Department of Cell Biology
Albert Einstein College of Medicine
New York, New York

INTRODUCTION

Comparisons of the amino acid sequences of many different myeloma proteins, including some which bind antigens, and of normal antibodies have shown an enormous amino acid sequence diversity in small areas of the NH_2-terminal portion of the immunoglobulin heavy and light chains (1–3). In the heavy chain, these "hypervariable" regions are usually found between residues 31 and 35, 50 and 65, and 95 and 107 (3). The areas of hypervariability in the light chain are roughly comparable in location (3). The importance of these hypervariable regions in antigen binding has been established by correlating amino acid sequence and specificity (3), affinity labeling with antigen (4) and studies of the three-dimensional structure of antibody molecules (5,6).

In spite of the large amount of information on the structure of antibodies and on the biology of the immune response, little is known about the exact molecular events and biochemical mechanisms responsible for the generation of hypervariability. Suggestions range from the germ line theory, which proposes that genes for each of the many sequences have evolved over a long period of time and are inherited in the germ line, to the somatic theory which assumes a very limited number of germ line genes which diversify in structure during

99

the development of the individual. While many refinements and modifications of these theories have been proposed, it has been difficult to generate direct experimental approaches to answer the questions posed by the sequence studies. Information such as that presented in this volume on the organization and structure of immunoglobulin genes should further define the problem and should provide some of the answers. However, it will still be necessary to describe the biochemical mechanisms involved.

One experimental approach is to assume that at least some of the sequence diversity found in antibodies is generated somatically and to try to explore the mechanism in continuously cultured plasma cells. The obvious difficulty with this approach is that cultured cell lines, such as those derived from mouse myeloma tumors, are usually already highly differentiated, malignant cells carrying tumor viruses. It will therefore be difficult to relate events observed in such cells to those which occur normally. On the other hand, such mouse myeloma cell lines provide a homogeneous population of cells producing large amounts of a well characterized immunoglobulin molecule. A number of reports have appeared which show that the expression of immunoglobulin genes is very unstable in both mouse myeloma cell lines and in tumors. For example, we have shown that a number of mouse myeloma cell lines synthesizing a variety of classes and subclasses of immunoglobulin spontaneously lose the ability to synthesize heavy chains at a rate of approximately 10^{-3}/cell/generation (7). This means that one in every thousand cell divisions results in a variant in immunoglobulin expression. Certain mutagens increase the frequency of variants to 2–6% of the surviving clones (7,8). While many of the spontaneous and mutagen-induced variants have lost the ability to produce one or both immunoglobulin chains, approximately 40% of the mutagen-induced variants produce heavy chains which differ structurally from the parental heavy chains (9,10). Milstein and his colleagues have used nucleic acid and protein sequence studies to show that frameshift, missense, and nonsense mutations occur spontaneously in the immunoglobulin produced by a cultured cell line (11). We have shown that the genetic instability of immunoglobulin production is not due to a general instability of mouse myeloma cells since these same cells spontaneously generate mutants resistant to 6-thioguanine, bromodeoxyuridine, and ouabain at frequencies of approximately 10^{-6}–10^{-7}/cell/generation and with mutagenesis at frequencies no higher than 10^{-5} (7).

The enormous genetic instability in the expression of immunoglobulin by cultured mouse myeloma cells suggested that this might be a good system to study the somatic generation of antibody diversity. However, all of the immunoglobulin structural variants of cultured cells which had been characterized appeared to be in the constant region of the molecule, which is highly conserved in normal antibodies, rather than in the hypervariable regions which are the expected target of the generator of diversity. This was easily explained in our own studies by the fact that we screened for variants with antibodies directed against constant region antigenic determinants (7–10). However, Cotton et al. (12) screened 7000 clones by isoelectric focusing and found four constant region mutants but apparently did not detect any mutants with changes in the variable region.

There are two obvious strategies to screen directly for variants with changes in the variable region. The first is to use a cell line which is producing an immunoglobulin that binds a particular antigen. Cells are then cloned in soft agar and overlaid with antigen. The immunoglobulin secreted by the clones diffuses into the agar and precipitates with antigen, producing a visible antigen–antibody precipitate around the parental clones. Clones which are not surrounded by a visible precipitate are presumptive variants which may have lost the ability to synthesize, assemble, or secrete the antibody or they may be producing immunoglobulins that have a decreased ability to bind or precipitate antigen.

A second approach to looking for variable region variants is a slight modification of the technique we used to quantitate and identify constant region variants (7). Myeloma cells are cloned in soft agar and overlaid with anti-idiotypic antibody made specific for the variable regions of the particular immunoglobulin produced by that myeloma. Clones which are not surrounded by a visible antigen–antibody precipitate are identified. Since both approaches identify variants of many possible phenotyes, the presumptive variants must be recovered from the agar and characterized in detail.

In this paper we will describe our attempts to use both techniques to identify and determine the frequency of variable region variants and compare this with the characteristics and frequency of variants in the constant region of mouse immunoglobulins.

VARIANTS WITH CHANGES IN ANTIGEN BINDING

As already described above, the most direct approach to looking for mutations in the variable, and hopefully hypervariable regions, is to seek variants producing immunoglobulin molecules with changes in their ability to bind antigen. The S107 cell line was chosen for these studies. It produces an IgA kappa immunoglobulin which binds the hapten phosphocholine (PC) (13). The sequence of the variable region of the heavy chain of S107 has been determined and compared with partial or complete sequences of other PC binding mouse myelomas as well as with other nonPC binding myelomas (3,14). The sequences of the light chains of S107 and the other PC binding myelomas are known through the first hypervariable region (3). S107 has the same variable region serology (idiotype) as the T15 and HOPC-8 PC-binding myelomas and as most of the natural antibodies made in response to PC immunization (15). In addition, the three-dimensional structure of the antigen binding site of McPC 603, a closely related PC-binding myeloma, has been determined by X-ray diffraction (16) and can serve as a guide to the amino acid residues of S107 which may come in contact with hapten.

The S107 cell line was cloned in soft agar and a freshly isolated clone was recloned and overlaid with PC-KLH. The majority of the clones were surrounded by small amounts of antigen–antibody precipitate, but some "unstained" clones were detected. However, the difference between "stained" and "unstained" clones was marginal and attempts were made to increase the amount of antigen–antibody precipitate. The technique at which we ultimately arrived was to clone the cells in the presence of small amounts of antibody against the IgA constant region. Clones containing two to eight cells were surrounded by small amounts of IgA–anti-IgA precipitate. At this stage, the clones were overlaid with PC-KLH. Those clones producing antibodies with strong PC binding reacted with antigen and the amount of precipitate increased over the next 5–10 days. The clones producing immunoglobulin which did not bind well to PC-KLH did not form visible precipitates with PC-KLH and the barely visible precipitates between secreted IgA and the "subliminal" amounts of anti-IgA dissolved in antigen (IgA) excess as the clones increased in size. The exact amounts of the various reagents and the optimum time to score clones were determined empirically and reconstruction experiments were included each time variants were sought. Although the assay is complex, we have recovered a large number of presumptive variants and so far have not found one which was incorrectly identified on the plate assay.

As can be seen from Table I (experiments 1 and 2) there is a very high frequency of clones which were not surrounded by a visible precipitate. We have observed similar frequencies in a large number of independent experiments (17). This was especially surprising since

TABLE I
Frequency of Variant Clones

Experiment number	Subclone	Overlay	Unstained/ stained	%
1	S107.3.4	PC-KLH	4/1652	0.24
2	S_1	PC-KLH	16/3740	0.43
5	S_3	PC-KLH	10/1105	0.91
		Anti-IgA	4/1339	0.29

these variants arose spontaneously. Since it was possible that all of the variants had lost the ability to synthesize, assemble, or secrete immunoglobulin, cells from a recently isolated antigen binding subclone of S107 were cloned and one set of dishes was overlaid with antigen while the other was overlaid with antibody against the constant region of the IgA heavy chain. As can be seen in experiment 5, Table I, only one-third of the clones which did not react with antigen had lost the ability to secret immunoglobulin. This suggested that variants with changes in antigen binding were in fact arising at a very high frequency. In order to confirm this, a number of nonantigen binding variants were recovered from the agar, recloned, grown to mass culture, and screened in a preliminary way to confirm their phenotype. As expected from experiment 5 in Table I, we were unable to detect IgA heavy chains either in the medium or intracellularly, in approximately 30% of the variants. However, the majority of the variants synthesized and secreted IgA which did not react with PC-KLH by agar diffusion. The secretions from these variants contained approximately the same amount of IgA by radial immunodiffusion as the parent clone but had a much lower hemagglutination titer for PC-KLH. This latter observation was important because it indicated that the immunoglobulin produced by the variant still reacted with PC but had a lower avidity for antigen.

Such a change in avidity could occur if the variant differed in its assembly of heavy and light chains into H_2L_2 monomers or the polymerization of the monomers into the higher polymers typical of IgA. This possibility was examined by incubating the cells from the parent and a variant with radioactive amino acids, specifically precipitating the intracellular and secreted immunoglobulin with antibody, dissolving the precipitate in sodium dodecyl sulfate (SDS) and examining the labeled proteins on SDS gels. Such a comparison of the immunoglobulins secreted by the parent and a first generation antigen binding variant is presented in Fig. 1, panels a and c. Since the light and heavy chains of the IgA produced by BALB/c mice are not covalently linked, the SDS dissociates the light chains from the heavy chain dimers and polymers, as can be seen in Fig. 1. The degree of polymerization of the parent and first generation variant were very similar. This was also established by comparing the polymerization of parent and variant on ultrogel columns under nondissociating conditions. Panel b of Fig. 1 presents the gel pattern of the secreted immunoglobulin of an unusual sort of antigen binding variant. The secretion of this variant did not precipitate with antigen and spurred with the parent when reacted with antibody against IgA. As can be seen from the figure, there is a single rapidly migrating radioactive peak. No free light chains are seen. Upon reduction and subsequent electrophoresis, the peak was shown to contain normal sized light chains and heavy chains which were smaller than the parental heavy chains. We can conclude from this that this particular variant is producing a disulfide-linked half molecule between a deleted heavy chain and a wild-type light chain. Similar defective IgA's have been reported for a

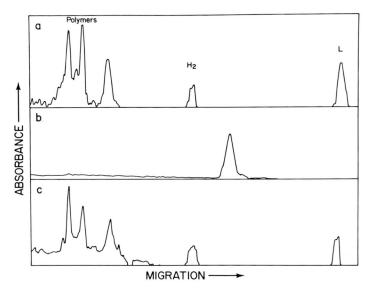

Fig. 1. Cells were labeled with amino acids, and secreted material was immune precipitated and analyzed on 5% polyacrylamide gels containing SDS in a phosphate buffer system. Panels a, b, and c are tracings of autoradiographs of unreduced material run on a slab gel; (a) wild-type S107 secretions, (b) S_1U_9 (half molecule variant) secretions, (c) variant U_1 secretions.

group of myelomas which have C-terminal deletions and produce half molecules (18,19). The apparent change in antigen binding could be due to the fact that the variant would be monovalent for PC and therefore could not form the lattice necessary to produce a visible antigen–antibody precipitate. So far we have identified only one variant of this sort.

The apparent change in avidity could also have resulted from changes in the amount of immunoglobulin produced by variant clones. Although we had dealt with this possibility by only testing secretions and cytoplasmic extracts of parental and variant clones which contained similar amounts of immunoglobulin, this possibility was examined more directly by injecting cells from variant clones into the peritoneal cavity of Pristane primed mice (20), removing the resultant ascites fluid, purifying the paraprotein on PC–Sepharose columns (21), and comparing the ability of identical amounts of purified protein to react with antigen by agar diffusion (Ouchterlony) and hemagglutination of PC-SRBC. Such a comparison for a first generation mutant, presented in Table II, confirms the results obtained with secretions and cell lysates. These results indicated that this variant and others like it had changes in the avidity of antigen binding.

A change in antigen binding was also demonstrated by attaching PC-KLH to polyvinyl microtiter plates, and comparing the amounts of parental and mutant protein required to prevent the binding of radioactively labeled parental protein. In this radioimmunoassay, it took ten

TABLE II
Characterization of Antigen Binding Variants

Generation	Reactivity with PC-KLH		Hemagglutination titer[a]	Relative binding[b]		
					Antiidiotypic ab	
	Overlay	Agar diffusion		PC-KLH	Site-specific	TI5
Parent	+	+	8192	100%	100%	100%
1	−	−	128	9	8.7	100
2	+	+	512	26	18	27
3	−	−	—	<0.4	n.d.	n.d.

[a] 250 μg of purified antibody is used as starting material.
[b] Competition between purified parental or variant antibody and labeled parent is examined in a solid phase radioimmunoassay. Relative binding is calculated as: ng parent required for 50% inhibition of binding of label/ng variant required for 50% inhibition of binding of label.

times as much protein from a first generation mutant protein as parental protein to inhibit by 50% the binding of labeled parental protein (Table II) (12).

All of these findings indicated that most of the variants which did not react with antigen in the plate assay had undergone changes in the conformation and/or charge of the antigen binding site. In order to obtain additional independent evidence for a change in the configuration of the antigen binding site, two types of antivariable region antibody were prepared. Rabbit antibody raised against the S107 protein was bound to a Sepharose-S107 column and eluted with a large excess of PC (22). This "site specific" antibody was shown in a radioimmunoassay to bind the parent better than the first generation mutant (Table II). So-called "T-15" anti-idiotypic antibody was prepared by absorbing a rabbit antiS107 antibody with other IgA myelomas including two (MOPC 511 and McPC 603) which bind PC but differ serologically from S107. This antiT15 antiserum did not distinguish between the parent and the first generation variant (Table II). These serological studies and antigen binding studies suggest that a subtle change has occurred in the structure of the antigen binding site.

The first generation variant described in Table I was cloned and overlaid with PC-KLH to look for revertants or clones with additional changes that increased antigen binding. Such clones arose spontaneously at a very high frequency (Table III). The phenotype of one such second generation variant is presented in Table II. It binds PC less well than S107 but better than the first generation variant from which it was derived. Since it also differs from both S107 and the variant in its variable region serology, this second generation variant is not a true revertant but rather appears to have undergone a secondary change which has increased its antigen binding (17). This second generation variant was recloned and then overlaid with PC-KLH, and a set of variants with decreased PC binding has been obtained from it. The

TABLE III
Frequency of "Revertant" Clones

Experiment number	Subclone	Overlay	Stained/ unstained	%
7	U_1U_1	PC-KLH	53/2332	2.28
8	$U_1U_1U_4$	PC-KLH	3/1075	0.28

phenotype of one of these third generation variants is presented in Table II. The antigen binding of this particular variant is so weak that it does not hemagglutinate PC-SRBC. Furthermore, it is the first variant we have seen that does not bind to a PC-Sepharose column.

These antigen binding and serological studies suggest that variants with changes in the antigen binding sites are arising spontaneously at an astonishingly high frequency. Since differences in antigen binding are found amongst PC-binding myelomas and are associated with changes in the sequence of the hypervariable regions of the heavy chain (3), it seemed reasonable to assume that the variants would also differ from the parent in the primary sequence of the hypervariable regions or in framework residues that would affect the folding of the antigen binding sites. In fact an analysis of the valine, threonine, and leucine-containing tryptic–chymotryptic peptides of the parental heavy chain and a first generation variant with a tenfold decrease in binding revealed small but reproducible changes in a few low yield peptides (17). A comparison of the lysine and arginine-containing tryptic peptides of the parental heavy chain also confirmed the differences (W. Cook, unpublished data). Both sorts of analysis of the light chains did not reveal any differences (17, and unpublished data). Since such peptide analysis does not examine all of the peptides and may not reveal conservative amino acid substitution, detailed sequence studies are essential. Dr. Stuart Rudikoff of the NIH is in the process of carrying out such studies.

Variants with apparent changes in their variable regions arise frequently in at least two other cell lines. We have prepared anti-idiotypic antibody to the IgG_{2b} MPC-11 protein, overlaid clones with this antiserum and identified a large number of variants which do not react with this antibody in the overlay assay (23). These are now being examined in more detail. Dr. Sherie Morrison and her colleagues have identified variants of J558 with changes in dextran binding which also arise spontaneously at a high frequency (24). In addition, a nonantigen binding variant of the MOPC-104E tumor has arisen *in vivo* (25).

CONSTANT REGION MUTANTS

It is reasonable to assume that the antigen binding variants of S107 (17) and J558 (24) will prove to have changes in their amino acid sequences within their hypervariable regions or in framework residues affecting the folding of the antigen binding site. If such changes do occur and are restricted to the hypervariable regions, this might suggest that the mechanism responsible was related in some way to the normal generation of antibody diversity. On the other hand, if some of the antigen binding variants have changes in framework residues of the variable region, or in the constant region, then it will be difficult to relate these findings to normal events. In fact, we already know that many mouse myeloma cell lines generate structural variants in the constant region at a very high frequency. We have previously shown that variants with deletions in the heavy chains arise in the MPC-11 cell line at a high frequency of approximately 1% after mutagenesis. The deletions may be internal (26) or in the C-terminal part of the molecule (9). Although certain sized deletions appear more frequently than others (9), as can be seen in Table IV, variants representing what appears to be a continuum in the size of the heavy chain have been isolated (23). Since such deletions are often associated with defects in glycosylation (27,28) (Table IV), the size of the nonglycosylated heavy chain is presented in Table IV. This was determined by preincubating cells in the presence of high doses of glucosamine and then labeling with amino acids and examining the relative size of heavy chain on sodium dodecyl sulfate-containing acrylamide gels (27).

We have also identified a second type of constant region variant in which the heavy chain acquires the serological determinants of a subclass which was not expressed in the parental cell. These "subclass switch" variants arise frequently in the MPC-11 cell line which produces IgG_{2b} heavy chains. Such "2a" positive variants still contain the serological determinants of the MPC-11 variable region (29) and many of the tryptic-chymotryptic peptides of bonafide IgG_{2a} proteins (10). Similar recombinant-like heavy chains have been observed in mouse myelomas (30) and in man (31–33). Recently, Dr. Barbara Birshtein

TABLE IV
Deletion Mutants of MPC-11

Clone	Mutagen	Heavy chain MW	Normal assembly	Normal glycosylation	Normal secretion
45.6	—	52,000	+	+	+
BD30	—	49,000	+	+	+
BD25	ICR191-OH	47,000	±	−	−
BD23	ICR191	45,000	±	−	−
BD19	ICR191	42,000	−	−	−
BD6	ICR191	40,000	−	−	−

and her colleagues have generated and characterized a large group of such 2a variants and shown that they contain all or part of the amino acid sequence of the IgG_{2a} subclass (29,34,35). In addition, Dr. Sherie Morrison and her colleagues have carried out a series of very interesting studies on this subclass switch which will be described elsewhere in this monograph.

In the context of this discussion we would merely like to use the subclass switch as a type of constant region variant whose frequency can be determined directly in the plate assay described in the previous section. Briefly, a fresh subclone of the MPC-11 IgG_{2b} producing line is cloned in soft agar, overlaid with antiserum made specific for the IgG_{2a} subclass, and then the plates are screened for clones surrounded by a visible antigen–antibody precipitate. As can be seen in Table V, such constant region variants arise at a frequency of between 0.15 and 0.34%. In view of the high frequency of the 2b to 2a switch, we have looked at a variety of other cell lines to see if other class or subclass switches such as IgM to IgG occur with or without mutagenesis. We have not found any other examples of this phenomenon. If such variants do arise, it is with a lower frequency than the 2b to 2a switch (Table V). This difference in frequency may be due to the large degree of sequence homology between IgG_{2a} and IgG_{2b} or reflect some special relationship in the organization of the constant region genes or messenger RNA. However, the main point to be made here is that changes in the constant region can also occur spontaneously at a very high frequency. Since the serological probes we are using to examine the constant region are probably less subtle than antigen

TABLE V
Subclass Switches[a]

Cell line (subclass)		Antiserum specific for	Stained/ unstained	Frequency (range)
MPC-11	(IgG_{2b})	IgG_{2a}	50/17,865	0.28%(0.15–0.34)
Cl	(IgG_{2a})	IgG_{2b}	0/13,000	<0.008
P_3	(IgG_1)	IgG_{2b}	0/35,445	<0.003
MOPC104	(IgM)	$IgG_{1,2a,2b}$	0/14,449	<0.007
S107	(IgA)	$IgG_{1,2a,2b}$	0/12,000	<0.008

[a] Cells were cloned in soft agar and overlaid with antiserum of the indicated specificity. In each experiment approximately equal numbers of mutagenized and unmutagenized cells were examined. Since there was no significant difference, the data from both types of cells was pooled.

binding, it is not reasonable to compare even the observed frequencies of presumed constant and variable region instability. Nevertheless we have to conclude that structural changes are occurring throughout the molecule and will probably be found in both the hypervariable and framework residues of the variable region, as well as in the constant region.

CONCLUSIONS

It is clear from the results described in this paper and the work of others that the expression of the immunoglobulin genes of mouse myeloma cells is extraordinarily unstable and that such cells spontaneously generate variants with changes in the sequence of the immunoglobulin molecule at a very high rate. This instability results in the frequent loss of heavy and light chain synthesis and in the somatic generation of antigen binding diversity, subclass switches, constant region deletions, and changes that resemble frameshift, nonsense, and missense mutations (9–11). Using the mouse myeloma cells, it should be possible to determine the mechanism(s) responsible for the genetic instability since the changes are occurring at such a high frequency in a homogeneous population of cultured cells. It is possible that identical events occur during the differentiation of normal plasma cells. Since such cells go through a limited number of cell divisions, only a rare clone would undergo the sort of constant region mutations observed in the myeloma cells. Even these rare events might well go unnoticed since many of the deleted molecules are not secreted and, those that are, are often degraded rapidly in the serum (36). It is also possible that some of the variation, for example that in the variable region, is mediated through normal mechanisms and that these changes predispose to secondary variation which is expressed because of the large number of cell divisions in the malignant as opposed to normal cells. There is a precedent for this in yeast where small N-terminal deletions in cytochrome c can lead to an increased frequency of C-terminal deletions (37). It is also possible that the genetic instability we are observing does not occur in normal cells but could reflect an unusual structure or organization of the immunoglobulin genes which is required for the evolutionary or somatic generation of antibody diversity or for the maintenance of diversity once it is established. Whatever the explanation, the genetic instability of the immunoglobulin genes in the mouse myeloma cells is so great that the mechanism demands further investigation.

ACKNOWLEDGMENTS

We gratefully acknowledge the expert assistance of Terri Kelly, Lucille Frank and Regina Flynn. WDC is supported by a scholarship from the Young Men's Philanthropic League. BD is a trainee of the National Cancer Institute. (CA 09173). The work was supported by Grants PCM 75-13609 from the National Science Foundation and AI5231 and AI10702 from the National Institutes of Health.

REFERENCES

1. Wu, T. T., and Kabat, E. A. (1970) *J. Exp. Med.* **132**, 211–250.
2. Dayhoff, M. O., ed. (1972) "Atlas of Protein Sequence and Structure," 5th ed. Natl Biomed. Res. Found., Washington, D.C.
3. Kabat, E. A., Wu, T. T., and Bilofsky, H. (1976) "Variable Regions of Immunoglobulin Chains," p. 115. Bolt, Beranek & Newman, Cambridge, Massachusetts.
4. Givol, D. (1974) *Essays Biochem.* **10**, 73–103.
5. Davies, D. R., Padlan, E. A., and Segal, D. M. (1975) *Annu. Rev. Biochem.* **44**, 639–667.
6. Poljak, R. J. (1975) *Nature (London)* **256**, 373–376.
7. Baumal, R., Birshtein, B., Coffino, P., and Scharff, M. D. (1973) *Science* **182**, 164–166.
8. Preud'homme, J.-L., Buxbaum, J., and Scharff, M. D. (1973) *Nature (London)* **245**, 320–322.
9. Birshtein, B., Preud'homme, J.-L., and Scharff, M. D. (1974) *Proc. Natl. Acad. Sci. U.S.A.* **71**, 3478–3482.
10. Preud'homme, J.-L., Birshtein, B., and Scharff, M. D. (1975) *Proc. Natl. Acad. Sci. U.S.A.* **72**, 1427–1430.
11. Adetugbo, K., Milstein, C., and Secher, D. S. (1977) *Nature (London)* **265**, 299–304.
12. Cotton, R. G. H., Secher, D. S., and Milstein, C. (1973) *Eur. J. Immunol.* **3**, 135–140.
13. Cohn, M., Notani, A., and Rice, S. A. (1969) *Immunochemistry* **6**, 111–123.
14. Rudikoff, S., and Potter, M. (1976) *Proc. Natl. Acad. Sci. U.S.A.* **73**, 2109–2112.
15. Potter, M., and Lieberman, R. (1970) *J. Exp. Med.* **132**, 737–751.
16. Padlan, E. A., Davies, D. R., Rudikoff, S., and Potter, M. (1976) *Immunochemistry* **13**, 945–949.
17. Cook, W. D., and Scharff, M. D. (1977) *Proc. Natl. Acad. Sci. U.S.A.* **74**, 5687–5691.
18. Mushinski, J. F. (1971) *J. Immunol.* **106**, 41–50.
19. Robinson, E. A., Smith, D. F., and Apella, E. (1974) *J. Biol. Chem.* **249**, 6605–6610.
20. Potter, M., Pumphrey, J. G., and Walters, J. L. (1972) *J. Natl. Cancer Inst.* **49**, 305–308.
21. Claflin, J. L., and Davie, J. M. (1974) *J. Exp. Med.* **140**, 673–686.
22. Claflin, J. L., and Davie, J. M. (1975) *J. Immunol.* **114**, 70–75.
23. Dharmgrongartama, B., and Scharff, M. D. (1978) In preparation.
24. Matsuuchi, L., and Morrison, S. L. (1978) *Fed. Proc., Fed. Am. Soc. Exp. Biol.* **37**, 1763.
25. Folds, J. D. (1977) *Immunol. Commun.* **6**, 385.
26. Morrison, S. L., (1979) "Cells of Immunoglobulins," Academic Press. pp. 113–126.
27. Weitzman, S., and Scharff, M. D. (1976) *J. Mol. Biol.* **102**, 237–252.

28. Weitzman, S., Nathenson, S., and Scharff, M. D. (1977) *Cell* **10**, 679–687.
29. Francus, T., Dharmgrongartama, B., Campbell, R., Scharff, M. D., and Birshtein, B. K. (1978) *J. Exp. Med.* **147**, 1535–1550.
30. Warner, N. L., Herzenberg, L. A., and Goldstein, G. (1966) *J. Exp. Med.* **123**, 707–721.
31. Kunkel, H. G., Natvig, J. B., and Joslin, F. G. (1969) *Proc. Natl. Acad. Sci. U.S.A.* **62**, 144–149.
32. Natvig, J. B., and Kunkel, H. G. (1974) *J. Immunol.* **112**, 1277–1284.
33. Werner, B. G., and Steinberg, A. G. (1974) *Immunogenetics* **1**, 254–271.
34. Francus, T., and Birshtein, B. K. (1978) *Biochemistry* **17**, 4324–4331.
35. Koskimies, S., and Birshtein, B. K. (1976) *Nature (London)* **246**, 480–482.
36. Weitzman, S., Palmer, L., and Grennon, M. (1979) *J. Immunology* **122**, 12–18.
37. Sherman, F., and Steward, J. G. (1974) *Genetics* **78**, 97.

Constant Region Mutants
of Mouse Immunoglobulins

SHERIE L. MORRISON

Department of Microbiology
College of Physicians and Surgeons
Columbia University
New York, New York

INTRODUCTION

It has been estimated that the mouse has the capacity to produce over 10^6 different antibody molecules which recognize and interact with the antigens encountered during the lifetime of the animal. An individual antibody-producing lymphoid cell makes antibody of a single antigenic specificity (1) and idiotype (2); however, as it differentiates it may synthesize immunoglobulins of several classes (3–6). Differentiation of the lymphocyte may also be accompanied by increased production of Ig. The molecular mechanisms which determine the structure of the Ig molecule and regulate differentiation of the Ig producing cell have not yet been defined.

One method of studying the molecular biology of antibody synthesis is to isolate cells mutant in their production of Ig. Potentially cells with a mutation affecting any aspect of Ig biosynthesis can be identified; variants which have either lost the ability to produce H (7,8), L (9), or both chains (9,10), or which are synthesizing different quantities of H or L chains have been recovered (10–14). However, some of the most interesting variants identified to date have been those synthesizing an Ig with a structurally altered chain.

Among the first structurally abnormal immunoglobulins identified were the deleted heavy chains present in patients with human heavy chain disease (for review, see Frangione and Franklin, 15,16). In heavy chain disease, neoplastic cells synthesize heavy chains which do not have light chains bound to them; in α and γ chain disease there is a failure to synthesize light chains. Studies showed that the heavy

113

chains with the deletion were synthetic products, not the result of the synthesis of normal sized chains which are degraded (17).

With the development of the cultured mouse myeloma cell lines, a more systematic investigation of mutation of Ig production was possible. The obvious advantage of this system over the observation of spontaneous mutants in patients was that the parental cell from which the mutant was derived could be identified and characterized.

Two approaches have effectively been used to isolate cells producing mutant immunoglobulin. In the first, clones were isolated at random and the products of these clones analyed by isoelectric focusing to identify cells producing an altered Ig. Using this methodology, deletion, missense and nonsense mutants of Ig were recognized (18). In the second approach, cells were cloned in soft agar, and developing clones overlaid with either an antiserum to or the antigen recognized by the Ig produced by the cell line. Using this technique clones synthesizing Ig altered either in its antigenicity or in its ability to react with antigen (8 – 21)have been identified (see also M. D. Scharff, this volume). Among the clones synthesizing antigenically altered heavy chains were some synthesizing chains with deletions, and others synthesizing normal sized heavy chains which were structurally altered. In particular, mutants synthesizing γ_{2a} heavy chains were derived from the γ_{2b} cell line 45.6 (22). With the exception of one variant with γ_{2a} determinants and a molecular weight of 75,000 (23), the γ_{2a} variants initially isolated were all 55,000 daltons, the same size as the parental heavy chain. All γ_{2a} variants studied so far retain the idiotype of the parental 45.6 cell line (24); however, heterogeneity of heavy chain sequence in the variants is indicated by different kinetics of H_2L_2 assembly, migration in agarose gels, and peptide map analysis.

Experiments were undertaken in our laboratory to determine the mechanism of the change in the constant region of the Ig produced by the 45.6 cell line. These experiments began with the isolation of a clone of 45.6 which was synthesizing fewer L chains than the parental line. From this clone, called B50, we isolated a spontaneous mutant (10-1) producing an internally deleted heavy chain. This internal deletion in the CH_1 domain served as an additional genetic marker when analyzing γ_{2a} clones derived from 10-1. Analysis of the γ_{2a} mutants obtained from 10-1 in either one or two steps (see Table I and Fig. 1) has not yet defined the mechanism of the constant region change. However, the γ_{2a} mutants occur at a high frequency, exhibit many different isoelectric focusing patterns, come in two discrete molecular weights (55,000 and 47,000) and may provide a model system for analyzing variation in Ig production. Most γ_{2a} mutants can be ex-

TABLE I
Properties of Representative Mutant Clones

Mutant	Serology	Heavy chain molecular weight	Parent	Remarks
B50	γ_{2b}	55,000	45.6	Synthesizes fewer L chains
10–1	γ_{2b}	47,000	B50	Internal deletion
G403	γ_{2b}	47,000	10–1	Synthesizes no L chain
G251	—	40,000	10–1	
I17	—	35,000	10–1	
G301	γ_{2a}	55,000	10–1	
G270	γ_{2a}	55,000	10–1	Distinctive isoelectric focusing pattern
G551	γ_{2a}	55,000	10–1	
G501	γ_{2a}	55,000	10–1	
I16	γ_{2a}	55,000	10–1	
K23	γ_{2a}	55,000	I17	Lacks many MOPC-173 peptides
K3	γ_{2a}	55,000	I17	
K24	γ_{2a}	47,000	I17	
K25	γ_{2a}	47,000	I17	

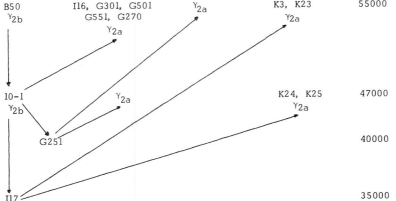

Fig. 1.   Diagram of the interrelationships of the immunoglobulin mutants described.

plained by traditional genetic mechanisms. However, one mutant, K23, can be explained by classical genetic mechanisms only if multiple changes are postulated.

ISOLATION AND CHARACTERIZATION OF 10-1, A MUTANT CELL LINE SYNTHESIZING AN INTERNALLY DELETED HEAVY CHAIN

The 45.6 cell line was adapted to continuous growth in tissue culture from the MPC-11 myeloma tumor by Laskov and Scharff (11); it synthesizes a γ_{2b} heavy chain and kappa light chains. Among the variants isolated from 45.6 was B50, which was delayed in its assembly of immunoglobulin (25). The heavy and light chains synthesized by B50 were identical by peptide analysis to those synthesized by 45.6; however, B50 synthesized fewer L chains than 45.6 and, unlike other Ig variants, reverted at high frequency to wild type.

B50 was cloned in soft agar, 257 subclones recovered, grown to mass culture and characterized. One of these clones, 10-1, (26) was distinctive (Figs. 2 and 3) in that it was producing a 47,000 dalton heavy chain instead of the 55,000 dalton heavy chain characteristic of 45.6. The deleted heavy chains of 10-1 form dimers but do not form any disulfide bonds with L chains (Figs. 2 and 3). 10-1 is serologically γ_{2b}, like its parent, and in Ouchterlony analysis no spurring between 10-1 and 45.6 is observed using either anti-γ_{2b} or anti-γ_2 antiserum. 10-1 retains its reactivity with antiserum prepared against the parental idiotype.

CNBr cleaves the 45.6 H_2L_2 molecule into a 100,000 dalton (Fab)$_2$ and a 27,000 dalton Fc. The H_2 molecule from 10-1 is cleaved by CNBr into ~27,000 dalton and ~40,000 dalton fragments (Fig. 4). To verify the identity of 27,000 dalton fragments from 45.6 and 10-1, labeled secreted products of 10-1 and 45.6 were prepared by growing cells for 24 hr in the presence of either ^{3}H- or ^{14}C-VTL. The H_2 of 10-1 and the H_2L_2 of 45.6 were isolated as discrete peaks following chromatography of the secretions on Sephadex G150 (8 M urea, 0.1 M formic acid). The isolated peaks were cleaved with CNBr and the ~27,000 dalton fragments isolated by chromatography on Sephadex G150 (8 M urea, 0.1 M formic acid). The ^{3}H and ^{14}C peaks were mixed, completely reduced in 8 M urea, 0.01 M Tris, 0.15 M 2-mercaptoethanol, pH 8.2, alkylated with 0.18 M iodoacetamide and chromatographed on G75-superfine (8 M urea, 0.1 M formic acid). Coincidence of the peaks from 45.6 and 10-1 was observed (Fig. 5). The Fc pieces were also analyzed by peptide mapping and no differences were observed. In addition,

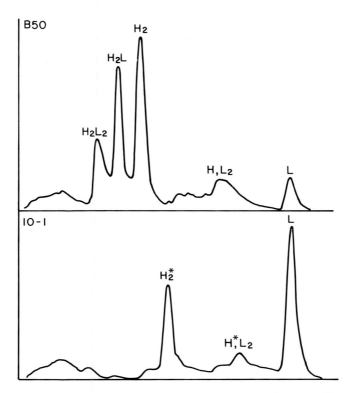

Fig. 2. Cytoplasmic immunoglobulins of cell lines B50 and 10-1. Cells were incubated in the presence of ^{14}C-valine, threonine, and leucine (VTL) for 30 min, cytoplasmic lysates prepared using 0.5% NP-40, and the immunoglobulins immune precipitated. Immunoglobulins were dissolved in 2% SDS, boiled, and analyzed on 5% SDS polyacrylamide gels. Position of the peaks was determined by scanning an autoradiogram with a Joyce–Loebel densitometer. Migration is from left to right.

amino acid sequence analysis of the piece derived from the C terminus of the Fc showed no differences from the parent (27). The Fc region of 10-1 thus appears to be identical to the Fc of its parent, 45.6.

The deletion in the H chain of 10-1 almost certainly involves the Fd region of the molecule. Sequence analysis of the CNBr fragment commencing at residue 21 shows identity between 45.6 and 10-1 (28). This identity coupled with preservation of idiotypic reactivity in 10-1 places the most probable site of the deletion in the CH_1 domain. The fact that the 10-1 heavy chain is aberrant in its disulfide bond formation and does not covalently bond its light chain in consistent with this location. Thus the 10-1 heavy chain has an internal deletion which can

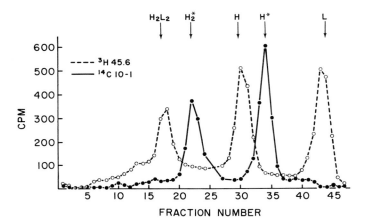

Fig. 3. Relative size of the heavy chain of 10-1. Intact, and reduced and alkylated ^{14}C-H_2^* were mixed with intact, and reduced and alkylated ^3H-H_2L_2 from 45.6. Samples were boiled in 2% SDS and analyzed on 5% SDS polyacrylamide gels. The gel was fractioned into scintillation vials using a Gilson Gel Crusher, and the position of the peaks determined with a Beckman Liquid Scintillation Counter.

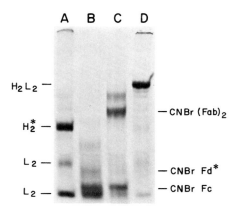

Fig. 4. SDS gel analysis of CNBr fragments of 10-1 and 45.6. The secreted Ig of 10-1 and 45.6 were labeled by growing the cells in the presence of ^{14}C-VTL for 24 hr. CNBr cleavage was by standard procedures. Fragments were analyzed on 5% SDS-polyacrylamide gels. Position of the peaks was determined by autoradiography. (A) 10-1 secretion, (B) 10-1 secretions treated with CNBr, (C) 45.6 secretions cleaved with CNBr, and (D) 45.6 secretions.

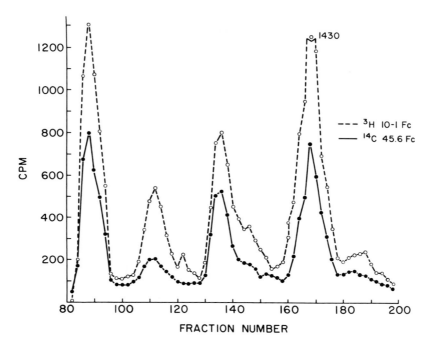

Fig. 5. Chromatography of CNBr-Fc. ^{3}H- and ^{14}C-CNBr Fc were prepared from 10-1 and 45.6, respectively, mixed, reduced in 8 M urea, 0.01 M Tris, 0.15 M β-ME, pH 8.2, and alkylated with 0.18 M iodoacetamide. Chromatography was on G75-superfine in 8 M urea, 0.1 M formic acid. Position of the peaks was determined with a Beckman Liquid Scintillation Counter.

serve as an additional genetic marker to aid in the interpretation of mutations which occur in immunoglobulin production.

MUTANTS DERIVED FROM THE 10-1 CELL LINE

Using the 10-1 cell line synthesizing an internally deleted heavy chain, we now sought to define the spectrum of mutants which could be derived from it.

Cell lines producing heavy chains but not light chains had been isolated from the P_3 γ_1 producing cell line (9) and the MOPC-460 IgA cell line (29). Though extensive analysis had been made of the 45.6 cell line, no mutants producing only heavy chains had been observed. This lack of heavy chain-producing variants from 45.6 could have resulted from a genetic constraint in the 45.6 cell line which made this type of mutant impossible: alternatively, because of heavy chain insolubility, production of heavy chain in the absence of L chain could be a lethal mutation in this cell line. If the second alternative were true, it would be expected that mutants producing only H chain could be isolated from 10-1 since the H_2 from this molecule was soluble in the absence of L chain. Also the human heavy chain disease proteins provided precedents for the synthesis of deleted heavy chains in the absence of L chains. In fact a mutant producing a deleted H chain and no L chain (G403) was isolated (Fig. 6). The lesion is in the synthesis of the L chain, not its synthesis and degradation, because even a short pulse (3 min) failed to show the presence of L chain. Cells producing only the 10-1 heavy chain secrete it as a H_2 dimer.

To determine if additional structural alterations in the 10-1 chain were possible, 10-1 was cloned in soft agar, and clones no longer secreting an immunoglobulin reactive with anti-γ_{2b} were identified, recovered, and characterized. Two mutants synthesizing heavy chains smaller than the heavy chain of 10-1 were isolated (Fig. 6). These were G251, synthesizing a heavy chain of about 40,000 daltons, and I17 synthesizing a heavy chain of about 35,000 daltons. Neither of these heavy chains reacts with any subclass specific antiserum and neither is secreted.

One of the most interesting mutational events observed in the 45.6 cell line is the switch from the synthesis of the γ_{2b} heavy chain to the

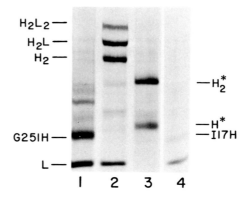

Fig. 6. Cytoplasmic immunoglobulins of cell lines. Cells were incubated for 30 min with ^{14}C-VTL, cytoplasmic lysates prepared, and the immunoglobulins immune precipitated. Electrophoresis was carried out on 5% SDS polyacrylamide slab gels and the positions of the peaks determined by autoradiography. Migration is from top to bottom. (1) G251, (2) B50, (3) G403, and (4) I17.

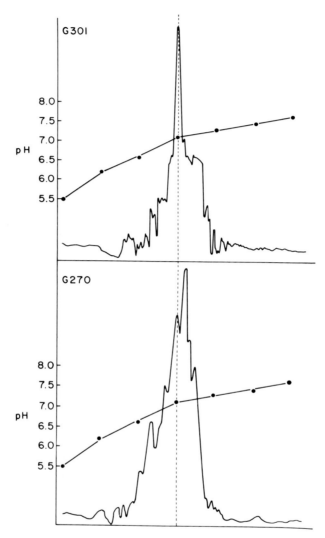

Fig. 7. Isoelectric focusing analysis of γ_{2a} synthesizing clones derived from 10-1. Cells were incubated for 3 hr in the presence of ^{14}C-VTL; secretions were prepared and dialyzed overnight against 8 M urea. Isoelectric focusing was carried out in 5% acrylamide gels, and the position of the peaks was determined by scanning an autoradiogram with the Joyce-Loebel Microdensitometer. The pH gradient was determined by eluting 1 cm gel slices with water.

synthesis of a γ_{2a} chain with the same variable region (22). To determine if heavy chains with an internal deletion can also undergo this switch in subclass, 10-1 was cloned and subclones secreting H chain reactive with γ_{2a} specific antiserum identified. Five such clones (G301, G270, G551, G510, I16) were isolated from different subclones of 10-1; since they were isolated from different subclones, the independence of their occurrence was assured. All five clones were synthesizing γ_{2a} heavy chains with molecular weights of approximately 55,000. Isoelectric focusing patterns of four of the clones (I16, G501, G551, G301) were identical; however, a fifth clone, G270, had a unique isoelectric focusing pattern (Fig. 7).

SUBCLASS SWITCH MUTANTS FROM G251 AND I17

Since the heavy chains synthesized by G251 and I17 are not secreted, it is difficult to obtain sufficient quantities for detailed structural analysis. In order to obtain additional information about the phenotype of these mutants, they were cloned in soft agar and cells identified which were secreting a heavy chain reactive with γ_{2a} and γ_{2b} antiserum (Table II). Although the assay would have detected γ_{2b} positive clones, none were identified. All 22 γ_2 positive clones recovered from I17 and G251, were serologically γ_{2a}. The isolated clones were synthesizing heavy chains of either ~55,000 daltons or ~47,000 daltons. The 55,000 dalton heavy chains were assembled in H_2L_2 molecules and secreted. The 47,000 dalton heavy chains, which could not be distinguished in molecular weight from 10-1, formed dimers, which were secreted; no covalent bonds were formed between the γ_{2a} 47,000 dalton chains and light chains. Though the γ_{2a} heavy chains were of one of two discrete molecular weights, they exhibited several different apparent amino acid sequences, as indicated by isoelectric focusing (Fig. 8).

TABLE II
Revertants Secreting Heavy Chains

Parental line	Frequency of clones secreting H chain[a]
I17	29/88603
G251	18/23641

[a] Number of clones reactive with γ_2 antiserum/total number of clones tested.

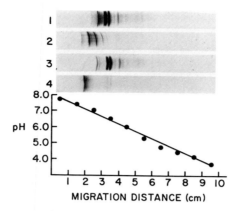

Fig. 8. Isoelectric focusing analysis of 55,000 dalton γ_{2a} clones derived from I17. Methods are as previously described, except that the position of the peaks was determined by autoradiography.

To determine if the Fc of the subclass switch mutants was identical to the Fc of the γ_{2a} myeloma, MOPC-173, ^{3}H-VTL Fc was prepared from MOPC-173. This ^{3}H-Fc was mixed with ^{14}C-VTL H chain from mutant clones, the mixture digested with trypsin and chymotrypsin, and the peptides analyzed using a Technicon P-2 column.

If the Fc of the mutant heavy chain were identical to the Fc of MOPC-173, all of the MOPC-173 peptides except one (the one adjacent to the papain cleavage point) should be present in the mutant heavy chain. Using this method the heavy chains produced by four different γ_{2a} mutants, two producing chains of ~47,000 daltons (K24, K25), and two producing chains of 55,000 daltons (K3, K23), were analyzed. Indeed three of the four heavy chains did contain all but one of the MOPC-173 Fc peptides (see Table III); thus these three mutants

TABLE III
Comparison of Fc Regions of Subclass Switch Mutants

Cell line	Heavy chain molecular weight (daltons)	MOPC-173 Fc peptides contained	MOPC-173 Fc peptides missing
K23	55,000	16	5
K3	55,000	20	1
K24	47,000	20	1
K25	47,000	20	1

appear to have an Fc identical to the Fc of MOPC-173. They differ from other subclass mutants of this type (30) in that two of them (K24, K25) are synthesizing deleted heavy chains. However, the fourth mutant (K23) even though synthesizing a full sized H chain appears to lack many of the peptides of the MOPC-173 Fc (see Table III).

MECHANISMS OF SUBCLASS SWITCH

Several possible mechanisms for the switch in subclass of H chains synthesized by myeloma cells are listed in Table IV. Each mechanism makes certain predictions about the constant region mutants which can be isolated.

TABLE IV
Possible Mechanisms for $\gamma_{2b} \rightarrow \gamma_{2a}$ Subclass Switch

1. V_H gene associated with different C_H. In this model all the genetic information necessary to code for the V_H or the C_H is assumed to be handled as a unit.
    A. Predicts all the γ_{2a} clones should have the same sequences.
    B. Predicts that even starting with a deletion in CH_1 all chains should show the wild-type molecular weight (or if deletion extended into V_H all chains should be of small, but identical size).

2. Deletion or nonutilization of part of the structural genes and the intervening genetic material between tandem constant region genes resulting in the fusion of the two genes; the V_H and the fused C_H are then transcribed and translated.
    A. Allows many different amino acid sequences and sizes of heavy chains depending on where deletion begins and terminates.
    B. Predicts that once chain begins γ_{2a} sequence, all sequences carboxy terminal to that point should be γ_{2a}.

3. Recombination between γ_{2a} and γ_{2b} genes on homologous chromosomes or sister chromatids.
    A. Allows many different amino acid sequences.
    B. If genes line up in register should get two different size heavy chains depending on the position of the recombination event.
    C. Predicts that in the majority of the heavy chains, once the γ_{2a} sequence begins, all residues carboxy terminal should be γ_{2a}; however, does allow for the intermixture of γ_{2b} sequences in the γ_{2a} sequence in the case of multiple crossovers.

4. Reassortment of small genetic units, i.e., smaller than V_H or C_H.
    A. Predicts two discrete sizes if a single genetic unit contains the deletion.
    B. Allows many but finite number of sequences, depending on the number of genetic elements; independent reassortment of discrete units should independently yield same sequences.

It is impossible at this time to decide among mechanisms 2, 3, or 4. However, our data are not compatible with mechanism 1, the subclass switch resulting from the association of an entire V_H gene with a different C_H gene. If this mechanism were operative, all mutants should have identical amino acid sequences and molecular weight; neither of these conditions was satisfied since we observed two different sized H chains and many different isoelectric focusing patterns.

Both mechanisms 2 and 3, deletion and recombination, are consistent with the observations of two discrete sizes of heavy chains; in both cases, depending on which genetic material was deleted or on the position of the crossover, the original deletion from the parental 10-1 could be maintained. The existence of two discrete sizes of H chains is also compatible with mechanism 4, the reassortment of genetic elements. If the deletion were of part or all of one element, two sizes would result. If the deletion extended into two or more elements, more than two discrete sizes would be possible. It is to be noted that several independently arising clones exhibit identical isoelectric focusing patterns; this observation suggests hot spots for recombination or deletion, or alternately, the existence of discrete elements which reassort. Amino acid sequence data and possibly nucleic acid sequence data will be necessary to distinguish among the alternatives. The internal deletion in the CH_1 domain will provide a valuable marker since all hypotheses predict that 47,000 dalton chains result if the switch occurred carboxy-terminal to the deletion, and 55,000 dalton chains result if the change occurred amino-terminal to the deletion. Structural data will indicate if all mutants follow this prediction, or if exceptions exist which suggest alternative mechanisms.

ACKNOWLEDGMENTS

This research was supported by grants ES 01293 and CA 16858 from the National Institutes of Health. S.L.M. is an Irma T. Hirschl Fellow. William Dackowski and Letitia Wims have furnished excellent technical assistance during the course of these studies.

REFERENCES

1. Nossal, G. J. V., Pike, B. L., Stocker, J. W., Layton, J. E., and Goding, J. W. (1976) *Cold Spring Harbor Symp. Quant. Biol.* **41**, 237–243.
2. Pernis, B., Brouet, J. C., and Seligmann, M. (1974) *Eur. J. Immunol.* **4**, 776–778.
3. Fu. S. M., Winchester, R. J., and Kunkel, H. G. (1974) *J. Immunol.* **114**, 250–252.

4. Cooper, M. D., Kearney, J. F., Lydyard, P. M., Grossi, C. E., and Lawton, A. R. (1976) *Cold Spring Harbor Symp. Quant. Biol.* **41**, 139–145.
5. Vitteta, E. S., and Uhr, J. W. (1976) *Eur. J. Immunol.* **6**, 140–143.
6. Pernis, B., Forni, L., and Luzzati, A. L. (1976) *Cold Spring Harbor Symp. Quant. Biol.* **41**, 175–183.
7. Baumal, R., Coffino, P., Bargellesi, A., Buxbaum, J., Laskov, R., and Scharff, M. D. (1971) *Ann. N.Y. Acad. Sci.* **190**, 235–249.
8. Coffino, P., Laskov, R., and Scharff, M. D. (1970) *Science* **167**, 186.
9. Morrison, S. L., and Scharff, M. D. (1975) *J. Immunol.* **114**, 655–659.
10. Coffino, P., and Scharff, M. D. (1971) *Proc. Natl. Acad. Sci. U.S.A.* **68**, 219–223.
11. Laskov, R., and Scharff, M. D. (1970) *J. Exp. Med.* **131**, 515–541.
12. Laskov, R., and Scharff, M. D. (1974) *J. Exp. Med.* **140**, 1112–1116.
13. Baumal, R., and Scharff, M. D. (1976) *J. Immunol.* **116**, 65–74.
14. Morrison, S. L., and Scharff, M. D. (1978) In preparation.
15. Frangione, B., and Franklin, E. C. (1973) *Semin. Hematol.* **10**, 53–64.
16. Franklin, E. C., and Frangione, B. (1975) *Contemp. Top. Mol. Immunol.* **4**, 89–125.
17. Buxbaum, J. N., and Preud'homme, J.-L. (1972) *J. Immunol.* **109**, 1131–1137.
18. Milstein, C., Secher, D. S., Cowan, N. J., Harrison, T. M., Cotton, R. G. H., and Brownlee, G. G. (1974) *In* "Cellular Selection and Regulation in the Immune Response" (G. M. Edelman, ed.), pp. 245–264. Raven, New York.
19. Milstein, C., Adetugbo, K., Cowan, N. J., Kohler, G., Secher, D. S., and Wilde, C. D. (1976) *Cold Spring Harbor Symp. Quant. Biol.* **41**, 793–803.
20. Adetugbo, K., Milstein, C., and Secher, D. S. (1977) *Nature (London)* **265**, 299–304.
21. Cook, W. D., and Scharff, M. D. (1977) *Proc. Natl. Acad. Sci. U.S.A.* **74**, 5687–5691.
22. Preud'homme, J.-L., Birshtein, B. K., and Scharff, M. D. (1975) *Proc. Natl. Acad. Sci. U.S.A.* **72**, 1427.
23. Koskimies, S., and Birshtein, B. K. (1976) *Nature (London)* **64**, 480–482.
24. Francus, T., Dharmgrongartama, B., Campbell, R., Scharff, M. D., and Birshtein, B. K. (1978) *J. Exp. Med.* **147**, 1535.
25. Morrison, S. L., Baumal, R., Birshtein, B. K., Kuehl, W. M., Preud'homme, J.-L., Frank, L., Jasek, T., and Scharff, M. D. (1974) *In* "Cellular Selection and Regulation of the Immune Response" (G. M. Edelman, ed.), pp. 233–244. Raven, New York.
26. Morrison, S. L. (1978) *Eur. J. Immunol.* (in press).
27. Birshtein, B. K., and Morrison, S. L., unpublished observations.
28. Francus, T. (1978) *Fed. Proc., Fed. Am. Soc. Exp. Biol.* **37**, 1763.
29. Bailey, L. K., Hannestad, K., and Eisen, H. N. (1973) *Fed. Proc., Fed. Am. Soc. Exp. Biol.* **32**, 1013.
30. Francus, T., and Birshtein, B. K. (1978) *Biochemistry* **17**, 4324.

Differentiation of Leukemic B Lymphocytes in Man

S. M. FU, N. CHIORAZZI, J. N. HURLEY,
J. P. HALPER, AND H. G. KUNKEL
The Rockefeller University
New York, New York

INTRODUCTION

Chronic lymphocytic leukemia (CLL) in man has been proved to be a disease due to clonal proliferation of B cells. Although immunofluorescent studies indicate that the majority of the lymphocytes from patients with CLL bear IgM and IgD as their surface immunoglobulins (Ig), it has been shown in our studies and those of others (1) that very little intracellular Ig was demonstrable in these cells. It appears that a differentiation block is present in the majority of the CLL cases. However, this block has been proven to be incomplete in certain patients (2). In the present paper, studies from our laboratory will be reviewed which demonstrated that the leukemic B cells in these patients were capable of maturation to plasma cells *in vivo*. New evidence will be presented to show that this maturation process can be accelerated markedly *in vitro*. In addition, a T cell helper function defect is documented in these patients.

IN VIVO DIFFERENTIATION

Despite the fact that the majority of the patients with CLL have decreased or normal levels of immunoglobulin in the serum, elevated serum immunoglobulin levels have been associated with monoclonal bands in some cases (3). The relationship between the monoclonal serum proteins and the leukemic lymphocytes was obscure. Previous

127

studies (2) led to the conclusion that the leukemic lymphocytes were the precursors of plasma cells responsible for the production of the serum band.

The first patient with CLL and a monoclonal band (Ei) studied in our laboratory was an 84-year-old woman. On her initial clinical presentation, the white cell counts were greater than 100,000/mm³. A serum monoclonal band was present at a concentration of 4 mg/ml. Figure 1 shows the electrophoretic pattern of the Ei serum. Serum immunoelectrophoresis revealed that the monoclonal protein was IgM K. This IgM K protein was isolated by Pevikon zone electrophoresis. An idiotypic antiserum was made against the protein. This antiserum identifies the specific marker for the variable regions of this IgM. The specificity of the idiotypic antiserum is shown in Table I. After extensive absorbtions with pooled IgG, IgM, IgA, and normal human serums, the antiserum agglutinated IgM Ei-coated erythrocytes readily to a dilution of 1/640. This agglutination was inhibited by 0.25 μg/ml of IgM Ei but not by normal sera, other IgM proteins, or pooled IgG at a concentration of 10 mg/ml.

In the first experiment on Ei in February, 1974, her white count was 23,000/mm³ (Table II). Twenty-three percent of her mononuclear cells formed sheep erythrocyte rosettes and 7% ingested latex particles. Thus about 70% of the mononuclear cells were of the B cell population. Rhodamine-conjugated F (ab')₂ antibodies specific for μ, δ, and K

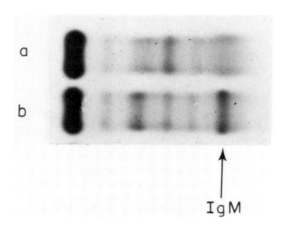

Fig. 1. Cellulose acetate electrophoresis of a normal serum (a) and the serum of patient Ei (b), showing a monoclonal IgM band.

TABLE I
Hemagglutination Inhibition Assay System for Detecting the IgM (Ei)
Idiotype Antigen[a]

Proteins	Concentration of inhibitory (mg/ml)						
	10	1	0.001	0.0005	0.00025	0.000125	0.000062
Pooled IgG	2[b]	2	2	2	2	2	2
IgM k	2	2	2	2	2	2	2
IgA	2	2	2	2	2	2	2
Normal serum	2	2	2	2	2	2	2
IgM (Ei)	0	0	0	0	0	2	2

[a] Test system: rabbit antiserum 616 absorbed with pooled IgG, IgM, IgA, and normal human serums and red cells coated with IgM (Ei).

[b] Hemagglutination is graded "0" to "4". "0" indicates no agglutination whereas "4" indicates big agglutinated red cell masses are present.

TABLE II
Immunofluorescent Analysis of Peripheral Mononuclear Cells of Patients
Ei and Se with Antiserums to Different Igs

Patient	Date	WBC	Surface Ig (%)					
			Se Id	Ei Id	IgM	IgD	K	λ
Ei	2/74	23,000[a]	—	68	67	56	68	5
	6/77	135,000[b]	—	85	87	—	80	—
Se	3/78	12,000[c]	34	—	44	—	33	2

Patient	Date	Intracellular Ig (%)					
		Se Id	Ei Id	IgM	IgD	K	λ
Ei	2/74	—	2.8	2.5	0	2.8	0
	6/77	—	0.2	0.2	0	0.2	0
Se	3/78	0.2	—	0.2	0	0.2	0

[a] Twenty-three percent of the mononuclear cells formed sheep erythrocyte rosettes and 7% ingested latex particles.

[b] Eight percent of the mononuclear cells formed sheep erythrocyte rosettes and 3% stained positively for peroxidase granules.

[c] Forty-two percent of the mononuclear cells formed sheep erythrocyte rosettes and 17% stained positively for peroxidase.

stained 67, 56, and 68% of the mononuclear cells, respectively, and only a few or none of the cells stained with the antisera specific for γ, α, and λ determinants. Sixty-eight percent of the cells also stained with the idiotypic antiserum. The staining with the idiotypic antiserum was blocked by Ei serum but not by normal sera. Thus, almost all the Ig-bearing leukemic cells showed the idiotypic specificity on their surface. Similar observations were made in several additional experiments. Furthermore, it was shown by the use of the idiotypic antiserum that IgM and IgD on Ei leukemic cells shared similar variable regions (4).

In addition, rhodamine-conjugated antisera specific for the idiotypic, μ and κ determinants identified 1–3% of the mononuclear cells in the peripheral blood of patient Ei as typical plasma cells. These cells were stained strongly for intracellular immunoglobulins by these antisera (Table II). Antisera specific for γ, α, and λ determinants failed to stain any cells intracellularly. In several experiments with both a fluorescein-conjugated anti-μ antiserum and the rhodamine-conjugated idiotypic antiserum as intracellular staining reagents, all the cells producing IgM as identified by the anti-μ antiserum also stained with the idiotypic antiserum. Thus, the idiotypic antiserum identified the same population of plasma cells as the anti-μ antiserum.

During the late stage of her disease, her white cell count increased to 135,000/mm^3 and 85% of her lymphocytes stained with the idiotypic antiserum (Table II). Only 0.2% of the mononuclear cells stained brightly for intracellular IgM and a similar percentage of cells stained intracellularly with the idiotypic antiserum.

Recently, a second patient, Se, was studied in a similar manner. An idiotypic antiserum raised against her IgM K monoclonal band stained the majority of B cells in the peripheral blood. Similar to the case of Ei, the idiotypic antiserum also stained a small population of cells brightly for intracellular Ig.

The relationship between the serum IgM band and leukemic lymphocytes is summarized in Fig. 2. An anti-idiotypic antiserum against the monoclonal IgM band stained the membrane IgM on the leukemic lymphocytes. In addition, it identified a small number of the cells to be plasma cells. Thus, the IgM on the membrane of the lymphocytes, the intracellular IgM in the plasma cells and the monoclonal IgM protein in the serum were idiotypically identical. It appeared that a small number of the leukemic lymphocytes matured by a process of differentiation *in vivo* to plasma cells which synthesized the serum monoclonal IgM band.

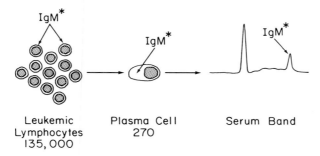

Leukemic   Plasma Cell   Serum Band
Lymphocytes   270
135,000

Fig. 2. Relationship between leukemic B lymphocytes and the serum monoclonal IgM band in patient Ei. The surface IgM on leukemic lymphocytes, the intracellular Ig in the plasma cells, and the serum IgM band shared a similar idiotypic specificity. * Designates the same idiotype.

INDUCTION OF *IN VITRO* DIFFERENTIATION OF LEUKEMIC B LYMPHOCYTES

As shown in Fig. 2, only 270 plasma cells were identified with the idiotypic antiserum in the peripheral blood of patient, Ei, although there were 135,000 leukemic lymphocytes/mm³ in her blood. It was apparent that the *in vivo* differentiation of the leukemic cells was proceeding at a low rate. Recent studies (5) were carried out to determine if this rate of differentiation could be accelerated *in vitro* by the addition of various stimulatory substances.

A series of stimulatory substances such as pokeweed mitogen, concanavalin A, phytohemagglutinin, lipopolysaccharide, streptokinase–streptodornase, and tetanus toxoid were added to the cultures of isolated leukemic B cells of the first patient, Ei. No increase in plasma cells was observed.

It has been known that T cell helper activity is needed for the differentiation of B cells. Potent T cell helper factors are generated in the mixed lymphocyte reaction. This phenomenon has been termed the allogeneic helper effect [reviewed in Katz (6)]. Therefore, isolated T cells from normal individuals were added to the cultures of leukemic B cells. A marked increase in plasma cells was seen in the cultures to which allogeneic T cells were added.

Two representative experiments of this type showing the effects on the maturation of the leukemic B cells from the patient Ei by the allogeneic effect factors generated in the mixed lymphocyte culture reaction are shown in Table III. In these experiments, T cells from

TABLE III
Maturation of Ei Leukemic Lymphocytes under the Influence
of Allogenic Helper Factors[a]

Ei B Cells	Allogeneic T cells	No. of plasma cells/culture	IgM Ei secreted (μg)
Exp. 1			
2.0×10^6	none[b]	1×10^4	0.1
2.0×10^6	2.0×10^6	5.5×10^5	1.6
Exp. 2			
2.0×10^6	none[b]	5×10^3	0.1
2.0×10^6	2.0×10^6	6.2×10^5	3.2

[a] Cells were cultured in Linbro Tissue Culture Plates (16-mm wells) in 2 ml of RPMI 1640 supplemented with 0.2 mM glutamine, 100 μ/ml penicillin, 100 meg/ml streptomycin, 1% trypticase soybroth, and 10% pooled human serum. After incubation for 6 days at 37°C in a humidified, rocking chamber containing a 5% CO_2 atmosphere, plasma cells were identified by immunofluorescence with an idiotypic antiserum and IgM Ei secretion was estimated by hemagglutination inhibition with the idiotypic antiserum.

[b] 2×10^6 syngeneic T cells were added to these cultures.

normal individuals were isolated by a selection procedure using neuraminidase-treated sheep red blood cells. The rosette-forming T cells were recovered at the bottom of a Ficoll–Hypaque density gradient. T cells were obtained after the sheep red cells were lysed. Leukemic B cells were obtained by the depletion of rosette-forming T cells. In the first experiment only 1×10^4 plasma cells were seen after a 6-day culture of 2×10^6 leukemic B lymphocytes. In contrast, 5.5×10^5 plasma cells were detected in a similar culture to which 2×10^6 allogeneic T cells from a normal individual were added. This represents a fifty-fivefold increase in plasma cells. In the second experiment, over a one hundredfold increase was observed.

IgM Ei secreted into the culture superatant was assayed directly by passive hemagglutination inhibition involving the idiotypic determinant (Table I). Even though the cultures were carried out in medium supplemental with normal AB serum, direct assaying for specific IgM Ei secretion was feasible. Very little IgM Ei secretion was found in the superatant when the leukemic B cells were cultured alone. In the first experiment, sixteenfold increase in IgM Ei secretion was detected in the culture of Ei cells to which allogeneic T cells were added. In the

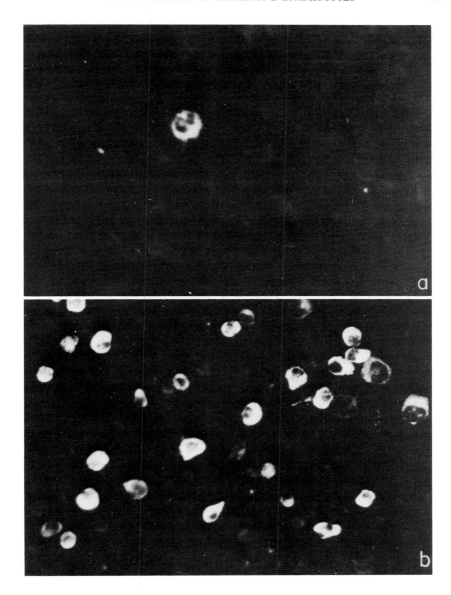

Fig. 3.   Staining of plasma cells generated *in vitro* by an idiotypic antiserum against IgM Ei. (a) A rare plasma cell in the control culture containing only Ei leukemic B cells; (b) Plasma cells in a culture of Ei leukemic B cells to which allogeneic normal T cells were added.

TABLE IV
Effect of Pokeweed Mitogen on the Differentiation of
Leukemic B Lymphocytes[a]

Se B cells	Se T cells	No. of plasma cells/culture	IgM Se secreted
1.0×10^6	None	2×10^3	0.1 μg
1.0×10^6	0.5×10^6	4×10^5	6.4 μg
1.0×10^6	1.0×10^6	3.2×10^5	6.4 μg

[a] Culture conditions and assay systems were identical to those described in Table III. Pokeweed mitogen was added to a final dilution of 1 : 100.

second experiment, a thirty-twofold increase was observed (Table III).

The staining of plasma cells by the rhodamine-conjugated idiotypic antiserum is shown in Fig. 3. Washed cultured cells were flattened onto the slide by cytocentrifugation. The cells were fixed to render the plasma cell membrane permeable to the staining agent. In this procedure only plasma cells with abundant intracellular IgM Ei stained brightly with the anti-idiotypic antiserum. A rare plasma cell was seen in a control culture in which less than 0.5% of cells stained brightly with the anti-idiotypic antiserum (Fig. 3a). In contrast, many plasma cells were seen in the culture to which allogeneic T cells were added. A representative field of such a culture is shown in Fig. 3b.

The second patient Se was studied in a similar manner. Leukemic B cells from Se also differentiated in response to allogeneic helper activity. However, this patient differs from the first patient Ei in that isolated B cells differentiated to plasma cells when autologous T cells and pokeweed mitogen were added to the culture. Over 40% of Se lymphocyte matured to plasma cells under these conditions (Table IV). As little as 5×10^5 autologous T cells were sufficient to allow maturation of significant numbers of leukemic B cells from Se in the presence of pokeweed mitogen. In contrast, as many as 1×10^7 autologous T cells in the case of Ei failed to help her leukemic B cells to differentiate under identical culture conditions.

In a limited number of cases of CLL without monoclonal Ig bands, pokeweed mitogen, allogeneic T cells and other stimulatory substances did not induce further differentiation of these leukemic lymphocytes.

EPSTEIN–BARR VIRUS TRANSFORMATION OF LEUKEMIC B LYMPHOCYTES

The Epstein–Barr virus (EBV) has been reported to be a polyclonal B cell activator for human B cells (7,8). EBV preparations were able to activate B cells from both Ei and Se. Multiple lymphoblastoid cell lines were obtained by EBV transformation in collaboration with Dr. M. Scharff and his co-workers (9). Certain characteristics of some of the cell line are shown in Table V. Of the seven lines derived from lymphocytes of the patient Se, only cells from the line SeD reacted with the idiotypic antiserum specific for IgM Se. Sixty-seven percent of the cells stained for surface Ig and 24% for intracellular Ig. This cell line has been cloned and seven clones studied showed similar characteristics. It is apparent that the SeD line was derived from the leukemic B cells. Furthermore, immunofluorescence involving double fluorochromes showed that the plasma cells which stained brightly for intracellular Ig had no detectable surface Ig in this line. The plasma cells and lymphoblast with surface Ig represent cells at different phases of the cell cycle. These cultured cells could also be considered to be at different stages of differentiation regarding the expression of intracellular Ig.

DEFECTIVE T CELL HELPER FUNCTION IN PATIENTS

Because of the above observation that the provision of appropriate T helper activities markedly increased the rate of differentiation of certain leukemic B cells *in vitro*, a reduction of helper T cell function might be responsible partly for the lack of *in vivo* differentiation in these CLL patients. The helper function of purified T cells from patients with CLL was examined. The system employed for assaying the helper activity of a given T cell population was the generation of plaque-forming cells by normal tonsillar B cells against sheep red cells co-cultured with the T cells (10). In such a system, few plaques were generated in a culture containing 2×10^6 B cells without the addition of allogeneic T cells from normal individuals (Table VI). In contrast, 1200 plaques were seen when T cells from a normal person were added. The addition of an equal number of purified T cells from three patients with CLL, Ei, Se, and Ya generated no additional plaques. Ya is a patient without a monoclonal band in his serum. Six additional cases of CLL without monoclonal Ig bands have been studied in detail

TABLE V

Percentage of Cells in Different Se and Ei Cell Lines Showing Membrane Ig and Cytoplasmic Ig as Detected by Fluorescence with Various Ig Antisera[a]

Line	Surface Ig (%)							Intracellular Ig (%)						
	Se Id[b]	Ei Id[c]	IgM	IgD	IgG	K	λ	Se Id	Ei Id	IgM	IgD	IgG	K	λ
SeD	67	0	72	37	0	67	0	24	0	29	9	0	30	0
SeA1	0	0	80	22	0	33	0	0	0	43	0	0	40	0
Se21	0	0	96	0	0	39	0	0	0	42	0	0	38	0
SeA2	0	0	0	0	0	0	0	0	0	0	0	28	20	0
Ei 26	0	75	80	0	0	15	0	0	46	51	0	0	49	0
Ei 39	0	4	4	0	0	2	0	0	27	22	0	0	26	0
Ei 81	0	0	0	0	0	0	0	0	34	35	0	0	24	0
Ei 151	0	0	0	0	0	0	0	0	0	0	0	27	0	25

[a] No cell lines were stained with an anti-IgA reagent.

[b] Antiserum specific for the idiotypic determinants of the IgM K paraprotein from patient Se.

[c] Antiserum specific for the idiotypic determinants of the IgM K paraprotein from patient Ei.

TABLE VI
Lack of Allogeneic Helper
Activity of Isolated T cells from
Patients with CLL, Using
Tonsillar B Cells as Test System[a]

Source of T cells (2×10^6)	No. of plaque-forming cells against sheep erythrocytes
None	6
Normal	1200
Ei	6
Se	3
Ya	3

[a] 2×10^6 Tonsillar B cells were cultured either alone or with T cells under identical conditions as described in Table III.

in a similar manner (11). Isolated T cells from all these patients lacked allogeneic helper activities irrespective of the stages of their disease. In two instances, monoclonal lymphocytosis was the only manifestation of the disease. In contrast, isolated T cells from three patients with Waldenstrom macroglobulinemia and two patients with multiple myeloma possessed allogeneic helper activity.

DISCUSSION AND CONCLUSION

Two patients Ei and Se with CLL and a monoclonal IgM band were studied. Idiotypic antiserums prepared in rabbits and rendered specific for the bands proved that the surface Ig on the leukemic lymphocytes and the serum IgM bands shared similar variable regions in both cases. In addition, the antiserums also identified a small population of the mononuclear cells to be plasma cells. It appeared that the leukemic lymphocytes were the precursor cells of the plasma cells responsible for the secretion of the Ig band. Although the rate of differentiation of leukemic lymphocytes to plasma cells was low *in vivo*, the block in differentiation observed in these cases of CLL was incomplete.

In vitro differentiation in the two cases studied could be markedly accelerated by the use of stimulatory agents. An increased rate of differentiation to plasma cells by the leukemic cells in both cases was documented when allogeneic helper activity was provided. Leukemic cells from patient Se also responded to pokeweed mitogen when sufficient numbers of autologous T cells were present. The lack of response to pokeweed mitogen by the leukemic B cells from patient Ei was perhaps due to the absence of appropriate T cells responsive to the mitogen. Evidence was also obtained that there was no excessive spontaneous or inducible suppressor activities in the mononuclear cell preparations from these patients (7). Thus, the lack of sufficient helper T cells appeared to be partly responsible for the reduced rate of differentiation observed *in vivo*.

Repeated attempts to induce differentiation of leukemic B cells from CLL cases without monoclonal bands have not been successful in the present studies. However, by a more sensitive method, Maino *et al.* (12) have demonstrated increased rate of light chain synthesis by the leukemic cells when phytohemagglutinin was added to the cultures. Perhaps these leukemic B cells also will mature to plasma cells when appropriate T cell helper activities are identified and provided.

A defect in T cell helper function was identified in the majority of the CLL cases studied. Isolated T cells from patients with this disorder cannot generate allogeneic helper factors as measured by the generation of plaque-forming cells against sheep red cells from a normal allogeneic B cell population. This defect was present during the early stages of the disease and may play some role in its pathogenesis. The lack of helper T cell activities may contribute to the accumulation of leukemic lymphocytes at their early stages of maturation.

ACKNOWLEDGMENTS

We thank Ruth Brooks and Mary Margaret Zansitis for their assistance. S. M. Fu is a scholar of the Leukemia Society of America. N. Chiorazzi is supported by a Fellowship from the Arthritis Foundation. J. P. Halper was supported by a Fellowship from the Arthritis Foundation. This investigation was supported by United States Public Health Service Grants RR-102, AI-10811, CA-24338, and a grant from the National Leukemia Association.

REFERENCES

1. Seligmann, M., Preud'homme, J. L., and Brouet, J. C. (1973) *Transplant. Rev.* **16**, 85.

2. Fu, S. M., Winchester, R. J., Feizi, T., Walzer, P. D., and Kunkel, H. G. (1974) *Proc. Natl. Acad. Sci. U.S.A.* **71**, 4487.
3. Azar, H. A., Hill, W. T., and Osserman, E. F. (1957) *Am. J. Med.* **23**, 239.
4. Fu, S. M., Winchester, R. J., and Kunkel, H. G. (1975) *J. Immunol.* **114**, 410.
5. Fu, S. M., Chiorazzi, N., Kunkel, H. G., Halper, J. P., and Harris, S. (1978) *J. Exp. Med.* **148**, 1570.
6. Katz, D. H. (1977) "Lymphocyte Differentiation, Recognition and Regulation." Academic Press, New York.
7. Rosen, A., Gergely, P., Jondal, M., Klein, G., and Birtton, S. (1977) *Nature (London)* **267**, 52.
8. Luzzati, A. L., Hengartner, H., and Schreier, M. H. (1977) *Nature (London)* **269**, 419.
9. Hurley, J. N., Fu, S. M., Kunkel, H. G., McKenna, G., and Scharff, M. D. (1978) *Proc. Natl. Acad. Sci. U.S.A.* **75**, 5706.
10. Chiorazzi, N., Ferrarini, M., Montazeri, G., Hoffman, T., and Fu, S. M. (1978) *In* "Antibody Production in Man: *In Vitro* Synthesis and Clinical Implications" (A. S. Fauci and R. E. Bailieux, eds.). Academic Press, New York (in press).
11. Chiorazzi, N., Fu, S. M., Montazeri, G., Kunkel, H. G., Rai, K., and Gee, T. (1979). *J. Immunol.* (in press).
12. Maino, V. C., Kurnick, J. T., Kubo, R. T., and Grey, H. M. (1977) *J. Immunol.* **118**, 742.

Intracellular Events in the Differentiation of B Lymphocytes to Pentamer IgM Synthesis

RICHARD A. ROTH, ELIZABETH L. MATHER,
AND MARIAN ELLIOTT KOSHLAND

Department of Bacteriology and Immunology
University of California
Berkeley, California

The immunocompetent B cell responds to its first antigenic stimulus by synthesizing and secreting pentamer IgM antibody. This differentiation process involves not only the covalent assembly of monomer IgM subunits, but also the incorporation into the pentamer structure of a third polypeptide, the J chain (1). Our laboratory has been investigating the *in vivo* polymerization of IgM with two purposes in mind: (1) to identify the intracellular activation events, and (2) to determine the control mechanisms involved.

As a first approach to the problem, the changes in intracellular J chain and monomer IgM and the secretion of pentamer IgM were followed as a function of time after mitogen stimulation. The experiments were performed with small cell populations isolated from rabbit spleen by 1 g velocity sedimentation (2,3). Previous studies in our laboratory (4) have indicated that B lymphocytes sedimenting between 2.7 and 3.5 mm/hr are not synthesizing J chain. Although low levels of intracellular J chain were detected in such cell fractions, the amounts present could be explained by the 0.1–0.2% activated B cells that were found to remain in the population. This deduction was supported by our recent analyses of two mouse B cell lymphomas, WEHI 231 (5) and 38C-13 (6,7). No intracellular J chain could be detected, indicating that less than 120 molecules were present per cell.

141

The experimental protocol used in the activation studies is given in Fig. 1. The small spleen cell fractions were cultured with pokeweed mitogen at cell densities known to selectively promote pentamer IgM synthesis (9). At 24-hr intervals after stimulation, the cells and culture supernatants were harvested, the cells were lysed with Nonidet P40, and their J chain and IgM contents were determined by radioimmunoassay. This method was chosen rather than radiolabeling because it allowed quantitation of the total intracellular pools. The limit of sensitivity for the J chain assay was 0.1 ng, and for the IgM assay 0.3

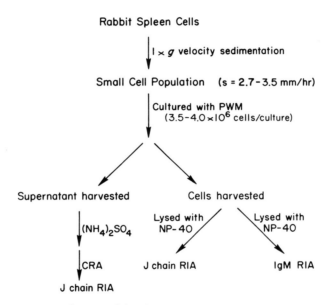

Fig. 1. Experimental protocol for the analysis of B cell activation events. Suspensions of rabbit spleen lymphocytes were depleted of red blood cells by treatment with 0.85% NH_4Cl, passed through a glass wool column to remove debris, and then separated according to size by 1 g velocity sedimentation (2). The lymphocytes which sedimented at 2.7–3.5 mm/hr were cultured with 10 μl pokeweed mitogen (Grand Island Biological Co.) in 1 ml of supplemented (8) RPMI 1640 at a density of 3.5–4.0 × 10⁶ cells/ml. Harvested cells were washed with RPMI 1640, lysed with 1% Nonidet P40, 0.1 M iodoacetamide in phosphate buffered saline, and centrifuged at 43,000 g for 30 min. The amount of cellular J chain, IgM, and IgG was determined by radioimmunoassay; varying amounts of the cell lysate were used to inhibit the binding of radioiodinated J chain, IgM, or IgG to their respective antisera. Culture supernatant fluids were concentrated by ultrafiltration and $(NH_4)_2SO_4$ precipitation (37%) and then made 10 M in urea and 60 mM in dithioerythritol for 2 hr at 37°C to effect complete reduction. Iodoacetic acid (150 mM) was added and after 30 min the supernatant fluids were dialyzed and assayed for J chain by radioimmunoassay.

ng. For the determinations of extracellular J chain and IgM, the culture
supernatant proteins were concentrated by ammonium sulfate precipitation, completely reduced and alkylated, and examined by radioimmunoassay. Because J chain was not detected free in the culture
supernatant and one J chain was known to be bound per pentamer (1),
the amount of covalent J chain released by reduction and alkylation
could be used to calculate the amount of pentamer IgM secreted.

The results of such experiments are shown in Fig. 2. It can be seen
from the left hand frame that the initial cell population contained the
usual small amount of J chain, ranging from 0.15 to 0.2 ng per culture.
Within 12 hr after pokeweed mitogen stimulation, the intracellular
level increased two- to threefold; it then doubled in each succeeding
24 hr interval to achieve a twenty- to forty-fold increase in 4½ days.
Extracellular J chain was detected at 36 hr in amounts significantly
lower than those within the cell. The secreted J chain then rapidly
accumulated until by 4½ days there were 25 ng per culture.

The right hand frame of Fig. 2 gives the comparable data for intracellular and secreted IgM. It is evident that the IgM content of the
population did not change dramatically over the sampling period. The
initial level of 44 ng per culture was maintained for 36 hr after stimula-

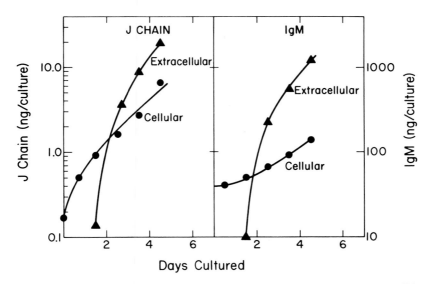

Fig. 2.   Response of rabbit B cells stimulated with pokeweed mitogen. Small lymphocytes were cultured and assayed as described in Fig. 1. Control experiments showed
that intracellular IgG decreased from 1.9 ng/culture at 0 hour to <0.07 ng/culture by 4½
days.

tion and rose only 3.5-fold in 4½ days. These values, however, do not provide an accurate index of the IgM synthesized for export. Because only a fraction of the B cell population responds to mitogen (10), the measurements include the membrane IgM on the remaining unactivated cells. To correct for the membrane contribution, the IgM content of cells grown in the absence of mitogen was subtracted from the total IgM content of the pokeweed stimulated population. The results of this correction are shown in Fig. 3. The data indicate that pokeweed mitogen effected a large increase in the IgM content of responding cells and the kinetics of the response paralleled that observed for the J chain.

From the findings of these radioimmunoassays it was possible to analyze the relationships between intracellular IgM and J chain and the secreted pentamer product. The results of such an analysis are presented as a bar diagram in Fig. 4. The total height of the bars represents the average intracellular IgM or J chain content within the time period indicated on the abscissa. The content is expressed in molecules per culture. The solid bars represent the average number of J chain or pentamer IgM molecules secreted per hour and the crossed bars the number secreted per 2 hours. The secretion rates were calculated from the amounts of J chain or IgM that accumulated in the supernatant in each time period and from the assumption that the secretion rate was constant over that time period. The 1 and 2 hour values were chosen because they constituted the lower and upper

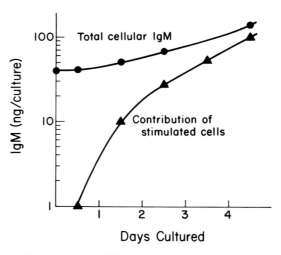

Fig. 3.   Adjusted increase in cellular IgM after pokeweed mitogen stimulation.

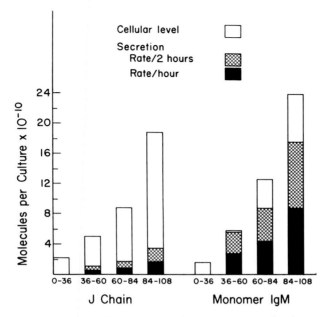

Fig. 4. Comparison of cellular levels and secretion rates of J chain and IgM.

limits for the average transit of the IgM monomer from the ribosome to the external medium (11).

From a comparison of the various bar heights it can be seen that relatively little monomer IgM accumulated within the stimulated cells. If internal transit takes 2 hr, almost all the IgM present could be accounted for as product destined for export. In contrast, the J chain content of the stimulated cells was clearly in excess of that secreted by a factor of five. These data suggested that the amount of monomer synthesized determines the amount of pentamer IgM secreted.

The most remarkable result of these analyses, however, was the one-to-one correspondence found in the number of intracellular J chain and IgM molecules. This relationship held over the entire time period studied. For example, from 0 to 36 hr, both the J chain and IgM content averaged 2×10^{10} molecules; from 36 to 60 hr, the values were 5 and 6×10^{10}, respectively; and from 84 to 108 hr, the values were 1.9 and 2.4×10^{11}. Moreover, a one-to-one correspondence was obtained in similar analyses of IgM-synthesizing myeloma cells such as the MOPC 104E plasmacytoma.

The presence of excess intracellular J chain could be explained in two different ways. *In vitro* polymerization studies have indicated that pentamer IgM assembly proceeds by a series of disulfide interchanges (12). Since this reaction has an equilibrium of one, efficient polymerization requires an excess of a starting component and/or the rapid removal of product. The high intracellular J chain content may then simply serve to drive the polymerization process, and in fact, a fivefold excess of J chain over monomer was found to be the optimum ratio for maximum polymerization *in vitro* (13). Alternatively, it is possible that one J chain molecule becomes covalently associated with each monomer IgM as an export signal. For example, the hydrophilic properties of the J chain might prevent the monomer from being incorporated into the plasma membrane as a receptor. Once the monomer–J chain complexes are assembled in the Golgi or the inner surface of the plasma membrane, polymerization would take place in such a way that four J chains are discarded, and only one remains covalently bonded to the secreted pentamer. Experiments are under way to distinguish between these two possibilities.

As a second approach to understanding the biochemical events in B cell differentiation, studies were undertaken of the role of disulfide interchange enzyme in IgM assembly. Della Corte and Parkhouse (14) have reported that disulfide interchange enzyme, as well as J chain, is essential for the *in vitro* polymerization of mouse IgM. The physiological significance of this finding was difficult to evaluate, however, because the enzyme was only partially purified from beef liver and high concentrations, 2.5 mg/ml, were required to effect IgM assembly. To resolve this question, our laboratory has purified disulfide interchange enzyme from mouse liver and used the preparation as a standard to determine the content of the enzyme in activated B cells and its contribution to IgM polymerization.

The purification of the mouse enzyme was accomplished by the scheme shown in Fig. 5 (15). The final product was homogeneous by electrophoretic criteria and exhibited high interchange activity as measured by two standard assays, the reactivation of scrambled ribonuclease (16) and the splitting of insulin into its component chains (15). Moreover, the molecular weight, isoelectric point, and amino acid composition of the mouse enzyme were in good agreement with the published values for the purified beef liver preparation (15). Antibodies were then raised against the mouse enzyme so that its tissue distribution could be quantitatively determined by radioimmunoassay. Interchange enzyme was found to be a component of all cell types examined including MOPC 104E plasmacytoma cells which synthesize pentamer IgM. The amounts present in the various cell types

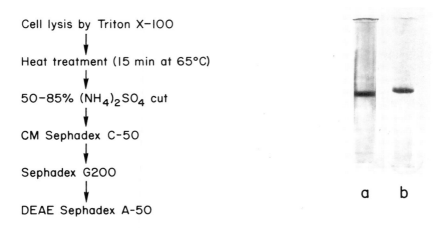

Cell lysis by Triton X-100

↓

Heat treatment (15 min at 65°C)

↓

50-85% $(NH_4)_2SO_4$ cut

↓

CM Sephadex C-50

↓

Sephadex G200

↓

DEAE Sephadex A-50

a   b

Fig. 5. Purification of mouse liver disulfide interchange enzyme (DSI). The enzyme was purified by the procedure of Carmichael, Morin, and Dixon (15), and the purified product was analyzed by applying 20 μg to: (a) 7.5% polyacrylamide gel (pH 9.5), and (b) 5% polyacrylamide SDS gel.

ranged from 0.05 to 0.5% of the total intracellular protein with MOPC 104E cells falling in the upper part of this range.

In order to evaluate the polymerizing capacity of the disulfide interchange enzyme present in lymphoid tissue, extracts of MOPC 104E cells were prepared by procedures similar to those used in the isolation of the liver enzyme, i.e., detergent solubilization of the membrane fraction, 50% ammonium sulfate precipitation, and chromatography on DEAE Sephadex A-50. Successive fractions from the DEAE column eluate were then incubated with reduced mouse monomer IgM and J chain and the extent of polymerization was assessed by SDS agarose gel electrophoresis. For comparison, polymerization assays were carried out using graded amounts of the purified liver disulfide interchange enzyme. The results of the assays (Fig. 6) were surprising. Several fractions of the MOPC 104E eluate were found to be thirty- to fiftyfold more active on a weight basis than the purified liver enzyme. For example, MOPC 104E fractions containing 0.1 mg/ml of protein effected 50% polymerization of the IgM, whereas the purified liver enzyme at concentrations of 2 mg/ml gave only 25% polymerization. These results suggested that MOPC 104E extracts contained a second component capable of promoting IgM polymerization.

Further evidence for such a promoter component was obtained by

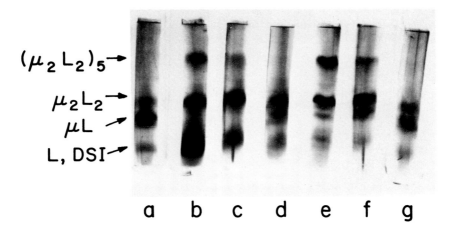

$(\mu_2 L_2)_5 \rightarrow$

$\mu_2 L_2 \rightarrow$

$\mu L \nearrow$

L, DSI $\nearrow$

a   b   c   d   e   f   g

Fig. 6. Comparison of the polymerizing activity of MOPC 104E cell extracts and purified DSI enzyme. For the assay, pentamer IgM (0.135 mg) was reduced with 3 mM dithioerythritol for 1 hr at 22°C and then chromatographed on a Sephadex G-25 column (in 0.02 M Tris-HCl, pH 7.5, 0.15 M NaCl, and 0.02% azide) to remove the reducing agent. Aliquots containing 25 μg of the reduced IgM and J chain were incubated for 1 hr at 37°C with either: the above buffer (a); 2, 0.7, 0.2 mg/ml of purified liver DSI, (b), (c), and (d), respectively; and 0.1, 0.03, 0.01 mg/ml of MOPC 104E lysate after DEAE chromatography, (e), (f), and (g), respectively. The reaction was stopped by alkylation with 50 mM iodoacetamide and the samples were run on SDS agarose gels (13).

monitoring the MOPC 104E eluate from the DEAE column for both polymerizing and disulfide interchange capacity. As the analyses in Fig. 7 show, the two activities were not coincident; material with high polymerizing capacity eluted ahead of the peak of disulfide interchange enzyme as measured by its ability to reactivate scrambled ribonuclease. Moreover, a comparable peak of polymerizing activity was not detected in extracts of mouse liver cells under similar conditions of DEAE chromatography.

Finally, the material with polymerizing activity and disulfide interchange enzyme could be distinguished by their immunological properties. These data are presented in Table I. When the MOPC 104E fractions with polymerizing activity were absorbed with anti-liver enzyme antibody, the content of disulfide interchange enzyme was decreased to undetectable levels as measured either by insulin degrading activity or radioimmunoassay. From the radioimmunoassay data it was determined that the disulfide interchange enzyme concentration was reduced at least two-hundredfold. Despite this depletion the polymerizing capacity of the preparation remained unchanged, av-

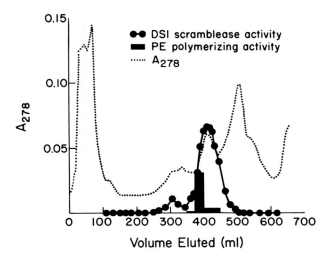

Fig. 7.   DEAE chromatography of MOPC 104E extracts. Fifty MOPC 104E tumors (total wet weight of 13 g) were homogenized and the isolated membrane fraction was solubilized with 0.25% deoxycholate. The preparation was brought to 50% saturated $(NH_4)_2SO_4$ and the resulting precipitate removed by centrifugation. The supernatant (containing about 30 mg protein) was extensively dialyzed against 30 mM Tris-HCl, pH 8, and applied to a 10 ml DEAE-Sephadex A-50 column equilibrated in the same buffer. The column was washed with 200 ml of 100 mM Tris-HCl, pH 8, and then a 0 to 0.5 M NaCl linear salt gradient was applied. The column eluate was tested for scramblease activity (16) and polymerizing activity as described in the legend to Fig. 6. The protein was monitored by the absorbance at 278 nm on a Zeiss PMQII spectrophotometer.

TABLE I
Separation of DSI and PE by Antibody Absorptions

PE preparation	PE activity[a] (units/ml)	DSI[b] (mg/ml)	DSI activity[c] (units/ml)
DEAE eluate	20	0.1	23
Anti-DSI absorbed	20	<0.0005	<5
Anti-PE absorbed	0	n.t.	n.t.
DSI Control	5	2.0	601

[a] The polymerizing (PE) activity was measured as described in the legend to Fig. 6 and one polymerizing unit was defined as the amount of material capable of polymerizing 10 μg of IgM under the conditions described for the assay.
[b] DSI was measured by a radioimmunoassay for the enzyme.
[c] DSI activity was measured by insulin degradation (15).

eraging 20 units/ml before and after absorption. The polymerizing activity could be quantitatively removed, however, by absorption with antisera raised against the active MOPC 104E extracts.

On the basis of these findings it would appear that the assembly of pentamer IgM in B cells is promoted by a polymerizing enzyme which differs from disulfide interchange enzyme both in substrate and antigenic specificity. Although the polymerizing enzyme has yet to be purified, it was calculated from the specific activity of the enriched extracts that less than one mole of enzyme per mole of monomer IgM promotes 50% pentamer assembly. These data indicate that the polymerizing enzyme acts catalytically whereas recent data (13) on disulfide interchange enzyme indicate that if it is active in *in vivo* IgM assembly, it merely provides a source of mixed disulfide.

In summary, our studies of IgM polymerization have succeeded in delineating some of the early intracellular events in B cell differentiation. By comparing the contents of virgin and activated B cells, evidence has been obtained that J chain synthesis is initiated as a consequence of antigen signaling. With this information it will be possible to probe whether the activating event involves unblocking J chain mRNA, processing its nuclear form, or transcribing the J chain gene. In addition, preliminary evidence has been obtained that activated B cells synthesize an enzyme that catalyzes the polymerization of monomer IgM and J chain. It will be of considerable interest to determine whether the expression of this enzyme depends on antigen signaling and thus can be used as a second tool for analyzing B cell differentiation. Finally, the relationships observed between internal and secreted IgM and J chain indicate that production of pentamer antibody depends on the amount of monomer synthesized and is optimized by a precisely controlled excess of J chain. These findings provide valuable clues for pursuing the regulatory mechanisms involved.

ACKNOWLEDGMENTS

This investigation was supported by Research Grant AI 07079 and AI 05417 from the National Institute of Allergy and Infectious Diseases, United States Public Health Services and by Grant Number CA 9179, awarded by the National Cancer Institute, DHEW. The cell lines 38C-13 and WEHI 231 were developed by Drs. Nechama Haran-Ghera and Noel Warner, respectively, and both were obtained from the Salk Institute. The authors thank Joan Fujita, Judy Benson, Milly Leung, and Richard Thomas for technical assistance.

REFERENCES

1. Koshland, M. E. (1975) *Adv. Immunol.* **10**, 51–69.
2. Miller, R. G., and Phillips, R. A. (1969) *J. Cell. Physiol.* **73**, 191–201.
3. Andersson, J., Lafleur, L., and Melchers, F. (1974) *Eur. J. Immunol.* **4**, 170–180.
4. Mather, E. L., and Koshland, M. E. (1977) *In* "Immune System: Genetics and Regulation" (E. E. Sercarz, L. A. Herzenberg, and C. F. Fox, eds.), Vol. 6, pp. 727–733. Academic Press, New York.
5. Warner, N. L., Harris, A. W., and Gutman, G. A. (1975) *In* "Membrane Receptors of Lymphocytes" (M. Seligmann, J. L. Preud'homme, and F. M. Kourilsky, eds.), pp. 203–216. Am. Elsevier, New York.
6. Bergman, Y., and Haimovich, J. (1977) *Eur. J. Immunol.* **7**, 413–417.
7. Bergman, Y., Haimovich, J., and Melchers, F. (1977) *Eur. J. Immunol.* **8**, 574–579.
8. Mishell, R. I., and Dutton, R. W. (1967) *J. Exp. Med.* **126**, 423–442.
9. Kearney, J. F., and Lawton, A. R. (1975) *J. Immunol.* **115**, 671–676.
10. Andersson, J., and Melchers, F. (1974) *Eur. J. Immunol.* **4**, 533–539.
11. Choi, Y. S., Knopf, P. M., and Lennox, E. S. (1971) *Biochemistry* **10**, 668–678.
12. Chapuis, R. M., and Koshland, M. E. (1974) *Proc. Natl. Acad. Sci. U.S.A.* **71**, 657–661.
13. Wilde, C. E., III, and Koshland, M. E. (1978) *Biochemistry* **17**, 3209–3214.
14. Della Corte, E., and Parkhouse, R. M. E. (1974) *Biochem. J.* **136**, 597–606.
15. Carmichael, D. F., Morin, J. E., and Dixon, J. E. (1977) *J. Biol. Chem.* **252**, 7163–7167.
16. DeLorenzo, F., Goldberger, R. F., Steers, E., Givol, D., and Anfinsen, C. B. (1966) *J. Biol. Chem.* **241**, 1562–1567.

PART III

MEMBRANE IMMUNOGLOBULINS

Receptor-Mediated Triggering and Tolerance in Murine B Cells

JONATHAN W. UHR AND ELLEN S. VITETTA

Department of Microbiology
University of Texas Southwestern Medical School
Dallas, Texas

Based on radioiodination studies of murine splenocytes, we suggested that a major class of murine immunoglobulin which had previously not been detected because of its susceptibility to proteolysis and the absence of a specific antiserum was the counterpart of human IgD (1). Because it was observed that murine IgD developed in neonatal mice after cell surface IgM (2) and at a time that such mice were markedly increasing their immune competence (3), we thought that IgD might be involved in the triggering of B lymphocytes.

Figure 1 summarizes our hypothesis that places IgD in the framework of B cell differentiation and speculates about its function (4,5). The major features are that IgM-positive cells acquire IgD and become cells bearing both isotypes. Some of these cells then lose their IgM to become cells that bear IgD only. It was postulated that the interaction of antigen with IgM-predominant $(\mu - p)$ cells induces tolerance whereas interaction with the cells bearing both isotypes $(\mu^+\delta^+)$ (in the presence of a T signal) stimulates the primary thymus-dependent IgM response. It was proposed that IgD positive cells carry immunologic memory.

Subsequent to this proposal, it was shown by others (6–8) and confirmed by ourselves (9,10) that there are cells which bear IgG and, also, IgD + IgM. Thus, one pathway of developing IgG-positive cells would be the one shown in the above model with the addition of cells bearing both IgD and IgG and, finally, cells bearing only IgG. Addi-

155

DIFFERENTIATION OF B CELLS

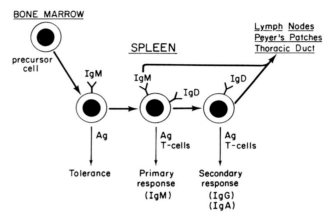

Fig. 1. A model for the differentiation of B lymphocytes (4).

tional studies confirm the existence of these subsets and, indeed, indicate additional ones (11,12). It should be emphasized that the relationship of these various subsets in differentiation is not known and it will be a formidable task to prove these relationships and thereby establish the pathways of differentiation of B cells.

THE ROLE OF SURFACE Igs IN B CELL TOLERANCE

As mentioned above, a highly speculative feature of our early model was that cells found in neonates, which bear predominantly IgM (μ − p), are readily tolerized after interaction with antigen. We began experiments to test this hypothesis by comparing the ability of TNP-human gamma globulin (TNP-HgG) to tolerize adult and neonatal spleen cells in an *in vitro* system (13,14). In this model (15), we were able to tolerize B cells in the absence of T cells and to assess tolerance by measuring an *in vitro* response of the tolerized cells in the presence of T-helper cells (15). Further, we assessed the ability of TNP-HgG to tolerize cells responsive to TD (TNP-sheep red blood cells [TNP-SRBC]) and TI (TNP-*Brucella*) forms of the antigen (16). We demonstrated that macrophages are not limiting in the system, that there is excess T help, and that suppressor T cells play no role in the induction of tolerance (17).

The results of a representative experiment, summarized in Fig. 2,

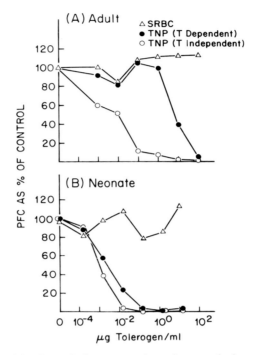

Fig. 2. Effect of the dose of tolerogen on the induction of tolerance in adult (A) and neonatal (B) splenic B cells responsive to thymus-dependent (TNP-SRBC) and thymus-independent (TNP-*Brucella*) forms of the trinitrophenyl determinant. Control responses are expressed as PFC/10^6 viable recovered cells. Adult responses: SRBC response, 3968; T-dependent TNP, 979; T-independent TNP, 571. Neonatal responses: SRBC, 1130; T-dependent TNP, 570; T-independent TNP, 685 (16).

demonstrated the following: (1) Tolerance is antigen-specific since the response to the control antigen (SRBC) was not depressed in either neonatal or adult cells tolerized to TNP. (2) Doses of tolerogen required to tolerize adult cells responsive to the TD form of TNP were approximately 1000-fold higher than those required to tolerize neonatal cells. Thus, neonatal cells responsive to TNP on a TD carrier are exquisitely susceptible to the induction of tolerance. Similar results were obtained by Metcalf and Klinman (18) using the Klinman system (19), and by Nossal and Pike (20) using adult bone marrow cells (3). Doses of tolerogen required to tolerize adult and neonatal cells responsive to TNP on a TI carrier were similar and very low, i.e., in the same range as doses required to tolerize neonatal TD responders. Based on these observations, Cambier *et al.* (16) suggested that the TI

responder in neonates *and* adults is a μ-p cell which is highly susceptible to tolerance induction. In contrast, the TD responders in neonates, but not adults, are also highly susceptible to tolerance induction.

It was possible to test the concept that acquisition of IgD affects
resistance to induction of tolerance by treating adult splenocytes
(primarily $\mu^+\delta^+$) with low doses of papain (21). We had previously
shown that IgD can be selectively removed by such treatment (22).
Thus, using iodinated splenocytes, papain removes IgD but not IgM or
four other surface molecules, H-2, Ia, Lyb 2, and CR. After removal of
IgD, cells were tolerized and assayed for a PFC response to TNP-
SRBC and TNP-*Brucella*.

As shown in Fig. 3, removal of IgD had no effect on the ability to
tolerize TI responders, further suggesting that these are μ-p cells or
that the IgD is not needed for $\mu^+\delta^+$ cells to respond to TI antigens. In
contrast, removal of IgD from adult TD responders greatly increased
their susceptibility to tolerance induction. In addition, if cells were
allowed to regenerate their surface IgD prior to induction of tolerance,
they regained resistance to induction of tolerance.

These results support the contention that acquisition of IgD changes

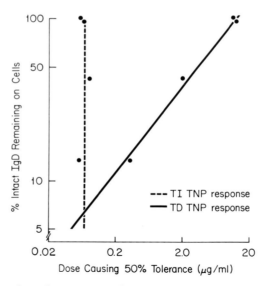

Fig. 3. Relationship of percentage of IgD remaining on murine splenocytes after
papain treatment to the tolerogen dose required to suppress plaque responses 50% ([T_{50}]
[●]). For TD response regression line, (——), r = 0.98. For TI regression line, (- - -),
r = 0.66 (21).

a cell bearing IgM from a tolerizable cell to one that is readily triggered. Further testing of this idea was accomplished by treating $\mu^+\delta^+$ cells from adult spleens with excess anti-μ or anti-δ in order to cap off and thereby remove the respective isotype during the period of attempted induction of tolerance.

The results provide further support for our earlier hypotheses cited above. Thus, removal of IgD with anti-δ was shown to increase susceptibility to tolerance induction of treated TD responders but had no effect on TI responders, confirming earlier results with papain (Fig. 4). In addition, it was shown that treatment with anti-μ did not similarly increase the tolerizability of TD responders. This is a critical point because it could be argued that diminishing the concentration of *either* isotype would result in an increased susceptibility to tolerance induction. The present studies indicate that different reactivities are conferred on a $\mu^+\delta^+$ cell by IgM and IgD with regard to tolerance induction,

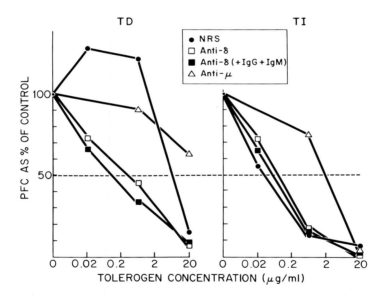

Fig. 4. The effect of removing IgM or IgD receptors on the ability to tolerize splenic B cells responding to TD (left panel) and TI (right panel) forms of TNP immunogen. The tolerogen was TNP$_{17}$HGG (15). The control SRBC plaque-forming cells (PFC) were unaffected by varying the dose of tolerogen as described previously (15,16). The TNP responses are expressed as direct PFC/10^6 viable recovered cells. TD control responses were: NRS, 810; $\alpha\mu$, 1098; $\alpha\delta$, 1149; $\alpha\delta(+\text{IgG}+\text{IgM})$, 1286; TI control responses were NRS, 412; $\alpha\mu$, 440; $\alpha\delta$, 517; $\alpha\delta(+\text{IgG}+\text{IgM})$, 435. This is a representative experiment of three that were done. Each point represents the average of the responses of duplicate cultures (22a).

i.e., these two isotypes can be responsible for conveying different signals to the same cell. The absence of a similar effect of anti-δ on TI responders argues that they lack IgD or that, if it is present, it does not determine tolerance susceptibility.

It was also observed that treatment of B cells with anti-μ decreased the susceptibility of TI responders to tolerance induction. This finding implies that interaction of tolerogen with IgM receptors is a necessary event for tolerance induction in TI responders and that removing such receptors by stripping and blocking with anti-μ prevents this interaction. It is provocative that the stripping induced with anti-μ antibody itself does not give a tolerogenic signal.

THE ROLE OF SURFACE Igs IN B CELL TRIGGERING (23,24)

Treated adult splenocytes were cultured with TNP-*Brucella* or TNP-SRBC in the presence of varying concentrations (0–1000 μg/ml) of the Ig fraction from the same antiserum used for capping. The effect of such treatment on the primary antibody response is shown in Fig. 5. The TD responses to both TNP and SRBC were virtually abolished by treatment with anti-μ, anti-δ, or anti-Ig at 100–1000 μg of Ig per ml. These results suggest that both IgM and IgD receptors are required for activation of responsive cells by TD antigens.

As also shown in Fig. 5, the primary TI response to TNP was blocked by anti-μ and anti-Ig, but not anti-δ at >100 μg of Ig per ml.

These results represent convincing evidence that the major precursor for the primary IgM antibody response to a TD antigen is a $\mu^+\delta^+$ cell. Previous studies in mice indicated that (i) splenocytes stained with *either* anti-μ or anti-δ and positively sorted on the fluorescence-activated cell sorter gave virtually all of the primary IgM response in an adoptively transferred host (10), (ii) elimination of μ^+ cells with anti-μ, complement, and azide abolished the primary IgM response, also in an adoptively transferred host (9), and (iii) either anti-μ or anti-δ alone was ineffective in preventing antigen-induced suicide of the cell giving rise to the primary IgM response (7). However, two critical experiments have not been performed: direct analysis of the contribution to the primary IgM response of $\mu^+\delta^+$ cells and determination of the effect of deleting δ^+ cells on the IgM response. The present observations that blocking with *either* anti-μ or anti-δ causes a reduction by over 90% of the primary response to TD antigens provide strong evidence that the precursor for the TD response bears both isotypes.

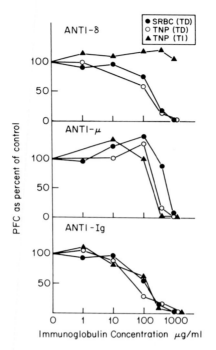

Fig. 5. Effect of antibody concentration on the inhibition of *in vitro* IgM responses to TD (●, SRBC; ○, TNP) and TI (▲, TNP) antigens. Cells were treated with the indicated antiserum and GARIg under capping conditions and cultured with an Ig fraction of the same antiserum used for capping. Responses of control cultures incubated without antibody, presented as PFC per 10^6 viable recovered cells, were as follows: anti-δ capped, SRBC 3408, TNP (TD) 434, TNP (TI) 342; anti-μ capped, SRBC 3905, TNP (TD) 445, TNP (TI) 215; anti-Ig capped, SRBC 2672, TNP (TD) 418, TNP (TI) 506 (23).

The above results also indicate that the precursor for the TI response to TNP-*Brucella* bears no functional IgD receptor. Earlier evidence that the precursor is a cell that bears predominantly IgM is as follows: (i) neonatal splenocytes that contain only μ-p cells (2,25) can give TI responses to certain antigens, and (ii) large cells from adult spleens that are μ-p (26) are enriched for TI responsiveness (27). The inability of anti-δ to block the primary IgM response argues either that no IgD is present on the precursor *or* that IgD is unnecessary for stimulation of the cell. Thus, the possibility that $\mu^+\delta^+$ cells are precursors but that the IgD receptor is not needed cannot be excluded.

The role played by each isotype in immune activation to TD anti-

TABLE I
Effect of Treatment with Anti-δ on *in Vitro* TD Responses

Age of donor (B cells)	% B cells that are δ⁺[a]	PFC/10⁶ viable cells			
		Anti-SRBC		Anti-TNP	
		Anti-δ	Control	Anti-δ	Control
49	83	208	5333	0	736
18	59	0	1476	0	284
7	3	0	302	0	20

[a] From Stocker (32).

gens is not known. One possibility is that each isotype gives an independent and necessary signal. Because T cells also provide an essential signal, triggering of TD-responsive B cells may require three signals. Another possibility is that the IgM and IgD receptors must interact with each other, possibly through additional membrane molecules to form a single triggering complex. Finally, the density of the receptors on TD responders may be relatively low, such that antigen interacting with either isotype is insufficient for delivering a signal; both must be involved in order to trigger.

There are several studies of embryonic or neonatal cells in culture that suggest that immune responsiveness to TD antigens develops *before* the acquisition of IgD receptors (28–32). Examination of the experimental protocols used in these studies indicates that, if ontogeny proceeds normally in culture, then immune responsiveness of fetal cells correlates with the expected time of appearance of surface IgD, 3–5 days after birth (25). For example, 17-day fetal liver cells that secrete antibodies after 8 days in culture would be analogous to B cells from 4-day-old neonates. Past studies are therefore consistent with the notion that receptor IgD is necessary for triggering virgin B cells with TD antigens. The present results (Table I) provide further direct evidence for this idea because removal of receptor IgD completely abrogated the primary IgM response of neonatal splenocytes to SRBC and TNP. We cannot exclude the possibility that there is a trace contribution to the TD response by a μ-p cell that is below the level of detection in our system.

ACKNOWLEDGMENTS

Supported by National Institutes of Health grants AI-11851, AI-12789, and AI-10867.

REFERENCES

1. Melcher, U., Vitetta, E. S., McWilliams, M., Phillips-Quagliata, J., Lamm, M. E., and Uhr, J. W. (1974) *J. Exp. Med.* **140**, 1427.
2. Vitetta, E. S., Melcher, U., McWilliams, M., Phillips-Quagliata, J., Lamm, M., and Uhr, J. W. (1975) *J. Exp. Med.* **141**, 206.
3. Spear, P. G., and Edelman, G. M. (1974) *J. Exp. Med.* **139**, 249.
4. Vitetta, E. S., and Uhr, J. W. (1975) *Science* **189**, 964.
5. Vitetta, E. S., and Uhr, J. W. (1978) *Immunol. Rev.* **37**, 50.
6. Mason, D. W. (1976) *J. Exp. Med.* **143**, 1122.
7. Coffman, R. L., and Cohn, M. (1977) *J. Immunol.* **118**, 1806.
8. Okumura, K., Julius, M. H., Tsu, T., Herzenberg, L. A., and Herzenberg, L. A. (1976) *Eur. J. Immunol.* **6**, 467.
9. Yuan, D., Vitetta, E. S., and Kettman, J. (1977) *J. Exp. Med.* **145**, 1421.
10. Zan-Bar, I., Strober, S., and Vitetta, E. S. (1977) *J. Exp. Med.* **145**, 1188.
11. Black, S. J., van de Loo, W., Loken, M. R., and Herzenberg, L. A. (1978) *J. Exp. Med.* **147**, 984.
12. Cooper, M. D., Kearney, J. F., Lawton, A. R., Abney, E. R., Parkhouse, R. M. E., Preud'homme, J. L., and Seligmann, M. (1976) *Ann. Immunol. (Paris)* **127**, 573.
13. Kettman, J. R. (1974) *J. Immunol.* **112**, 1139.
14. Borel, Y. (1976) *Transplant. Rev.* **31**, 3.
15. Cambier, J. C., Kettman, J. R., Vitetta, E. S., and Uhr, J. W. (1976) *J. Exp. Med.* **144**, 293.
16. Cambier, J. C., Vitetta, E. S., Uhr, J. W., and Kettman, J. R., Jr. (1977) *J. Exp. Med.* **145**, 778.
17. Cambier, J. C., Uhr, J. W., Kettman, J. R., and Vitetta, E. S. (1977) *J. Immunol.* **119**, 2054.
18. Metcalf, E. S., and Klinman, N. R. (1976) *J. Exp. Med.* **143**, 1327.
19. Klinman, N. R. (1972) *J. Exp. Med.* **136**, 241.
20. Nossal, G. J. V., and Pike, B. L. (1975) *J. Exp. Med.* **141**, 904.
21. Cambier, J. C., Vitetta, E. S., Kettman, J. R., Wetzel, G. M., and Uhr, J. W. (1977) *J. Exp. Med.* **146**, 107.
22. Vitetta, E. S., and Uhr, J. W. (1976) *J. Immunol.* **117**, 1579.
22a. Vitetta, E. S., Cambier, J. C., Ligler, F. S., Kettman, J. R., and Uhr, J. W. (1977) *J. Exp. Med.* **146**, 1804.
23. Cambier, J. C., Ligler, F. S., Uhr, J. W., Kettman, J. R., and Vitetta, E. S. (1978) *Proc. Natl. Acad. Sci. U.S.A.* **75**, 432.
24. Ligler, F. S., Cambier, J. C., Vitetta, E. S., Kettman, J. R., and Uhr, J. W. (1978) *J. Immunol.* **120**, 1139.
25. Goding, J. (1977) *Contemp. Top. Immunobiol.* **8** (in press).
26. Goodman, S. A., Vitetta, E. S., Melcher, U., and Uhr, J. W. (1975) *J. Immunol.* **114**, 1646.
27. Gorczynski, R. M., and Feldmann, M. (1975) *Cell. Immunol.* **18**, 88.
28. Press, J., and Klinman, N. (1973) *J. Immunol.* **111**, 829.
29. Rosenberg, Y. J., and Cunningham, A. J. (1976) *J. Immunol.* **117**, 1618.
30. Phillips, R. A., and Melchers, F. (1976) *J. Immunol.* **117**, 1099.
31. Elson, C. J. (1977) *Eur. J. Immunol.* **7**, 6.
32. Stocker, J. W. (1977) *Immunology* **32**, 275.

Structure of Lymphocyte Membrane Immunoglobulin

A. FEINSTEIN, N. E. RICHARDSON, AND
R. A. J. McILHINNEY

A.R.C. Institute of Animal Physiology
Babraham, Cambridge,
Cambridgeshire, England

INTRODUCTION

This article is concerned with the structure of the immuno-globulins found on the surface of the B lymphocytes which are the precursors of cells involved in immunoglobulin secretion. The field was reviewed by Marchalonis (1) in 1976, and briefly discussed more recently by Vitetta and Uhr (2), and others in the same volume. The key questions which need to be answered can be summarized as follows:

1. Which classes of immunoglobulin act as cell surface antigen receptors, and on which populations of B lymphocytes?

2. Do these surface immunoglobulins have essentially the same structure as their secreted counterparts? Are they transmembrane proteins, or do they interact with proteins which are integral to the membrane?

3. Does any such structural information suggest or rule out any mechanism through which interaction with antigens could contribute to a signal, leading to mitogenesis and Ig biosynthesis, or to tolerance?

Other contributors to this symposium will deal with the first question. In the present context we are concerned with those Ig classes which can be isolated from lymphocyte membranes sufficiently pure, and in sufficient quantity, for structural studies.

Early studies revealed that monomeric IgM was the major B cell surface Ig labeled when using enzymatic radioiodination (3,4). Later it was found that most human B lymphocytes carry IgD molecules (5,6)

165

and that mouse B lymphocytes also carry an Ig which is a presumed counterpart of human IgD (7,8). The presumed mouse δ chains appeared to be significantly smaller than the human δ chain, but this seems to be the result of proteolysis of a mouse chain initially similar to the human chain in size (9). Although other classes of Ig are detected on B cells, they have not been isolated for structural studies.

In comparison with IgM, the more recent discovery of surface IgD, its greater susceptibility to proteolysis, and the incomplete knowledge of its structure are all probably responsible for the large majority of surface Ig structural studies being confined to IgM when attempting to answer the questions listed under question 2 above. There are as yet no clearcut answers to these questions. In a recent review (10) the authors concluded that the available data were compatible with the attachment of IgM to the cell surface occurring through a μ chain C-terminal hydrophobic polypeptide, or through covalently bound lipid, or as a result of interaction with an integral membrane protein. The surface and secreted μ chains are probably similarly glycosylated and are of similar apparent molecular weight in SDS gel electrophoresis, though surface μ chains may appear a little larger. In relation to the question of whether surface IgM might be a transmembrane protein, it has been shown (11) that whereas other human B cell surface proteins were labeled when the cytoplasmic membrane surface of inside-out vesicles was radioiodinated using lactoperoxidase, surface IgM was not. Secreted μ chains have a C-terminal tyrosine, and we have presented evidence that surface μ chains also terminate in a tyrosine residue (12). If this tyrosine can be shown to be iodinatable under the conditions used by Walsh and Crumpton (11), then the failure to iodinate IgM at the cytoplasmic surface might be taken as evidence for surface μ chains not being transmembrane. However, the C-terminal region could be masked sterically in the membrane, for example by interaction with another protein.

In the studies to be presented here, we have extended our findings by looking for more extensive homology between the C-terminal regions of secreted μ chains and those on the surface of mouse and human B lymphoma cells.

METHODS

PREPARATION OF IgM

Mouse IgM was purified from the serum of mice bearing the plasmacytoma MOPC 104E (13) by means of the method described by

Milstein *et al.* (14). Human IgM was isolated from the serum of patient Qu as described (15).

PARTIAL REDUCTION OF IgM

Cleavage of interchain disulfide bridges (partial reduction) was performed by treating IgM solutions, under N_2, with 5 mM dithiothreitol (DTT) for 1 hr at room temperature in 0.3 M NaCl–0.2 M Tris-HCl buffer, pH 8.0, containing 10 mM EDTA. Reduced samples were then alkylated with either 33 mM iodoacetamide or 33 mM iodoacetate for 1 hr at room temperature, and finally dialyzed against phosphate-buffered saline.

TUMOR LINES

Murine lymphocytoma McPc 1748 (16) (a gift from Dr. D. I. Stott) was passaged ascitically in the intraperitoneal cavity of normal female BALB/c mice. Murine B lymphoma line WEHI-231 (a gift from Dr. A. Harris) was maintained in Dulbecco's MEM containing 10% fetal calf serum and 5×10^{-5} M 2-mercaptoethanol. Human lymphoblastoid cell line Bristol 8 (Bri-8, obtained from G. D. Searle, High Wycombe, U.K.) was maintained in RPMI-1640 containing 10% fetal calf serum.

CELL PREPARATION

Ascitic fluid was removed from mice bearing McPc 1748 tumors and the cells washed with phosphate-buffered saline (PBS), or RPMI-1640. Washed cells were suspended at the required cell density and their viability determined by trypan blue exclusion; only cell suspensions of greater than 90% viability were used in this study.

Cell Surface Iodination. The following adaptation of the method of Marchalonis *et al.* (17) has been used. Cells (2×10^6) were incubated for 7 min at 30°C in 100 μl PBS, 200 μCi Na ^{125}I, 5 μl 5×10^{-5} M KI, 5 μg lactoperoxidase (LPO), and 0.015% H_2O_2. Alternatively the same number of cells was iodinated using a hydrogen peroxide generating system as described by Walsh and Crumpton (11). After radioiodination the cells were washed twice with 10 ml PBS and lysed at 4°C for 20 min in 1 ml PBS containing 1% NP-40, 1 mM phenyl methanesulfonyl fluoride (PMSF), 0.1 M iodoacetamide, and 0.01% NaI. After centrifugation (30,000 g; 30 min) and dialysis for 8 hr at 4°C twice against 1 liter PBS containing 0.01% NaI, the lysate was immunoprecipitated and further analyzed by SDS polyacrylamide gel electrophoresis.

Incorporation of ³H-amino Acids. Cells (1×10^7/ml) were incubated for 4 hr at 37°C in leucine-free or tyrosine-free RPMI-1640 containing either L-[4,5 − ³H]leucine (50μCi/ml;) or L-[3,5 − ³H]tyrosine (100 μCi/ml) (Radiochemical Centre, Amersham). Following this the cells were washed and incubated in complete RPMI for a further 6 hr. Lysis of the cells was performed as above except that dialysis was in four changes of PBS over a period of 72 hr.

Membrane Preparation and Iodination. Washed cells were suspended in 10 mM Tris-HCl, pH 7.5, at 10^8 cells/ml and then disrupted by passage under pressure, past a spring-loaded valve, using an apparatus similar to that of Wright *et al.* (18) and Crumpton and Snary (19). Membranes were isolated according to the method of Crumpton and Snary (19).

Both lactoperoxidase (LPO) and chloramine-T were used to iodinate the membranes. When LPO was used conditions employed were those described above using H_2O_2 for cells, except that the membranes (100 μg) were suspended in 50 mM phosphate buffer pH 7.2 (100 μl). For chloramine-T iodinations identical conditions were used except that LPO and peroxide were replaced by one addition of 25 μl of chloramine-T (25 mM). After 5 min at room temperature the reaction was terminated by the addition of 20 μl sodium metabisulfite (20 mM). The subsequent lysis and dialysis were performed as described above.

ANTISERA AND IMMUNE PRECIPITATION

Antisera against murine IgM λ and human IgM κ were raised in sheep immunized with purified myeloma IgM from the serum of mice carrying plasmacytoma MOPC 104E, or purified IgM from the serum of a patient (Ma) and then absorbed with Sepharose-coupled antigens until the antisera were monospecific for μ chains.

Immune precipitations were performed by the addition of the appropriate serum to aliquots of cell lysates followed by incubation at 4°C for 1 hr. IgM (20 μg) was then added and precipitation allowed to proceed at 4°C overnight. In all cases a control precipitation was performed using sheep anti-ovalbumin and ovalbumin as the precipitating system.

The precipitates were washed once with 1 ml of cold PBS containing NP-40 (1%) and twice with cold PBS and then dissolved for SDS gel analysis by incubation at 37°C for 30 min, and 100°C for a further 1 min in 8 M urea containing 2% SDS, 10% 2-mercaptoethanol, and 62.5 mM Tris-HCl, pH 6.8. When samples were electrophoresed without reduction, the mercaptoethanol was replaced by 0.1 M iodoacetamide.

POLYACRYLAMIDE GEL ELECTROPHORESIS

SDS-polyacrylamide gel electrophoresis was performed in rods and slabs according to the method of Laemlli (20). After electrophoresis the rod gels were sliced into 2 mm thick portions and each slice analyzed for radioisotope. Slab gels were fixed and stained for 1 hr after electrophoresis in Coomassie Brilliant Blue R-250 and then destained. The slab gels were dried using a Bio-Rad Gel Slab Dryer (Model 224) and subsequently radioautographed employing Kodak KD54-T X-Ray Film.

PEPTIDE "MAPPING"

Radiolabeled proteins were eluted from SDS-rod gel slices by incubation for 2 days at room temperature in 20 mM phosphate buffer, pH 7.2, containing 0.1% SDS and 0.05% sodium azide (300 μl). Purified IgM (100–200 μg) was added to the eluate, followed by a $\frac{1}{9}$ volume of 1 M Tris-HCl, pH 8.0, and a further $\frac{1}{9}$ volume of 0.1 M dithiothreitol. The stoppered tube was left at room temperature for 1 hr and then iodoacetamide or iodoacetate was added to a final concentration of 65 mM. Alkylation was allowed to proceed for a further 1 hr at room temperature, after which treatment varied according to whether the samples were to be treated with carboxypeptidase-A. Samples which were to be peptide "mapped" without carboxypeptidase treatment were precipitated at 4°C for 16 hr by the addition of trichloracetic acid (TCA) to 12%. The TCA precipitates were washed twice with acidified acetone (1 ml), dried *in vacuo*, and then dissolved in 100 μl of either formic acid–acetic acid, pH 2.1 (formic acid–acetic acid–water, 1 : 4 : 45, by vol.) for subsequent pepsin digestion, or 0.1 M ammonium bicarbonate, pH 8.5, for trypsin digestion. Enzyme was added to give a protein–enzyme ratio of 50 : 1. Digestion was carried out at 37°C overnight, after which the peptides were dried *in vacuo*.

Alternatively, some iodoacetamide alkylated preparations that were to be carboxypeptidase treated were dialyzed against 1% sodium bicarbonate containing 1.6% SDS (1 liter) after the alkylation step described above. The dialyzed samples were then split into two equal aliquots and one was treated with carboxypeptidase-A for 30 min at 37°C as described by Ambler (21) and the other aliquot was incubated at 37°C in parallel without the addition of enzyme. The protein–enzyme ratio was 5:1. After digestion the samples were placed on ice and acidified with HCl to 1 N. TCA was then added to 15% and after 20 min the samples were centrifuged. The pellet was washed once with 10% TCA (1 ml) and twice more with acidified acetone (1 ml) and finally dried *in vacuo*. Pepsin digestion was then performed as described above.

The peptides were mapped by a modification of the method used by Mole (22), as follows. After extraction of the digests with water–acetic acid–pyridine electrophoresis buffer, pH 3.5 (189:10:1, by vol.) the soluble peptides were applied at positions 9 cm and 11 cm from one side of a 20 × 20 cm plastic-backed silica gel sheet (BDH Ltd., Poole, U.K.) at a distance 6 cm from the intended anodic end. Centrally, between the samples a marker mixture was applied containing E-DNP-lysine and Thymol FF and the sheet was then sprayed with the same buffer, the two origins having been protected by a polythene strip. After spraying, the polythene strip was removed and the origins wetted with buffer by allowing careful diffusion from both sides. Excess buffer was removed by blotting the silica gel, and electrophoresis carried out for 5 hr at 400 V and 25–30 mA in a Desaga 121221 thin layer electrophoresis apparatus (Uniscience Ltd., Cambridge, England). Subsequently the plate was air-dried at room temperature, and guillotined into two halves along the electrophoresis axis, each half then being subjected to ascending chromatography in butan-1-ol:acetic acid:water:pyridine (15:3:12:10, by vol.) and dried for 30 min at 80°C. The peptide "maps" were then radioautographed useing Kodak KD-54T X-ray film. The R_f's and electrophoretic mobilities (relative to the electrophoretic mobilities of the E-DNP lysine and thymol FF markers) are indicated in the relevant figures.

RESULTS

CHARACTERIZATION OF MEMBRANE IgM OF CELL LINES

Cells of the mouse B-lymphoma lines McPc 1748, WEHI-231, and the human lymphoblastoid line Bri-8 were radioiodinated using lactoperoxidase. Subsequently the radiolabeled surface IgM in the cell lysates was analyzed by immune-precipitation and SDS polyacrylamide gel electrophoresis. Routinely, the proportion of radiolabel which was immune-precipitable as IgM compared to total TCA precipitable radiolabel for McPc 1748, WEHI-231, and Bri-8 was 2, 5–10, and 1.5%, respectively. Figure 1 shows the distribution of radiolabel obtained on various SDS polyacrylamide gels when we analyzed the immune-precipitated IgM from the lysates of each cell line. The gels showed in each case that nearly all of the radiolabel was present in monomeric IgM ($\mu_2 L_2$) with a minor amount as half-subunits (μL), when compared to selectively reduced secreted IgM markers. The $\mu_2 L_2$ band derived from mercaptoethylamine selective reduction of secreted IgM has a slower mobility in SDS slab gels than that derived from DTT selective reduction of secreted IgM, and the membrane IgM had a mobility very similar to the mercaptoethylamine-produced $\mu_2 L_2$. Reduced immune precipitates of the surface-labeled membrane IgM (Fig. 2) demonstrated that the majority of radiolabel was present in μ chains and L chains, but that in addition, especially in McPc 1748 and Bri-8 preparations, a third radioactive component was always present with a mobility midway between μ and L chains, which we have shown by peptide mapping to be membrane actin (see Fig. 9).

Cells from lines McPc 1748 and Bri-8 were cultured in the presence of ^{3}H-leucine for 4 hr and chased for 6 hr in unlabeled medium. SDS gel studies confirmed that McPc 1748 cells secrete very little IgM (16), whereas Bri-8 cells are essentially nonsecreting. Figure 3 shows the distribution of radiolabel obtained on SDS gels when the cold chased McPc 1748 cultured cells were analyzed, confirming that the membrane IgM on these cells was $\mu_2 L_2$. As in the surface radioiodinated experiments, we found a peak present in the reduced SDS gels of the internally labeled material which was presumably membrane actin. When treated with papain in order to remove cell surface proteins, 70% of the total radiolabel incorporated into the cells was removed, leaving the viability of the cells unchanged. Since an identical digestion removed 70% of the radiolabeled IgM present on the cells after surface labeling using lactoperoxidase and Na^{125}I, it appears that the 6-hr chase of McPc 1748 had resulted in all of the radioactive IgM present being membrane IgM.

We find that the apparent size in SDS slab gels of secreted μ chains from MOPC 104E cells is larger than that of the intracellular precursor μ chains, due to carbohydrate differences (23). The radioiodinated or internally radiolabeled membrane and secreted μ chains are similar in apparent size.

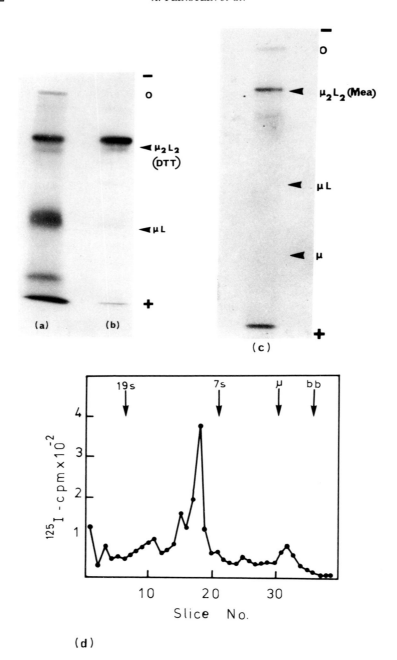

(a)   (b)

(c)

(d)

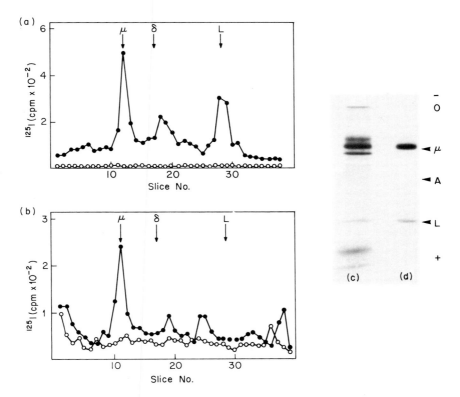

Fig. 2. Characterization of reduced surface-labeled IgM. The experimental details are as described for Fig. 1, except that immune precipitates were fully reduced before electrophoresis on SDS gels containing 10% polyacrylamide. (a) Rod gel profile, McPc 1748, ●——●; (b) rod gel profile, Bri-8, ●——●; (c) reduced total cell lysate, WEHI-231; (d) slab gel radioautograph, WEHI-231. The profile of the reduced ovalbumin-anti ovalbumin control is shown by ◆——◆. Marker proteins were mouse and human μ and L chains (μ and L), and pig actin (A, a gift from Dr. M. J. Crumpton).

Fig. 1. Characterization of IgM from surface-labeled cells of tumorlines: (a) radio-autograph, total cell lysate of WEHI-231 surface-labeled cells; (b) WEHI-231; (c) McPc 1748; (d) Bri-8. Cells were radioiodinated using lactoperoxidase, and IgM immune-precipitated using sheep anti-μ-chain sera as described in the Methods section. The precipitates were analyzed nonreduced on SDS gels. (b) and (c) Radioautographs of gels which contained 6% polyacrylamide; (d) profile of composite rod gel containing 2.5% acrylamide and 1.0% agarose. The markers were: human IgM (19 S); subunits derived from murine or human pentameric IgM by reduction with either dithiothreitol (DTT) or mercaptoethylamine (Mea); bb denotes the position of the bromophenol blue dye front.

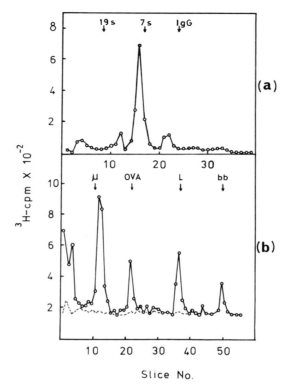

Fig. 3. Characterization of ³H-labeled IgM from theMcPc 1748 cell line. Cells were cultured in the presence of ³H-leucine for 4 hr, then chased in complete medium. After lysis, the IgM was immune-precipitated with sheep anti-mouse μ chain serum as described in the Methods section. The precipitates were analyzed either: (a) nonreduced in composite SDS rod gel with 2.5% polyacrylamide and 1.0% agarose or (b) reduced in SDS rod gel with 10% polyacrylamide. The dashed line in (b) denotes the profile obtained with the reduced ovalbumin anti-ovalbumin control precipitate. Marker proteins were: mouse IgM (19 S), $\mu_2 L_2$ subunit derived from mouse IgM by Mea reduction (7 S), sheep IgG and ovalbumin (OVA); bb indicates the position of the bromophenol blue dye front.

Studies of the C-Terminal Regions of Surface μ. The surface IgM of McPc 1748 and Bri-8 cells was internally labeled with ³H-tyrosine as described above and the isolated surface μ chains were digested with carboxypeptidase-A (12). These studies suggested that the membrane μ chain terminates in a tyrosine residue, as do secreted μ chains. The results are presented in Table I.

TABLE I

Carboxypeptidase Treatment of L[3,5-³H] Tyrosine Radiolabeled Membrane μ Chains

Cell line	Secreted μ chain carrier (nmol)	Residues tyrosine released from carrier IgM by CPA digestion (nmol)	Release of tyrosine residues from carrier μ (%)	Total radiolabel in digested sample (cpm)	Radiolabel released by digestion (cpm)	Release of radiolabeled tyrosine[a] (%)
McPc 1748	100.0	48.0	48	19,200	370	46
	21.0	9.0	43	57,450	850	36
	37.5	19.4	52	91,040	2,020	53
Bri-8	100.0	36.0	36	34,200	920	43
	65.0	25.4	39	66,360	1,230	30

[a] The release of radiolabel from preparations incubated in the absence of enzyme was found never to exceed 0.4% of the total radiolabel in the digested sample. From McIlhinney et al. (12).

PEPTIDE MAPPING STUDIES

Identification of Secreted μ Chain C-Terminal Peptide. MOPC 104E IgM was partially reduced and alkylated with either iodoacetate (carboxymethylation) or iodoacetamide (amidomethylation) prior to radioiodination. Peptic digests were examined by mapping on thin layer silica plates. Comparison of the maps using these two different methods of alkylation (Fig. 4a and b) showed that only two spots, later identified as being derived from the C-terminal peptide (μ4) of the μ chain, were altered in position. As we will show, this alteration is due to a charge effect resulting from carboxymethylation of a sulfydryl generated by cleavage of the μ4 interchain disulfide bridge. This C-terminal peptide only is affected because it is the only interchain bridge peptide having an iodinatable tyrosine residue (14). We will call this technique the carboxymethylation "shift" method. In order to confirm that the shifting peptides were indeed C-terminal, we isolated the ^{14}C-carboxymethylated C-terminal μ chain peptic peptides from MOPC 104E IgM using high voltage paper electrophoresis and paper chromatography. We have found in previous studies (14) that a variable number of spots derive from the C-terminal peptide, and this was attributed to modification of a methionine residue. Throughout the present studies a similar variability in multiplicity of C-terminal spots was found. Subsequent iodination of a portion of these isolated peptides and analysis by thin layer mapping demonstrated that the iodinated peptides had an altered position with respect to the ^{14}C-carboxymethylated peptides before iodination (Fig. 5). The measured R_f's and relative electrophoretic mobilities of the carboxymethylated iodopeptides (Fig. 5b) agreed with those of the shifted carboxymethylated peptides seen in Fig. 4b and d. This result confirmed that the shifting spots correspond to the C-terminal peptide using a technique which could later be applied to membrane IgM. A similar shift was obtained with human IgM (Qu) (Fig. 8a and b).

A second technique for identifying the C-terminal amidomethylated peptide in the peptide maps of μ chains is demonstrated in Fig. 6a and b. Figure 6b shows the peptide map of iodinated MOPC 104E μ chain which had been previously treated with carboxypeptidase-A, releasing C-terminal iodotyrosine (which was identified by TLC analysis). Comparison with the map in Fig. 6a shows that the treatment has resulted in the loss of a spot which must correspond to the C-terminal peptide and which agrees with the position identified by the above carboxymethylation "shift" method.

We now describe the application of both methods to membrane μ chains.

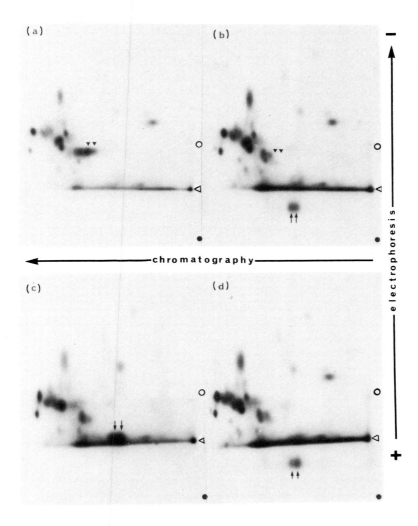

Fig. 4. Radioautographs of thin-layer peptic peptide maps derived from secreted mouse MOPC 104E IgM. IgM was partially reduced (see Methods) and amidomethylated (a), or carboxymethylated (b) and (d), prior to radioiodination using chloramine-T. In (c) IgM was radioiodinated as a pentamer. ▼ indicates position (whether present or absent) of amidomethylated μ chain C -terminal peptide (μ4). ↓ indicates the alternative positions of carboxymethylated μ4, depending upon the stage at which iodination took place. In this and subsequent map figures the origin of electrophoresis is indicated by ◁, while the positions of migration of markers during electrophoresis are shown as O (E-DNP lysine) and ● (thymol-FF).

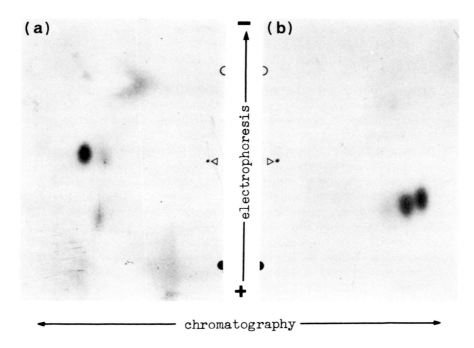

Fig. 5. Radioautographs of thin layer peptic peptide maps of ^{14}C-carboxymethylated MOPC 104E μ chain C-terminal peptides (μ4) isolated from paper [Milstein *et al.* (14)]; (a) untreated; (b) after radioiodination.

Identification of Membrane μ Chain C-Terminal Peptide. Iodinated membrane mouse μ chains were mapped after isolation from McPc 1748 cells (Fig. 6c) and WEHI-231 cells (Fig. 6e). The positions of the C-terminal peptides were identified as in Fig. 6a by demonstrating their disappearance or weakening in maps of carboxypeptidase-A-treated chains. With both cell lines, the R_f's and relative electrophoretic mobilities of the C-terminal peptides corresponded closely with those of the C-terminal peptides from the secreted μ chains.

Fig. 6. Radioautographs of thin layer peptic peptide maps of radioiodinated amidomethylated mouse μ chains: (b), (d), (f) previously carboxypeptidase-A treated; (a), (c), (e) without previous carboxypeptidase-A treatment. (a) and (b) from secreted MOPC 104E IgM; (c) and (d) from the membranes of McPc 1748 cells; (e) and (f) from the membranes of WEHI-231 cells. Radioiodination, isolation of μ chains, carboxypeptidase-A (CPA) digestion, and peptide mapping were performed as described in the Methods section. ▼ indicates the peptides removed by carboxypeptidase-A digestion.

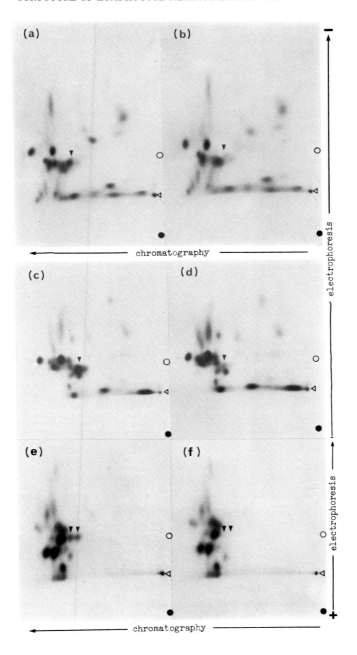

Examples of the application of the carboxymethylation "shift" method to McPc 1748 and Bri-8 membrane μ chains are shown in Figs. 7 and 8. Comparing amidomethylated chains (Fig. 7a) with carboxymethylated chains (Fig. 7c), the same effect of shifting peptides

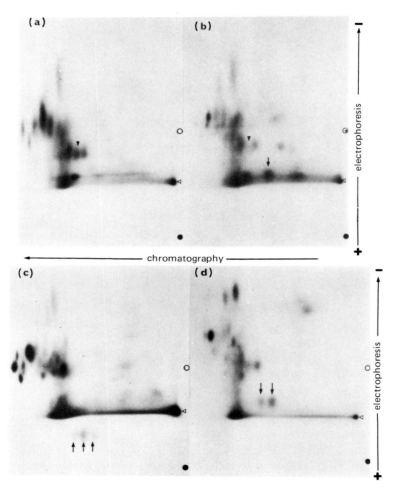

Fig. 7. Radioautographs of thin layer peptic peptide maps of mouse radioiodinated membrane μ chains from McPc 1748 cells: (a) fully reduced and amidomethylated; (b), (c), (d) fully reduced and carboxymethylated, showing the alternative positions of the μ chain C-terminal peptides (μ4). ▼ indicates presence of absence of amidomethylated μ4 peptides; ↓ denotes carboxymethylated μ4 peptides.

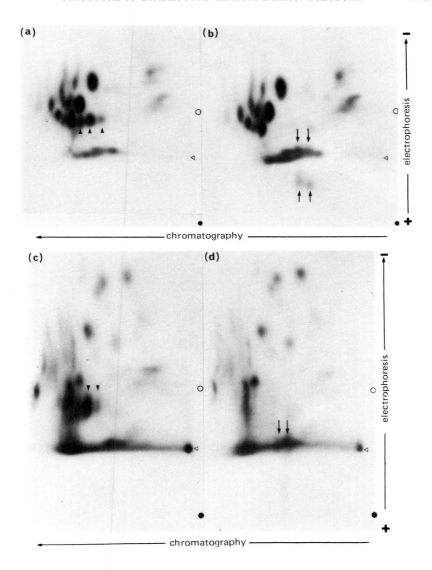

Fig. 8. Radioautographs of thin layer peptic peptide maps of human radioiodinated μ chains: (a) partially reduced and amidomethylated secreted human (Qu) μ chains; (b) as (a) except carboxymethylated after partial reduction; (c) fully reduced and amidomethylated Bri-8 membrane μ chains; (d) as (c) except carboxymethylated after reduction. ▼ indicates position of amidomethylated μ4 peptides; ↓ denotes position of carboxymethylated μ4 peptides.

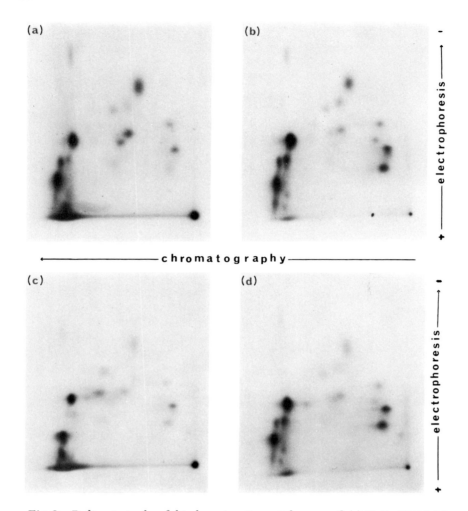

Fig. 9. Radioautographs of thin layer tryptic peptide maps of: (a) McPc 1748 IgM-associating protein, (b and d) McPc 1748 membrane major band, and (c) pig skeletal actin. The iodinated proteins were prepared and digested as described in the Methods section.

was seen as with secreted IgM (Fig. 4a, b, d) and the positions of shifting membrane μ chain spots agreed closely with those identified as corresponding to the C-terminal peptide in secreted μ chains. In many maps of carboxymethylated membrane μ chains the shifted spots appeared in the positions shown in Fig. 4c (see, for instance Fig.

7b, d, and 8d). This is the result obtained with μ chains from secreted IgM iodinated before reduction and carboxymethylation, moreover, it also corresponds closely to the position of the noniodinated carboxymethylated C-terminal peptide (Fig. 5a). Clearly an unknown modification occurs when iodination follows carboxymethylation, producing an enhanced shift.

IgM-Associating Membrane Protein. McPc 1748 membranes were radioiodinated, and after SDS-gel electrophoresis the major radiolabeled component was isolated. The close similarity of tryptic radiopeptide maps obtained with this major membrane component (Fig. 9d) and with pig skeletal actin (Fig. 9c) demonstrates that, as with human and pig lymphocytes (24), the major radioiodinatable component in the mouse lymphocyte membranes is actin. When the map (Fig. 9a) of isolated IgM-associating protein (see Fig. 2a) from McPc 1748 lymphocyte membranes is compared with that of the actin from the same preparation of iodinated membranes (Fig. 9b) they are very similar, with all the radiopeptides corresponding in position, though not always in intensity. This result was confirmed by peptic peptide maps. Thus the protein associating with membrane IgM in immune precipitates is membrane actin.

DISCUSSION

We have shown that the yield of tyrosine from carboxypeptidase-treated mouse and human membrane μ chains is similar to that simultaneously released from the C-terminus of secreted μ chains (12). In the case of secreted μ chains the neighboring residue is amidomethylcysteine, which is known to be only slowly released. Although no time course was followed, it seems unlikely that the carboxypeptidase was releasing tyrosine in such similar yield from a position far from the C-terminus of the membrane μ chains, so it appears that the μ chains of surface IgM have tyrosine at (or very near) the C-terminus. This is, of course, insufficient evidence to claim a similarity of sequence for the two types of μ chains in the C-terminal region.

More informative were the peptide maps, showing that peptic peptides having relative electrophoretic mobilities and R_f values very similar to those of the secreted μ chain C-terminal peptides, which were absent or weakened when the mouse chains were mapped after treatment with carboxypeptidase. This extends the earlier finding, since it shows that there was an iodotyrosine-containing peptic peptide released from the C-terminal region of iodinated surface μ chains, which has characteristics in the mapping system identical to that from the secreted μ chains. These observations make it clear that this peptic peptide from membrane μ chains is truly C-terminal, and cannot have arisen during digestion through a pepsin cleavage at a point C-terminal to this peptide, between it and an additional hydrophobic C-terminal polypeptide on the surface μ chain.

Although extremely unlikely, it might have been argued that the C-terminal peptic peptides of surface and secreted μ chains are unrelated structurally, despite the coincidence of their mobilities in both electrophoresis and chromatography. However, their identity was confirmed by their similar characteristics after modification in the peptide shift experiments. The fact that a charge modification could be achieved by carboxymethylation demonstrated the presence of a cysteine residue in the membrane C-terminal peptide. Moreover, since the C-terminal peptide was the only peptic peptide derived from secreted μ chain to contain both iodotyrosine and cysteine, this acted as an additional confirmation of the C-terminal position of the corresponding membrane peptide. The fact that the altered position of the modified membrane and secreted peptides also agreed with each other again confirmed their identity.

The above findings indicate that the following C-terminal sequences, previously known to be present on the μ chains of secreted IgM (14,25–27):

```
Pepsin
  ↓
-    Ile-Met-Ser-Asx-Thr-Gly-Gly-Thr-Cys-Tyr-COOH      Mouse
-    Val-Met-Ser-Asp-Thr-Ala-Gly-Thr-Cys-Tyr-COOH      Human
```

also probably form the μ chain C-termini of the surface IgM of B cells. This does not rule out the possibility that in surface IgM there is a hydrophobic insert, for example, somewhere within the stretch of nine residues between the end of most C-terminal μ chain domain (Cμ4), and the sequence forming the characterized C-terminal peptic peptide. Indeed, preliminary experiments by one of us (R. A. J. McIlhinney) suggest a greater binding of detergent to the membrane IgM than to secreted IgM. Further studies of the C-terminal region should identify such an inserted sequence, or alternatively a modification through covalent binding of lipid in this region.

We have looked for an integral membrane protein interacting with surface IgM, but have found only a single protein co-precipitating with surface IgM, which we have identified as actin. Since in control experiments we failed to bind actin in immune precipitates of non-membrane proteins formed under comparable conditions, there is some specificity in the surface IgM–actin interaction. This interaction could clearly be of considerable functional importance if IgM were a transmembrane protein, but less obviously so if it were not transmembrane, in view of the failure so far to identify an integral membrane protein which could mediate the interaction. However, one observation is of particular interest in this connection. We consistently find that actin is relatively well radioiodinated on the surface of McPc 1748 cells, but hardly at all on WEHI 231 cells (see Fig. 2c). This accounts for the absence of co-precipitated actin counts in Fig. 2d. Gel patterns stained for protein indicate that both McPc 1748 and WEHI 231 membranes have actin as the major component. Actin can also be radioiodinated on the surface of Bri-8 cells (11). The absence of radioiodinatable actin on the outer surface of WEHI 231 cells relative to McPc 1748 and Bri-8 cells is extremely interesting in view of the fact that whereas Bri-8 and McPc 1748 cells can be conventionally capped using fluorescent anti-Ig reagents, we cannot similarly cap WEHI 231 cells. This observation is compatible with an involvement in the capping of surface IgM of a species of actin which is radioiodinatable from the outside of the cell, and which is virtually absent in our WEHI 231 cell line.

Finally, considering the possible relation of structure to function, it has been proposed that the only function of surface Ig may be to bind antigen, which then in turn binds active factors (28). It has been pointed out that if this hypothesis were true, it would be difficult to imagine how it could benefit a cell to carry multiple classes of antibody (29), particularly since it is known that IgD and IgM on a single cell share idiotype and specificity (30–32). The contrary proposal, that surface IgM and IgD are responsible for mediating different signals, has been investigated by many workers, and the possibility that this involves their interacting with different membrane proteins, or differing in effective valency, has been discussed (2). Considering structural differences between secreted IgM and IgD which might apply to the surface molecules, and which could relate to antigen binding differences, IgD appears to have a hinge region separating the Fab and Fc regions (33), whereas IgM does not (26,27). From electron microscope studies we have suggested that the two Fab arms within each IgM subunit have limited movement with respect to each other (34–36), and this is borne out by other types of study (37). If this is equally true for surface IgM, two comments are appropriate. One is that cross-linking of surface IgM by antigens might depend considerably on the spacing of repeated determinants, but this dependency might be less for a more flexible IgD molecule (or for any other class of surface Ig having a flexible hinge region). Second, it is much easier to envisage the transmission to the membrane, along a relatively rigidly coupled IgM subunit, of effects due to the binding of Fab units to antigens.

Preliminary to a detailed study of surface Ig conformation, we have examined the assembly and structure of intracellular IgM subunits in secreting plasmacytoma cells (23), and have come to the conclusion that their structure is that seen in Fig. 10. Since the disulfide bridges and domain interactions resemble those seen in the subunits of secreted pentameric IgM molecules, the Fab arms could well be restricted in their independent movement, and this would be equally true for surface IgM if it follows the same assembly pathway. However, whereas intracellular IgM subunits are presumably assembled free of membrane, we cannot yet say whether surface IgM is so assembled. If surface IgM were to be assembled while the μ chains were membrane-bound, this could lead to important structural differences, particularly, for example, if disulfide bridge $\mu2$ were not formed on the membrane. We are looking into this problem.

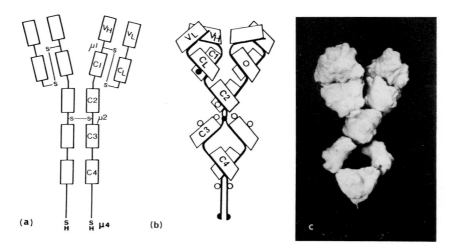

Fig. 10. Structure of mouse intracellular IgM. (a) Interchain disulfide bridge arrangement; (b) proposed domain interactions: ●, interchain disulfide bridge; ◖, cysteine residue; ○, site of attachment of oligosaccharide group. The interactions are those proposed for the IgM pentamer; (c) space-filling model. [From Richardson and Feinstein (23).]

ACKNOWLEDGMENTS

We thank Celia P. Milstein for maintaining the Bri-8 cell cultures, Edward V. Deverson for performing amino acid analyses, and Dr. G. Corte and Andrew Morgan for their help. R. A. J. McIlhinney is in receipt of a Cancer Research Campaign Fellowship.

REFERENCES

1. Marchalonis, J. J. (1976) *Contemp. Top. Mol. Immunol.* **5**, 125–160.
2. Vitetta, E. S., and Uhr, J. W. (1977) *Transplant. Rev.* **37**, 50–88.
3. Vitetta, E. S., Baur, S., and Uhr, J. W. (1971) *J. Exp. Med.* **134**, 242–264.
4. Marchalonis, J. J., Cone, R. E., and Atwell, J. L. (1972) *J. Exp. Med.* **135**, 956–971.
5. Knapp, W., Bolhuis, R. L. M., Rade, J., and Hijmans, W. (1973) *J. Immunol.* **111**, 1295–1298.
6. Rowe, D. S., Hug, K., Forni, L., and Pernis, B. (1973) *J. Exp. Med.* **138**, 965–972.
7. Abney, E. R., and Parkhouse, R. M. E. (1974) *Nature (London)* **252**, 600–602.
8. Melcher, U., Vitetta, E. S., McWilliams, M., Lamm, M. E., Phillips-Quagliata, J. M., and Uhr, J. W. (1974) *J. Exp. Med.* **140**, 1427–1431.
9. Sitia, R., Corte, G., Ferrarini, M., and Bargellesi, A. (1977) *Eur. J. Immunol.* **7**, 503–507.
10. Vitetta, E. S., and Uhr, J. W. (1977) *Immunol. Rev.* **37**, 50–88.
11. Walsh, F. S., and Crumpton, M. J. (1977) *Nature (London)* **269**, 307–311.
12. McIlhinney, R. A. J., Richardson, N. E., and Feinstein, A. (1978) *Nature (London)* **272**, 555–557.
13. McIntire, K. R., Asofsky, R. M., Potter, M., and Kuff, E. L. (1965) *Science* **150**, 361–363.
14. Milstein, C. P., Richardson, N. E., Deverson, E. V., and Feinstein, A. (1975) *Biochem. J.* **151**, 615–624.
15. Beale, D., and Feinstein, A. (1969) *Biochem. J.* **112**, 187–194.
16. Andersson, J., Buxbaum, J., Citronbaum, R., Douglas, S., Forni, L., Melchers, F., Pernis, B., and Stott, D. I. (1974) *J. Exp. Med.* **140**, 742–763.
17. Marchalonis, J. J., Cone, R. E., and Santer, U. (1971) *Biochem. J.* **124**, 921–927.
18. Wright, B. M., Edwards, A. J., and Jones, V. E. (1974) *J. Immunol. Methods* **4**, 281–296.
19. Crumpton, M. J., and Snary, D. (1972) *Contemp. Top. Mol. Immunol.* **3**, 27–56.
20. Laemlli, V. K. (1970) *Nature (London)* **227**, 68;–685.
21. Ambler, R. (1967) *In* "Methods in Enzymology" (C. H. W. Hirs, ed.), Vol. 11, pp. 155–166. Academic Press, New York.
22. Mole, L. E. (1975) *Biochem. J.* **151**, 351–359.
23. Richardson, N. E., and Feinstein, A. (1978) *Biochem. J.* **175**, 959–967.
24. Barber, B. H., and Crumpton, M. J. (1976) *FEBS Lett.* **66**, 215–220.
25. Frangione, B., Prelli, F., Mihaesco, C., and Franklin, E. C. (1971) *Proc. Natl. Acad. Sci. U.S.A.* **68**, 1547–1551.
26. Putnam, F. W., Florent, G., Paul, C., Shinoda, T., and Shimizu, A. (1973) *Science* **182**, 287–291.
27. Watanabe, S., Barnikol, H. U., Horn, J., Bertram, J., and Hilschmann, N. (1973) *Hoppe-Seyler's Z. Physiol. Chem.* **354**, 1505–1509.

28. Coutinho, A., and Moller, G. (1974) *Scand. J. Immunol.* **3**, 133–146.
29. Parkhouse, R. M. E., and Cooper, M. D. (1977) *Immunol. Rev.* **37**, 105–126.
30. Salsano, F., Froland, S. S., Natvig, J. B., and Michaelson, T. E. (1974). *Scand. J. Immunol.* **3**, 841–846.
31. Fu, S. M., Winchester, R. J., and Kunkel, H. G. (1975) *J. Immunol.* **114**, 250–252.
32. Pernis, B., Brouet, J. C., and Seligmann, M. (1974) *Eur. J. Immunol.* **4**, 776–778.
33. Jefferis, R., and Matthews, J. B. (1977) *Immunol. Rev.* **37**, 25–49.
34. Feinstein, A., Richardson, N. E., and Munn, E. A. (1976) *In* "Structure-Function Relationships of Proteins" (R. Markham and R. W. Horne, eds.), pp. 111–127. Elsevier, Amsterdam.
35. Beale, D., and Feinstein, A. (1976) *Q. Rev. Biophys.* **9**, 135–180.
36. Feinstein, A., and Beale, D. (1977) *In* "Immunochemistry: An Advanced Textbook" (L. E. Glynn and M. W. Steward, eds.), pp. 263–306. Wiley, New York.
37. Holowka, D. A., and Cathou, R. E. (1976) *Biochemistry* **15**, 3379–3390.

Role of Membrane Immunoglobulins in Lymphocyte Responses

BENVENUTO PERNIS
Departments of Microbiology and Medicine
Columbia University College of Physicians and Surgeons
New York, New York

LUCIANA FORNI
Basel Institute of Immunology
Basel, Switzerland

SUSAN R. WEBB
Department of Microbiology
College of Physicians and Surgeons
Columbia University
New York, New York

INTRODUCTION

Bone marrow-derived (B) lymphocytes carry on their membrane immunoglobulin molecules (MIg) that have a stable bond with the membrane itself. It appears likely, but not yet proved, that these immunoglobulin molecules have a direct connection with the lipid bilayer of the cell membrane and that they are therefore, true membrane proteins.

One given B lymphocyte may carry on its membrane actively synthesized (endogenous) immunoglobulin molecules or passively acquired molecules bound to the cell through the Fc receptor. Under normal conditions, most B lymphocytes have on their membrane only the endogenous immunoglobulins. An important rule is that the endogenous immunoglobulins that are present on the membrane of a single lymphocyte have uniform antibody combining sites; conversely, members of different clones have MIg with different antigen binding specificity.

189

This condition, together with the proven fact that the specificity of the antibody molecules secreted by the plasma cell is the same as that of the MIg of the parent lymphocyte, fulfills a prediction made by the clonal selection theory (1) and identifies the MIg molecules as functional receptors.

In fact several experiments have shown that lymphocytes cannot respond to antigens if they are exposed to anti-immunoglobulin antibodies that react with their MIg receptors [reviewed by Warner (2)].

This phenomenon is not due to any damage to the cell by the anti-immunoglobulin antibodies since it does not require complement and is reversible (3); it appears that the anti-immunoglobulin antibodies block the lymphocyte response to antigens by disturbing the establishment of a functional interaction between the antigen and the MIg receptors.

While there is no doubt on the fact that binding of antigen by the membrane immunoglobulins is essential for the activation of B cells and that the specificity of the response is the consequence of the clonal distribution of receptors with different combining sites, there is no clear understanding of the molecular mechanisms through which the immunoglobulin receptors perform their role. There are two main views of this problem. One view states that the interaction of the MIg with antigen delivers to the cell a definite signal (4) that will result in tolerance unless the cell receives a second signal from the "associative antibody" produced by the T lymphocytes. Another view ascribes to the MIg only the role of focusing the antigen on the membrane of specific lymphocytes, while the molecular triggering chain is started by a relatively nonspecific receptor that is identified as a receptor for mitogens. According to this second view, the antigen acts as a "mitogen" either directly or through the concentration of a physiological "mitogen" that is nothing else but the helper antibody synthesized by the T lymphocytes. In support of this second view is the fact that there are several different kinds of molecules that can directly activate B lymphocytes to proliferation and maturation to immunoglobulin-secreting cells, without apparently interacting with the MIg receptors; accordingly the B cell activation induced (*in vivo* or *in vitro*) by these agents is polyclonal and therefore nonspecific. These polyclonal B cell activators (PBA), on the other hand, precisely because they activate the B lymphocytes, apparently without involving their immunoglobulin receptors, offer a very interesting opportunity to study the possibility that the immunoglobulin receptors themselves may play a role in the physiology of B lymphocytes that is not limited to the focusing of the antigen molecules. In fact, if the MIg have no physiological role in modulating the reactivity of the B lymphocytes, it should be possible to interact with the MIg in various ways (with antigens or with anti-immunoglobulin antibodies) without influencing the reaction of these cells to a polyclonal activator.

Experiments on the effect of anti-immunoglobulin antibodies on the polyclonal stimulation of B lymphocytes by PBA (such as the lipopolysaccharides of Gram-negative bacteria) have been performed in different laboratories (5,6) with the main result that these antibodies block the maturation (but not the proliferation) of B lymphocytes obtained by short-term (6 days) cultures of these cells in the presence of mitogenic concentrations of lipopolysaccharides (LPS).

In this paper we wish to report an extension of these studies as well as preliminary results obtained with the use of *antigens* in a similar system. The first part of the work was performed at the Basel Institute of Immunology and the second at Columbia University.

EFFECT OF ANTI-IMMUNOGLOBULIN ANTIBODIES ON B LYMPHOCYTE MATURATION INDUCED BY LPS

These experiments were performed by adding the IgG fraction of rabbit antisera directed against the different mouse immunoglobulin classes and subclassed to cultures of mouse spleen by lymphocytes stimulated *in vitro* by LPS. After 7 days of culture the percentage of plasma cells containing immunoglobulins of the different classes and subclasses was determined by immunofluorescence examination of the cultured cells flattened on slides with a cytocentrifuge and subsequently fixed.

The culture conditions, the preparations of the antisera and their absorption, the conjugation with fluorochromes and staining procedures as well as the microscopic examination of the slides were as described by Pernis *et al.* (7). The F(Ab')$_2$ fraction of the rabbit antiserum specific for mouse μ chains was prepared by pepsin treatment of the absorbed rabbit IgG. It must be noted that the IgG fraction of the different specific rabbit antisera was added to the culture medium at the beginning of the culture at the concentration of 250 μg IgG/ml and that the antibodies were left in the culture fluid throughout the culture period; no complement was added to the cultures.

The results of the experiments on the effects of antibodies directed against mouse μ chains (complete IgG or F(Ab')$_2$ of the antibodies) as well as of antibodies directed against mouse γ_1, γ_{2a}, and γ_{2b} chains, are collected in Table I. The values reported in Table I give the number of

TABLE I
Effect of Different Anti-Immunoglobulin Antibodies on the Induction of
Plasmablasts and Plasma Cells Containing Different Immunoglobulin
Classes, in Mouse Lymphocyte Cultures Stimulated by LPS for
7 Days in Culture[a]

Antiserum in culture (250 μg IgG/ml	Total blasts	Cells with cytoplasmic IgM	Cells with cytoplasmic IgG_1	Cells with cytoplasmic IgG_{2a}	Cells with cytoplasmic IgG_{2b}
Anti μ intact Ig	82	6	3	7	3
F(Ab')$_2$ of anti μ	92	10	6	7	5
Anti γ_1	70	100	10	105	70
Anti γ_{2a}	110	125	110	12	110
Anti γ_{2b}	120	138	120	120	25

[a] The results represent one set of experiments. All experiments were repeated at least three times with similar results. The values express the percentage of a given response as compared to the companion control culture with normal rabbit IgG (see text).

total blasts and of blasts and plasma cells containing a given immuno-globulin class in cultures treated with the antibodies of different specificity, as compared with control cultures treated with the same concentration of normal rabbit IgG. For instance, if, in a typical experiment, 70% of all cells in a 7 day LPS culture with added normal rabbit immunoglobulins, contain intracytoplasmic IgM whereas in a comparison culture containing the immunoglobulins from a rabbit antiserum against mouse μ chains, only 7% of all cells show intracytoplasmic IgM, this result is interpreted as indicating that the IgM response in the treated culture is 10% of the control. The results summarized in Table I were obtained by pooling different experiments in which the effect of a given antiserum was always compared with a companion control culture containing normal rabbit IgG. In addition, it should be noted that in the whole series of experiments, the variation in the percentage of cells containing different immunoglobulins in day 7 *control* cultures varied within a relatively limited range.

The data of Table I confirm the results of Andersson *et al.* (5) inasmuch as they show that anti-immunoglobulin antibodies block the maturation but not the proliferation of B lymphocytes induced by LPS. In fact in the cultures treated with antibodies, there was a marked inhibition of the appearance of mature B immunocytes (plasmablasts and plasma cells) containing intracytoplasmic immunoglobulins as discussed below, but there was only a very limited reduction in the total number of "blasts." We also confirm the observations of Kearney *et al.* (6) that anti-μ antibodies block the maturation of cells synthesizing IgM as well as those synthesizing IgG, whereas anti-γ antibodies inhibit only the latter.

In addition, the data of Table I show that the effect of antibodies directed against the different IgG subclasses is quite selective since they appear to inhibit the appearance only of those cells that synthesize the corresponding immunoglobulin. This interesting observation is in agreement with the fact (7) that in LPS-stimulated cultures (as well as in normal mouse lymphoid tissues) there are no cells that simultaneously express IgG of different subclasses. This latter finding is valid also for the membrane IgG that appear very early (6 hr) after the stimulation *in vitro* with LPS (7) and suggests that the mechanism whereby the antibodies directed against the different IgG subclasses block the appearance of the corresponding plasma cells, is precisely an interaction with the membrane immunoglobulins of the same subclass at this early stage of lymphocyte activation.

Furthermore, the data of Table I show that the F(Ab′)₂ fragment of rabbit antibodies against mouse μ chains has the same effect as the intact molecules; this fact will be discussed later.

Finally we wish to point out that, whereas the anti-μ antibodies have a profound effect on cells that synthesize IgG of different subclasses, the reverse does not happen insofar as the different anti-γ antibodies induce, if anything, a slight increase of cells that contain intracytoplasmic IgM.

This is in spite of the fact that, after 6 hr of treatment with LPS, about one-half of all lymphocytes that have membrane IgM also have membrane IgG (and about one-third have IgG₁). It will be very interesting to separate these cells with anti-γ antibodies (either by rosetting or with a cell sorter) and investigate what may be their future development in culture with LPS, either in the absence or presence of anti-γ antibodies, with the aim of investigating the possibility that in the latter condition the cells may be diverted to maturation into plasma cells synthesizing IgM only.

EFFECT OF ANTIGEN ON B LYMPHOCYTE MATURATION INDUCED BY LPS

The simplest explanation of the blocking effect of anti-immunoglobulin antibodies on the maturation of B lymphocytes induced by LPS is that these antibodies determine a cross-linking of the membrane immunoglobulins (notably IgM), and that this condition somehow alters the responsiveness of the cells to LPS, an alteration that results in a block of maturation. We reasoned that if this is the case, polyvalent antigens should have the same effect and that exposure of the mouse spleen lymphocytes to one such antigen should selectively eliminate from the final population resulting after 7 days of culture the mature cells capable of secreting antibodies against the antigen added to the culture itself. We have therefore prepared a conjugate of trinitrophenol with keyhole limpet Hemocyanin (TNP-KLH) by treating the protein with TNP-sulfonate; the resulting conjugate had 800 TNP groups per 8×10^6 M.W. of the protein. We have then cultivated normal mouse spleen cells (BALB/c) in the presence of LPS; the culture conditions were as described by Kearney *et al.* (6) with the addition of different amounts of TNP-KLH. Numerous cultures were set up with final TNP-KLH concentrations ranging from 0.25 to 250 μg/ml. After 7 days of cultures the cells were harvested and the number of cells *secreting* antibodies against TNP or Fluorescein (FITC) was scored by counting hemolytic plaques with sheep erythrocytes conjugated with TNP (TNP-SRBC) or with Fluorescein isothiocyanate. The preparation of TNP-SRBC was done as described by Rittenberg and Pratt (8) and that of FITC-SRBC as described by Möller (9); the effectiveness of the conjugation with TNP was checked by hemagglutinations with a specific anti-TNP antiserum and that with FITC by examination of the conjugated SRBC under the fluorescence microscope. The number of anti-TNP or of anti-FITC plaques was calculated after subtraction of the number of plaques scored with untreated SRBC. In different experiments the number of direct plaques that we scored in 7 day LPS cultures of BALB/c spleen lymphocytes with our erythrocyte preparations showed relatively small variations in control cultures and was around 2500 plaques/10^6 cells with TNP-SRBC and around 5000 plaques/10^6 cells with FITC-SRBC; the background plaques with untreated SRBC were around 250/10^6 cells.

In the cultures with added TNP-KLH the values were practically the same, except when the concentration of added TNP-KLH was 250 μg/ml. In the latter cultures a reduction of the TNP-plaques of about 50% was noted, but this was accompanied by a comparable reduction of FITC plaques.

We conclude from these results that the addition of TNP-KLH did not influence the maturation of the TNP-specific B lymphocytes, induced by LPS, since the inhibition seen with the highest concentration of TNP-KLH appeared nonspecific (parallel inhibition of the FITC-plaques) and was probably due to a toxic effect on the cells.

It appears therefore that a large antigen molecule with numerous identical determinants (TNP-KLH) has no effect on the LPS-induced maturation of mouse B lymphocytes, and that in this respect, it differs from anti-immunoglobulin antibodies, in spite of the fact that both antigen and antibodies should induce comparable cross-linking of the membrane Ig receptors in the antigen-binding cells. We reasoned in fact that the wide range of antigen concentrations that we have used in our experiments should have provided adequate binding of the polyvalent antigen even with cell population with considerable differences in the affinity of their receptors for TNP.

Comparable results, that is, absence of an effect on maturation of antigen-specific cells in LPS-stimulated cultures performed in the presence of the antigen, have been obtained by G. Möller (personal communication). The antigens he has employed were (4-hydroxy-3,5-dinitrophenyl) acetyl (NNP) and FITC coupled with human gamma globulins.

The experiments with antigen appear therefore to rule out the possibility that simple cross-linking of the membrane immunoglobulins can block the maturation of the B lymphocytes induced by LPS. What is then the mechanism of the inhibitory action of anti-immunoglobulin antibodies in the same system? Several possibilities can be listed:

(a) The site of binding of the antibodies to the immunoglobulin receptors and of the antigen is not the same. If this is the explanation then the implication would be that the immunoglobulin receptors have some properties of an allosteric molecule or that the anti-immunoglobulin antibodies cover up some areas of the receptors that interact with other membrane proteins.

(b) The mechanism of the inhibitions by antibodies requires the endocytosis of the complexes and is mediated by the interaction between the antibody and the nascent immunoglobulin chains in some critical sites inside the cells. Clearly, the antigen would not do that since it would not be able to interact with sufficient affinity with the isolated chains.

(c) The anti-immunoglobulin antibodies that are immunoglobulin themselves, even when xenogeneic, deliver to the cell some sort of negative signal associated with their own immunoglobulin structure. This possibility appears unlikely in view of the above mentioned experiments of G. Möller, who used human gamma globulin as a carrier and failed to obtain inhibition. Furthermore, our experiments on the inhibitory effect of the $F(Ab')_2$ fragment of the anti-immunoglobulin antibodies appear to rule out a role of the Fc of these molecules, that might have reacted with the Fc receptor present on the membrane of most mature B lymphocytes.

In conclusion, it appears to us that the mechanism of the clear and specific inhibition of the LPS-induced maturation of B lymphocytes that is obtained with anti-immunoglobulin antibodies, remains to be investigated. Several experimental approaches can be devised on the basis of the working hypotheses that we have just listed, and it is reasonable to expect that this line of research will contribute to our understanding of the physiology of B lymphocytes.

SUMMARY

Addition of lipopolysaccharide (LPS) to mouse spleen lymphocytes in culture induces the proliferation and maturation of bone marrow-derived (B) lymphocytes. The maturation to immunoglobulin-secreting cells (but nôt the proliferation) is blocked by antibodies that react with the immunoglobulin receptors. It is shown in this paper that the antibodies directed against the different IgG subclasses specifically block the appearance of the corresponding plasma cells; anti-IgM antibodies block all. The $F(Ab')_2$ fragment of the antibodies is also efficient in blocking.

Conversely, no inhibition of LPS-induced maturation to antigen-specific plasma cells was obtained by added antigen (TNP-KLH) to the cultures. This suggests that simple cross-linking of the membrane immunoglobulin receptors is not the mechanism through which the anti-immunoglobulin antibodies exert their inhibitory effect on B lymphocyte maturation.

ACKNOWLEDGMENT

Supported in part by National Institutes of Health grant AI ROI 14398.

REFERENCES

1. Burnet, F. M. (1959) "The Clonal Selection Theory of Acquired Immunity." Cambridge Univ. Press, London and New York.
2. Warner, N. L. (1974) *Adv. Immunol.* **19**, 67.
3. Fuji, H., and Jerne, N. K. (1969) *Ann. Inst. Pasteur, Paris* **117**, 801.
4. Bretscher, P. A., and Cohn, M. (1970) *Science* **169**, 1052.
5. Andersson, J., Bullock, W. W., and Melchers, F. (1974) *Eur. J. Immunol.* **4**, 715.
6. Kearney, J. F., Cooper, M. D., and Lawton, A. R. (1976) *J. Immunol.* **116**, 1664.
7. Pernis, B., Forni, L., and Luzzati, A. L. (1977) *Cold Spring Harbor Symp. Quant. Biol.* **41**, 175.
8. Rittenberg, M. B., and Pratt, K. L. (1969) *Proc. Soc. Exp. Biol. Med.* **132**, 575.
9. Möller, G. (1977) *Cold Spring Harbor Symp. Quant. Biol.* **41**, 217.

PART IV

IMMUNOGLOBULINS AS
REGULATORY MOLECULES

Function of Surface Immunoglobulin of B Lymphocytes

EMIL R. UNANUE

Department of Pathology
Harvard Medical School
Boston, Massachusetts

One key point of interest for those studying B lymphocyte physiology is the delineation of the program of responses that ligands are capable of triggering when interacting with the cell. A full understanding of B cell responses, in our view, requires: (1) determining which specific or unique responses can ligands to surface Ig elicit; (2) determining how these specific responses compare or differ with the responses produced by ligands directed to other membrane structures; and (3) establishing the extent to which these responses are changed or modulated by the structure of the ligand and/or by extrinsic influences such as those brought about by the helper cells, i.e., macrophages and T cells.

We, as well as others, have been able to identify a series of discrete events taking place in B cells, resulting from the interaction of surface Ig with antigen. These events start, as expected, at the cell membrane, immediately produce cytoplasmic changes, some of which generate metabolic changes leading to proliferation and differentiation. Each discrete step in the process is complex and regulated in various ways. An important point is that the expression of each is highly conditioned to the state of development or maturation of the cell.

I would like to summarize briefly three aspects of the interaction of B cells with ligands that have been studied in our laboratory: (1) early surface–cytoplasmic changes popularly referred to as capping; (2) the process of receptor reexpression; and (3) the control of proliferation.

199

CAPPING

The first event that takes place in B cells is the redistribution of surface Ig–ligand complexes (1). Capping involves the selected segregation of the complexes to one area of the cell surface. It takes place extremely fast, within the first 5–10 min after ligand binding (1,2). Two major questions have been addressed by those studying this phenomenon. What is the mechanism of Ig capping? What is its function? The mechanisms of capping are of great interest to establish since it is one phenomenon in which the surface complexes interact directly or indirectly with the cytoplasm and in which both cytoplasm and membrane reciprocally influence each other. Capping of surface Ig is an expression of the activation of the cell's contractile proteins (3). This becomes evident when the reaction is closely examined. Capping of Ig complexes takes place within a few minutes after the ligand (antigen or anti-Ig) binds to the membrane. The small microclusters of complexes rapidly flow in a highly coordinated process to one pole of the cell. The rate of Ig complexes during capping is extremely fast and has been estimated to be about 10^{-8} cm^2 sec^{-1}, which is comparable to the rate of flow of lipids and somewhat faster than that estimated for proteins that are not cross-linked by a ligand (2). At the time that Ig complexes are redistributing, cytoplasmic actin and myosin also become concentrated to the area of the cap (3). The coordination between the capping of Ig and the redistribution of cytoplasmic myosin is impressive. Seconds after the cap has formed, an area of constriction develops around it; and at the same time, small ruffles appear on the membrane, always opposite the cap. The small ruffles also contain contractile proteins. This is the stage of translatory motion in which the lymphocyte, if attached to a substratum, now moves at random. The point to emphasize is that ligand–surface Ig interaction stimulates translatory motion in B cells (4). Indeed, we have found that B lymphocytes can move chemotactically to a gradient of molecules of anti-Ig antibodies (5).

How do the membrane-bound complexes of ligand–surface Ig interact with contractile proteins? The answers are not available. We have hypothesized that the interaction between both may be through some physical linkage perhaps involving a transmembrane protein (2,6). So far, the only structure on the membrane which is known to interact with surface Ig is the Fc receptor. This association was found during capping of Ig where the Fc receptor co-caps with it (7,8). The reverse is not true, however: capping of Fc receptors does not co-cap surface

Ig. Whether the Fc receptor is the transmembrane protein remains speculative.

Experiments using drugs have given some clues on how the Ig–contractile protein association may take place. Two drugs that we have used are the Ca^{2+} ionophore A23187 and the local anesthetics. Ca^{2+} ionophores interact with the membrane and induce a flow of extracellular Ca^{2+} into the cell. The local anesthetics are lyophilic chemicals that bind to acidic phospholipids and can displace membrane-bound Ca^{2+}. Both drugs stop formation of Ig caps. Most interestingly, their addition to B cells *after* caps have formed results in the breaking of the cap. The complexes then disperse as small clusters over the entire surface. At the time the complexes disperse, myosin no longer remains concentrated under the area of the cap. Other observations suggest that the mode of action of both drugs may be different. The dissolution of the cap by the ionophore can be stopped by drugs that affect energy metabolism; these same drugs have no effect on the cap disruption produced by the anesthetic. We have speculated that the Ca^{2+} ionophore, by increasing intracellular Ca^{2+}, results in a systemic activation of the contractile proteins that interfere with the discrete segmental activation during formation and maintenance of the cap. Indeed, cells treated with ionophore show myosin in large, irregular patches. In contrast, our speculation is that the anesthetics may sever the association between surface complexes and the actin–myosin network, which then allows the surface complexes to freely diffuse throughout the membrane (reviewed in Schreiner and Unanue, 2).

Recent studies by Braun *et al.*, have compared capping of various macromolecules in lymphocytes (9,10). Our conclusion is that, although all molecules redistribute, there are marked differences among them insofar as kinetics, number of ligands required to induce the reaction, and changes in translatory motion. Ig is the typical example of the molecule that caps fast, while H-2 antigens are the example of molecules that cap slowly and which require two ligands (an antibody to H-2 plus an antibody to the anti-H-2 antibody). The fast capping of some molecules like Ig results, in our view, from the direct or indirect association of the surface complexes with the cell's contractile protein, which will contribute to the reorganization of the surface complexes. The slow capping of other molecules results from the progressive coalescence with time of complexes of increasing size. The complexes are not associated with the cytoplasm. In fact, translatory motion is not triggered by this set of ligands (like H-2); and the ionophores or the anesthetics do not affect their capping. Hence, these drugs clearly

TABLE I
Comparison of Capping of Ig and H-2

	Ig	H-2
Kinetics	Fast	Slow
Need for two ligands	No	Yes
Co-segregation of myosin	Yes	No
Stimulation of motility	Yes	No
Effect of anesthetics	Inhibits capping breaks caps	Does not inhibit or break caps

separate the two sets of fast and slow capping molecules. Table I compares capping of Ig and H-2 antigens.

In summary, in our view, interaction of surface Ig with a ligand triggers the activation of the contractile elements which serve to organize the membrane and give polarization and orientation to the cell. This step of increased motility in B cells may be crucial in the cellular reorganization taking place in a lymphoid structure at the time of antigen stimulation.

ENDOCYTOSIS OF Ig–LIGAND COMPLEXES

After capping, most of the surface complexes are interiorized in vesicles, while only a small percentage is shed from the membrane. The interiorized complexes are degraded largely but not entirely to amino acids. These studies were made with radioiodinated IgG having antibodies to surface Ig. Less detailed studies were also done with labeled protein antigens (reviewed in Schreiner and Unanue, 2). Is this step important? Is it necessary to internalize and degrade the ligands? No clear answers are available, but experiments with antigens that are poorly degraded by natural enzymes suggest that metabolizability of the ligand may be a critical factor. The evidence comes from studies using haptens (such as dinitrophenyl, DNP) bound to synthetic peptides made of glutamic acid and lysine (GL). B cells exposed *in vitro* to DNP-GL made of d-amino acids are readily tolerized. These B cells will bind the compound, much of which appears to remain on the surface. The B cells will not show evidence of free receptors, even hours after a brief incubation with the antigen. In contrast, a similar compound but made of l-amino acids can be cleared from the cell and will not produce an impairment of receptor regeneration. Hence, interactions with antigens that cannot be degraded by the cell result in the persistence of the compound and in the functional inactivation of the cell. The mechanisms of cell inactivation remain unexplained.

RECEPTOR REEXPRESSION

After the interiorization of the ligand–surface Ig complexes, the B cell will be free of its antigen receptor—or depleted of it—for a few hours, after which there is full regeneration through a process that requires protein synthesis. I would like to analyze the lack of receptor reexpression found in several conditions but most strikingly in B cells from neonatal mice. B cells from neonatal mice show distinctly different characteristics from the cells of adult mice. These B cells have IgM on their membrane and lack IgD (11) and C3 receptors (12). The surface phenotype changes by about the tenth to fourteenth day of life when C3 receptors become apparent in a large percentage of the B cells. It is also by about this time that IgD is detectable by surface radioiodination methods. The B cells from young mice, when placed in culture with anti-Ig antibodies, cap at a slow rate but eventually clear their membrane of the complex. The striking effect, however, is the lack of regeneration of new surface Ig (13). Thus, incubation of B cells from 1 to 24 hr with anti-Ig antibodies followed by a 24–72 hr period in fresh medium results in little or no regeneration of surface Ig on their membranes. The cells are presumably still alive in the culture since they can be identified by the presence of Ia molecules. Treatment of B cells with pronase removes surface Ig—and presumably other membrane proteins—but will not produce a lack of Ig regeneration.

Hence, it appears that Ig–ligand interaction can trigger a negative response from B cells at a particular stage of their development. Essentially similar results were obtained by Raff et al. (14). Others have shown the greater sensitivity of B cells from neonatal mice to tolerance induction in vitro (15). Negative effects brought about by ligand–Ig interaction have been obtained in B cells from adult mice but never to the extent of suppression of Ig regeneration.

This lack of receptor regeneration raises the possibility that this may be the mechanism of tolerance induction during neonatal life. Perhaps the presence of antigen early in life deletes the specific antigen-binding clone of B cells, a process which may tip the fine balance between helper–suppressor idiotype reacting cells and eventually results in lasting B cell tolerance.

TABLE II
Anti-Ig Effects in B Cells from Neonatal and Adult Mice

	Neonate	Adult
Capping	Slow	Fast
Anti-Ig → Ig reexpression	Inhibition	+
Pronase → Ig reexpression	+	+
Anti-Ig (pulse) → continuous LPS	Inhibition of proliferation	Proliferation
Anti-Ig (continuous) plus 2-ME	No proliferation	Proliferation

The negative effects brought about by the ligand–Ig interaction in young B cells is also reflected in their lack of proliferation to anti-IgM antibodies *in vitro*. Mature murine B cells proliferate in culture in response to anti-IgM antibodies, in the presence of mercaptoethanol in the culture media (15–17). Under similar conditions, B cells from neonatal mice do not respond (16). These results imply that during normal development B cells go through a stage of high sensitivity to negative signals generated from the interaction between their receptor and antigen (Table II). This sensitivity has been found in B cells isolated from bone marrow which are readily tolerized upon exposure to antigen *in vitro* (18). Along these lines, observations of Ault and Unanue (19) in human B lymphocytes are of interest though puzzling. The observations are that peripheral blood B lymphocytes show, as the B cells from murine neonates, a lack of regeneration after clearing the membrane by anti-Ig but not by pronase treatment. B cells from tonsils and spleen, however, regenerate Ig readily. The peripheral blood B cells appear to be "mature" cells having IgD, IgM, and C3 receptors. Thus, the correlation between surface phenotype and lack of regeneration as criteria of maturity may not be strict.

MODULATION OF PROLIFERATION

The interaction between anti-Ig and surface Ig can regulate proliferation in either a positive or a negative way. This point has become particularly noticeable in the mouse. In some other species, most notably the rabbit, a prolonged interaction for 24–48 hr between anti-Ig antibodies and B cells usually results in stimulation of DNA synthesis (20). The main points that have been found in the mouse are summarized in Table III. The main conclusion is that interactions between surface Ig with anti-Ig antibodies result in stimulation of proliferation

TABLE III
Proliferation of Murine B Lymphocytes

---

1. Soluble polyvalent anti-Ig antibodies or anti-IgM antibodies generally will not stimulate proliferation and will inhibit LPS stimulation.
2. Anti-IgM stimulates proliferation in the presence of 2-ME or a 2-ME serum-derived factor.
   Antibodies to Fab determinants or to IgD stimulate poorly even in the presence of 2-ME.
3. Anti-IgM antibodies have an additive effect on the proliferation stimulated by LPS, in the presence of 2-ME. Under the same conditions, anti-IgM antibodies inhibit differentiation to PFC.
4. Anti-Ig antibodies bound to beads stimulate proliferation.
5. B cells from neonatal mice do not proliferate upon incubation with anti-IgM (plus 2-ME).
   B cells from aged mice respond to anti-IgM in the absence of 2-ME.

---

provided that certain conditions are met. The conditions that favor stimulation of proliferation include: (1) the presence of 2-mercaptoethanol (2-ME) in the culture medium; (2) the use of antibodies with specificity to anti-IgM; so far, we have obtained very poor results using antibodies to IgD or to Fab determinants; (3) the use of an F(ab')$_2$ fragment of antibody; and (4) the use of mature B cells. A brief comment on each of these points follows.

A reducing agent such as mercaptoethanol favors markedly the proliferative response. The effect of 2-ME is in great part exerted on a serum protein found in serum which, if reduced and alkylated, serves as the co-factor necessary to stimulate the response. In the absence of 2-ME, the interaction between anti-IgM and the B cell does not produce proliferation and, furthermore, results in the inhibition of the stimulatory effect. Thus, the 2-ME—or its serum-derived co-factor—determines whether the cell receives a negative or positive signal.

A second interesting point relates to the lack of stimulation by antibodies to IgD or to Fab determinants. It suggests to us that IgM serves as a receptor for receiving signals that affect DNA synthesis, while perhaps the IgD receptor may be involved in other regulatory functions. The poor stimulation by antibodies to Fab determinants is more difficult to explain. The interaction of the anti-Fab antibody with surface IgM is not inhibitory *per se* and will not reduce the stimulation produced by anti-IgM. It suggests to us that perhaps the way in which Ig molecules are on the membrane is such that cross-linking the heavy chains results in the crucial change required to trigger the cell, which presumably is mimicked physiologically by antigen.

The interaction between Fc receptor and surface Ig results in the generation of a most powerful negative signal. This conclusion derives from experiments using pepsin fragments of anti-Ig antibodies which, in the absence of 2-ME, are less inhibitory and, in the presence of 2-ME, are more stimulatory.

A final point of discussion concerns the relationship between proliferation and differentiation. Interaction of ligands with B cells usually does not result in differentiation unless the ligand in itself possesses other intrinsic properties such as those exhibited by endotoxins. With regular protein antigens or using anti-Ig antibodies, differentiation to a secretory step does not appear to take place. Nevertheless, anti-Ig antibodies can affect the differentiative process. We have been impressed by the observation that the interaction of B cells with anti-IgM plus LPS results in a marked stimulation of DNA synthesis; at the same time the regular differentiation that takes place in some cells from the proliferating population is abolished. Hence, while the stimulus for proliferation was in progress, that for differentiation was reduced. Our speculation is that perhaps a fine balance exists between both signals and that, for a full response to occur, as shown by clonal expansion and differentiation, a well-integrated interaction between proliferative and differentiative signals is required.

In summary, ligands to surface Ig can stimulate a number of important and complex responses in the B cells, only some of which have been started to be analyzed at a molecular level. The complexity of the B cell response is compounded by the contrasting effects that can be generated by a single ligand, by the ease with which extrinsic factors exert modulatory influences, and by the effects of cell development in the response.

ACKNOWLEDGMENTS

This paper summarizes the work of this laboratory, which has involved Jonathan Braun, George F. Schreiner, Kenneth A. Ault, and Charles L. Sidman.

REFERENCES

1. Taylor, R. B., Duffus, W. P. H., Raff, M. C., and de Petris, S. (1971) *Nature (London)*, *New Biol.* **233**, 225–228.
2. Schreiner, G. F., and Unanue, E. R. (1976) *Adv. Immunol.* **24**, 38–165.
3. Schreiner, G. F., Fujiwara, K., Pollard, T. D., and Unanue, E. R. (1977) *J. Exp. Med.* **145**, 1393–1397.

4. Unanue, E. R., Ault, K. A., and Karnovsky, M. J. (1974) *J. Exp. Med.* **139**, 295–305.
5. Ward, P. A., Unanue, E. R., Goralnick, S. J., and Schreiner, G. F. (1977) *J. Immunol.* **119**, 416–430.
6. Schreiner, G. F., and Unanue, E. R. (1977) *J. Immunol.* **119**, 1549–1551.
7. Abbas, A. K., and Unanue, E. R. (1975) *J. Immunol.* **115**, 1665–1671.
8. Forni, L., and Pernis, B. (1975) *In* "Membrane Receptors of Lymphocytes" (M. Seligmann, ed.), p. 193. North-Holland Publ., Amsterdam.
9. Braun, J., Fujiwara, K., Pollard, T. D., and Unanue, E. R. (1978) *J. Cell Biol.* **79**, 409–418.
10. Braun, J., Fujiwara, K., Pollard, T. D., and Unanaue, E. R. (1978) *J. Cell Biol.* **79**, 419–426.
11. Melchers, U., Vitetta, E. S., McWilliams, M., Lamm, M., Phillips-Quagliata, J., and Uhr, J. W. (1974) *J. Exp. Med.* **140**, 1427–1439.
12. Gelfand, M. C., Elfenbein, G. J., Frank, M. M., and Paul, W. E. (1974) *J. Exp. Med.* **139**, 1125–1139.
13. Sidman, C. L., and Unanue, E. R. (1975) *Nature (London)* **257**, 149–153.
14. Raff, M. C., Owen, J. J. T., Cooper, M. D., Lawton, A. R., Megson, M., and Gethings, W. E. (1975) *J. Exp. Med.* **142**, 1052–1067.
15. Metcalf, E. S., and Klinman, N. R. (1976) *J. Exp. Med.* **143**, 1327–1332.
16. Sidman, C. L., and Unanue, E. R. (1978) *Proc. Natl. Acad. Sci. U.S.A.* **75**, 2401–2405.
17. Sieckmann, D. G., Asofsky, R., Mosier, D. E., Zitron, I. M., and Paul, W. E. (1978) *J. Exp. Med.* **147**, 814–829.
18. Nossal, G. J. V., and Pike, B. L. (1975) *J. Exp. Med.* **141**, 904–919.
19. Ault, K. A., and Unanue, E. R. (1977) *J. Immunol.* **119**, 327–329.
20. Sell, S., and Gell, P. G. H. (1965) *J. Exp. Med.* **122**, 423–434.

The Role of Immunoglobulin in the Induction of B Lymphocytes

J. ANDERSSON

Department of Immunology
University of Uppsala
Uppsala, Sweden

A. COUTINHO AND F. MELCHERS

Basel Institute for Immunology
Basel, Switzerland

INTRODUCTION

Clonal growth and differentiation of lymphocytes are results of the interaction between ligands, mitogens, and their corresponding cell surface receptors. Bone marrow-derived (B) cells are thus induced by a variety of ligands, B-cell mitogens (1), mainly of bacterial origin such as lipopolysaccharide (2), lipoprotein (3), and dextran (4), to divide and differentiate into high rate immunoglobulin synthesizing and secreting cells, plasma cells. Complete knowledge of the structure of such mitogens (5,6) has not increased our understanding of the molecular nature of the functional receptors capable of binding these different mitogens.

Genetic analysis has shown that such mitogen receptors are not identical to surface Ig molecules and are not coded for by genes which code for Ig-heavy chain allotypes or products of the major histocompatibility complex (7–10). Mitogen receptors are, however, functionally associated with immunoglobulin molecules in the surface membrane of B lymphocytes since anti-immunoglobulin antibodies can be found which interfere with mitogen-induced growth and maturation of B cells (11–13). Thus, ligands binding to surface immunoglobulin may regulate growth and maturation of B cells only if such cells simultaneously interact with mitogens through their corresponding mitogen receptors.

209

Antibodies have been found which recognize mitogen receptors on B cells (14–16). Such antibodies are obvious tools in the analysis of the molecular structure and cell surface organization of mitogen receptors. We will present data which indicate that within the population of natural serum IgG there are molecules which recognize structures in the surface membrane of B cells which can serve as mitogen receptors. The functional implication of these findings will be discussed in terms of the development of B lymphocytes and the generation of diversity of B-cell receptor repertoires.

RESULTS

EFFECT OF ANTIBODIES AGAINST IMMUNOGLOBULIN CHAINS ON THE MITOGENIC STIMULATION OF SMALL, RESTING B CELLS

Different immunoglobulin populations with antibody activities against the various classes of heavy chains and types of light chains have been found to have different effects on resting B cells. A variety of antisera, their purified Ig fractions or their immunosorbent-purified specific antibodies raised in rabbits, goats, sheep, or guinea pigs against purified μ-, γ-, or α- and against purified κ- or λ- chains of mouse Ig, as well as a monoclonal mouse anti-mouse δ-H chain by themselves, do not activate small murine B cells from their resting state to either growth or to maturation to Ig secretion. Some can, however, influence a subsequent stimulation of such resting B cells by mitogens such as lipopolysaccharide (LPS) or lipoprotein (LP) [Table I]. Antisera against α- and δ-H chains and against λ-L chains have no effect. Antibodies against μ-H or κ-L chains have immediate effects, inhibiting *either* growth *and* development to Ig secretion *or only* development to Ig secretion but not growth induced by mitogens. Wherever stimulation to Ig secretion is inhibited it is so both for the development of IgM as well as for IgG secreting cells.

Antibodies against γ-H chains have no immediate effects but will inhibit mitogen-induced development of IgG secretion after an initial 12 hr period of mitogenic activation in the absence of any anti-Ig antibody. This indicates that γ-H chains are not yet expressed as functionally active molecules on resting B cells, but become effective in anti-Ig antibody-induced inhibition only after at least 12 hr of mitogenic activation. From the spectrum of specificities of inhibitory antibody molecules, it is likely that IgM molecules predominantly with κ-chains and, later, IgG molecules on B cells are involved in the inhibition. The failure to detect any effects with anti-λ antibodies may be

TABLE I

Inhibitory Effects of Antibodies against Immunoglobulin H and L Chains on the Induction of B Cells by Mitogens[a] to Growth and to Maturation into Ig-Secreting Cells

Antibodies	Growth[b]	Maturation[c]
I. Effective on IgM *and* IgG development		
Sheep anti-mouse IgG (γ,κ,λ)	−	+ IgM and IgG
Guinea pig anti-mouse IgG	+	+ IgM and IgG
Rabbit anti-mouse IgM (myeloma 104E, λ,μ)	−	−
Rabbit anti-mouse IgM (myeloma 104E, λ,μ)	+	+ IgM and IgG
Rabbit anti-mouse μ-chain (myeloma 104E, λ,μ)	−	+ IgM and IgG
Rabbit anti-mouse κ-chain (MOPC 46 myeloma)	−	+ IgM and IgG
Rabbit anti-mouse κ,λ L chains (from serum pool IgG)	+	+ IgM and IgG
Rabbit anti-mouse κ-L chain (myeloma MOPC41)	+	+ IgM and IgG
II. Effective on IgG development *only*		
Rabbit anti-F$_c\gamma$		
Washed out after 1 hr	−	−
Kept in culture	N.D.[d]	+ IgG only
Rabbit anti γ-H chain (Anti-MOPC 21 myeloma, absorbed with MOPC 104E IgM, MOPC 315 IgA and κ-L chains of serum pool IgG)		
Washed out after 1 hr	−	−
Kept in culture	N.D.[d]	+ IgG only
III. Ineffective		
Rabbit anti-α-H chains (Anti-MOPC 315 IgA, absorbed with MOPC 104E IgM, MOPC 21 IgG and κ-L chains from serum pool IgG)	−	−
Rabbit anti-λ chains (Anti-RFC 20 myeloma)	−	−
Mouse anti-mouse δ-H chain (Monoclonal antibodies, see Ref. Eur. J. Imm., 7, 1977, 684–690)	−	−
Rabbit anti-*E. coli* β-galactosidase	−	−

[a] Regularly with LPS (50 μg/ml).

[b] Measured either by thymidine uptake or by the increase in the number of cells in culture.

[c] Measured by the increase in the number of Ig-secreting, plaque-forming cells.

[d] N.D. = not determined

due to the fact that very small numbers of B cells express λ-μ on the surface membrane. On the other hand, the lack of detectable effects with anti-δ reagents, which certainly react with a large majority of B cells, would indicate that either surface δ molecules are not functionally involved as part of a mitogen receptor complex or that the available reagents are unable to induce structural changes in the mitogen receptor complex necessary for inhibition. Pepsin F(ab)$_2$ fragments, but not, or much less so, papain Fab fragments of the anti-μ- and anti-κ-antibodies will also inhibit. This rules out any involvement of the F$_c$ portions of these antibodies and their binding to F$_c$ receptors on B cells in the inhibition. It appears that cross-linking of Ig molecules may be important in this phenomenon.

The inhibitory action of anti-Ig antibodies appears to persist during several successive cell cycles even though excess antibody can be

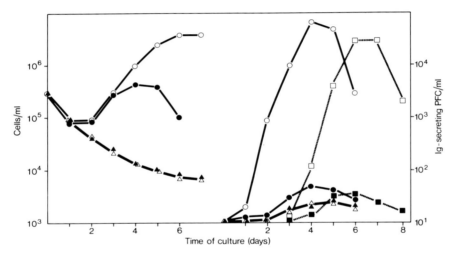

Fig. 1. Effect of anti-Ig antibodies on mitogen-induced growth and maturation. Small, resting spleen cells from C3H/Tif mice, purified by velocity sedimentation at 1 g, were cultured at 3×10^5 cells/ml in PRMI tissue culture medium containing 10% fetal calf serum (17,18).

Half the cultures received sheep anti-IgG antibodies (Type I in Table I) at a final dilution of 1/100 (full symbols). Thereafter the untreated (open symbols) as well as anti-Ig treated cultures were treated with the B-cell mitogen LPS at a concentration of 50 μg/ml. On each day of culture the number of cells/ml (left-hand part) as well as the number of Ig secreting plaque-forming cells (PFC) (right-hand part) was determined: $\triangle$, no mitogen; $\blacktriangle$, no mitogen + anti-Ig; $\bigcirc$, $\square$, LPS; $\bullet$, $\blacksquare$, LPS + anti Ig. In right-hand figure: straight line: IgM PFC; dotted line: IgG PFC.

removed by washing prior to exposure of the anti-Ig-treated B cells to mitogen. This is particularly evident in those cases of anti-Ig antibodies which inhibit activation to Ig secretion but which will allow the anti-Ig-treated mitogen-stimulated cells to grow (Fig. 1).

The negative effects of anti-Ig antibodies which persist in B cells upon subsequent stimulation with mitogen, are, on the other hand, reversible, as long as mitogen is not added. Thus, removal of the anti-Ig antibodies by proteases or by shedding *before* addition of the mitogen, restores the capacity of the B cells to be stimulated by mitogen to growth *and* to Ig secretion.

Addition of the mitogen *prior* to anti-Ig antibodies, finally, commits the B cells to grow and to mature to Ig secretion, even though anti-Ig antibodies may be added as early as 8–12 hr after the initiation of mitogenic stimulation. This indicates that mitogenic stimulation fixes the B cells to grow *and* mature when anti-Ig antibodies are absent at the time of the encounter of mitogen with the cells, as much as it fixes the B cells to grow but *not* to mature when anti-Ig antibodies are present at the time of encounter.

Taken together, these results suggest that a complex of Ig molecules and mitogen receptors exist on the surface of B cells. Binding of anti-Ig antibodies (or of antigen) to Ig molecules does not trigger, by itself, reactions which lead to growth and maturation. The triggering is done by mitogens via mitogen receptors. The state of occupancy of Ig molecules in the surface membrane, and then possibly the relative position to each other and to mitogen receptors, maybe through cross-linking, could determine whether B cells, upon mitogen encounter, will or will not grow and/or mature to secretion.

MITOGEN-DEPENDENT GROWTH OF B CELLS IN THE PRESENCE OF ANTI-Ig ANTIBODIES

When B cells are cultured at low cell densities under conditions which allow clonal growth for long periods of time, mitogen induces growth in equally many cells in the presence or absence of certain anti-Ig antibodies (Type I in Table I) for the first 3 days of culture whereafter anti-Ig treated cells cease to grow (Fig. 1). Non-anti-Ig treated cells, however, show exponential growth over longer periods of time (in the experiments shown on Fig. 1 up to day 5 of culture). The development of IgM and IgG secreting cells monitored in the same cultures, is inhibited by the anti-Ig antibodies although cells were growing in response to mitogen.

Since the same number of cells can be found growing during the first 3 days of culture whether treated or not with anti-Ig antibodies, we conclude that there cannot be a large difference in the total number of cells initiating growth in response to mitogens. It is, therefore, likely, although not formally shown, that mitogen stimulates the same cells to grow in the presence of anti-Ig, but that the antibodies selectively interfere with the mitogen-induced maturation to Ig secretion. This, in turn, suggests that the well-documented balance in B cells between growth and maturation to Ig secretion can be modulated by ligand binding to surface Ig molecules and, consequently, indicates that two chains of reactions may exist inside B cells which regulate these two response patterns of B cells.

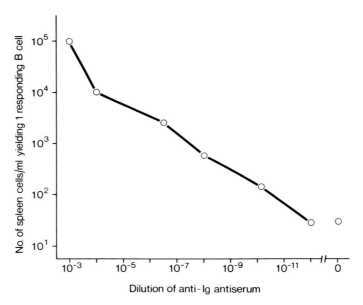

Fig. 2. Limiting dilution analysis on the effect of different concentrations of anti-Ig antibodies. Purified small spleen cells from C3H/Tif mice were cultured under our standard conditions from 10^5 cells/ml to 10^1 cells/ml in the presence of 3×10^6 rat thymus filler cells (17,18). Prior to stimulation with LPS (50 μg/ml) the cultures were treated with various concentrations of sheep anti-IgG antibodies (Type I, Table I) ranging from 10^{-3} to 10^{-12} final dilution of the original serum. At day 5 of culture, the total number of IgM secreting PFC was determined by the protein A plaque assay. A total of twelve individual cultures were assayed for each antiserum concentration at each cell concentration. The antiserum concentration allowing one B-cell clone to develop into IgM secreting cells out of the total number of cultured cells was computed.

EFFECT OF ANTI-Ig CONCENTRATION ON THE INHIBITION OF
LPS-INDUCED MATURATION

The inhibition of mitogen stimulation by anti-Ig is concentration dependent. If anti-Ig antibodies act directly on B cells by binding to surface Ig, and if this primary ligand–receptor interaction is of high affinity and is a prerequisite for inhibition to occur, then changes in the concentration of receptors, i.e., number of cells/ml, should result in altered requirements for anti-Ig antibody concentrations needed for inhibition.

The minimum concentration of anti-Ig antibodies required for (99.9%) inhibition of LPS-induced maturation of B cells was determined in limiting dilution assays under conditions where, in the absence of anti-Ig, mitogen will induce clonal growth and differentiation to plaque-forming cells in one-third of all cultured B cells. As can be seen in Fig. 2, diluting the cells over the range from 10^5/ml down to 10^1/ml allowed anti-Ig antibodies dilution from 10^3 to 10^{-12} to achieve the same inhibitory effect.

THE EFFECT OF SERUM Ig ON B CELLS

Mouse serum normally does not activate resting murine B cells. It is often even inhibitory for mitogenic activation of these B cells induced

TABLE II
Stimulation of Normal A/J Spleen Cells by the IgG Fraction of
Normal Mouse Serum

	Amount of protein added (μg/ml)[a]						
	0.125	0.5	2	25	75	150	300
Normal serum	3.7/1.2	3.3/0.5	2.5/0.4	1.8/0.3	1.2/0.09	0.9/0.06	0.7/0.02
Excluded fraction[b] (macroglobulin)	3.2/0.5	4.3/0.4	4.6/0.6	5.8/1.4	6.8/1.6	7.7/2.0	11.8/1.7
IgG fraction[b]	5.4/1.6	9.7/2.9	22.2/7.9	32.8/9.8	41.1/14.8	35.2/13.0	32.7/8.2

[a] Response measured as thymidine uptake on day 2 of cultures containing 2×10^5 spleen cells in 0.2 ml of RPMI medium containing 10% FCS (17) or a total number of Ig secreting cells in the protein A plaque assay (PFC, 20). Values given are thymidine uptake $\times 10^{-3}$/plaque-forming cell $\times 10^{-3}$.

[b] Pooled normal A/J serum was precipitated with 40% saturated ammonium sulphate and chromatographed on Sephadex G 200 in PBS. The excluded fractions and fractions corresponding to an apparent molecular weight of 120,000–180,000 was pooled, concentrated, millipore-filtered, and used in amounts indicated. Response of untreated cells was 3.5/0.2 and cells receiving LPS (50 μg/ml) was 33.4/15.0.

by LPS or LP. However, when it is separated into protein fractions of different molecular weights, either by sucrose gradient centrifugation, by gel filtration or by ion exchange chromatography, B-cell stimulating activities appear, particularly in the fractions which sediment near 7 S IgG and which have apparent molecular weights near 150,000 in gel filtration (Table II). This B-cell activation results in polyclonal growth and in maturation to IgM and IgG secretion, measured by hemolytic plaques in the protein-A plaque assay. The activating activities can be found in sera of different mouse strains, such as A/J, BALB/c, AKR, CSW, and CWB (Table III). Spleen cells of different mouse strains, such as A/J, BALB/c, C57Bl/6J, CSW, CWB, BALB/c, nu/nu, and C56Bl/6J nu/nu are activated. Mature T cells, therefore, are not re-

TABLE III

Effect of Normal Serum IgG and Purified Myeloma Proteins on Growth and Maturation of Normal Spleen Cells[a]

| | Spleen cells from | | | | | | | |
| | CSW | | CWB | | A/J | | AKR | |
Addition	PFC[b]	TdR[b]	PFC	TdR	PFC	TdR	PFC	TdR
0	1.7	3.5	0.9	4.2	0.5	1.3	0.1	0.8
LPS[c]	59.4	37.8	54.3	56.8	31.0	30.3	24.5	24.3
LP[c]	51.8	76.8	26.9	89.2	29.4	42.3	6.6	53.7
A/J IgG[d]	55.9	128.4	53.3	122.1	21.6	57.7	44.7	78.9
CSW IgG	1.7	10.4	1.8	20.8	0.7	4.7	0.3	4.0
CWB IgG	1.7	14.3	2.3	14.2	0.9	3.8	0.1	3.1
AKR IgG	0.8	7.7	0.6	8.4	0.6	2.3	1.1	1.7
BALB/c IgG	1.7	9.2	1.7	11.3	1.3	4.5	1.7	6.3
MOPC 21[e]	4.0	9.1	2.8	9.6	0.6	2.6	0.5	2.6
MOPC 104E	1.8	12.4	1.7	8.8	0.3	2.6	0.1	2.6
H 2020	1.0	4.0	1.3	4.0	0.4	1.3	0.2	1.1
RPC 5	1.3	3.7	1.2	4.3	0.5	1.1	0.1	1.1
FLOPC 21	0.4	3.1	0.9	4.1	0.5	0.9	0.02	0.7
MOPC 195	0.6	4.0	0.8	3.8	0.4	0.9	0.1	0.6
UPC 10	1.5	7.0	1.0	7.3	0.7	2.6	0.001	1.4
MOPC 41	2.1	5.0	1.0	4.9	0.4	1.6	0.3	1.5

[a] Spleen cells were cultured at 5×10^5 cells/ml in RPMI 1640 medium containing 10% FCS. 0.2 ml cultures in Microtiter II plates.

[b] IgM secreting cells (PFC) per $10^5 \times 10^{-3}$ cells determined by the protein-A plaque assay on day 4. Thymidine uptake (TdR) determined on day 2 of culture.

[c] Both at 50 μg/ml.

[d] 50 μg/ml for all normal serum IgG preparations.

[e] Purified myeloma proteins from Bionetics all at 50 μg/ml.

TABLE IV
Removal of the Stimulatory Capacity of IgG Fractions
after Passage through Immunosorbent Columns

Treatment of IgG[a]	Total IgM secreting cells[b] (PFC × 10^{-3})	
	−LPS	+LPS[c]
—	60	48
Anti-μ passed	70	52
Anti-κ passed	8	40
Anti-β-gal passed	60	48

[a] A total of 0.2 ml containing 3.3 mg/ml of protein from an IgG fraction of normal A/J serum was applied to immunosorbent columns of Sepharose-4B coupled gamma globulin fractions from rabbit antisera specific for κ-L or μ-H chains, as well as for *E. coli* β-galactosidase (11). Material not bound was eluted with 2.0 ml PBS, filtered and used in culture at a final protein concentration of 30 μg/ml.

[b] Measured at day 5 of culture. Response expressed as PFC per 10^5 cultured cells. Background response was 8000 and LPS induced 54.000 IgM PFC.

[c] 50 μg/ml.

quired for activation in the spleen cell suspensions. Small, resting B cells can be activated.

A series of experiments indicate that serum 7 S Ig molecules [most of them probably IgG (γ,κ)] are involved in this polyclonal stimulation of B cells. Thus, the mitogenic activity in these preparations is retained in immunoabsorbents with anti-γ-H or anti-κ-L chain specificity, but not with anti-μ-H or other nonIg specificities (Table IV).

DISCUSSION

Antisera raised in different species against mouse immunoglobulin molecules may show different activities on the induction of B lymphocytes by mitogens. One type of antisera specific for μ-heavy chains or κ-light chains *only* affects maturation to Ig secretion and does not inhibit B-cell growth induced by mitogen. Another type of antisera inhibits both growth and maturation of stimulated B cells. Yet a third type of antisera also specific for μ-H chains or μ-H and κ-L chains has no effect on mitogen-induced growth and maturation. Such noninhibitory antisera can be shown to contain antibodies which bind to B cells and precipitate radiolabeled surface immunoglobulin.

We will discuss these findings in the context of a mitogen–receptor complex, which may operate in the induction of B cells.

Since there are anti-Ig antibodies which, in a dose-dependent way, interfere with B-cell induction, it is possible that surface Ig is functionally linked and even structurally associated with mitogen receptors on the outer surface membrane of lymphocytes. Such a complex of structures can exist in different conformations in which it has increased tendencies to associate either with a series of molecules constituting chains of reactions leading to response or another series of molecules constituting chains of reactions leading to suppression of further stimulation.

Response of B lymphocytes manifests itself by growth and/or by maturation to Ig secretion. The difference in activity between the different antisera inhibiting either growth *and* secretion or *only* secretion may merely reflect a difference in occupancy of surface Ig molecules by the various anti-Ig antibodies. Thus, high occupancy could favor mitogen-induced reactions leading to suppression of both growth and maturation, whereas intermediate occupancy of Ig molecules in the membrane would only inhibit maturation to Ig secretion but would allow for induction of growth. The results (Table I), anyhow, suggest that reactions leading to maturation are different from reactions leading to growth and that they can be distinguished through the action of some anti-Ig antibodies.

Alternatively, the distinct properties of the various types of antisera may not be the result of an active process of inducing suppressive reactions, but rather to interference with B-cell induction at the membrane level—in which case both growth and maturation would be inhibited—or somewhere along the mitogen-induced pathway leading to Ig synthesis.

The finding that normal mouse IgG is stimulatory for normal, small, resting B cells, even in syngeneic conditions, is intriguing. A number of samples of IgG, obtained from sera of different strains of normal mice and prepared either by gel filtration methods or by ion exchange chromatography were all found to be mitogenic for B cells. The extent of stimulation however, did not correlate with the amount of IgG in the different preparation nor with the distribution of subclasses in the various IgG fractions. Therefore the mitogenic activity is not a property of every IgG molecule, but rather it is due to a particular component contained in the IgG fraction. Because of the absorption data (Table IV), we conclude that the stimulation is due to molecules containing

κ-light chainlike antigenic determinants and a molecular weight of 150,000. We suggest, therefore, that these are 7 S Ig molecules which are a regular component of normal mouse serum. Some, but not all, of the purified myeloma proteins tested were found to be mitogenic for B cells (Table II). This could be due to contaminating normal serum IgG, since the myeloma tumors were grown *in vivo* and the proteins were isolated from serum of tumor-bearing mice. On the other hand, if the stimulatory molecules of IgG are derived from normal background Ig secreting cells, it is possible that such cells could also be subject to malignant transformation into plasma cell tumors producing stimulatory molecules.

The presence of large numbers of Ig secreting cells (up to 1% of all lymphocytes) and high levels of serum Ig in normal or nude mice, bred under conventional or germfree conditions, indicates that activation of natural antibody secreting cells is not dependent on stimulation by antigen nor on internal T-cell activities. Our finding that molecules in normal serum IgG fractions can stimulate normal resting B cells to grow into clones of Ig producing cells would offer an explanation for the origin of such background, Ig secreting cells. Furthermore, the existence of stimulatory antibodies would provide a mechanism by which the B-cell system is competent of self-stimulation and thereby of controlling the development of its own clonal members.

Since the binding of normal serum 7 S Ig molecules to B cells is stimulatory, they are, by definition, specific ligands for mitogen receptors on B cells. Two general types of such molecules can be envisaged:

(1) Antibodies with combining sites specific for mitogen receptors
(2) Molecules with structures, other than the combining site, complementary to mitogen receptors—such as subgroup specific determinants or idiotypes, or even constant region determinants

If stimulatory molecules are, in fact, antibodies to mitogen receptors, the epitopes recognized may be of two distinct categories which are important to distinguish from a genetic point of view:

(1) Mitogen receptors encoded by germlike genes of the mouse, such as the receptor for LPS, mapped on chromosome 4
(2) Viral products, encoded by episomal genes of a virus, being expressed on the B-cell membrane and behaving functionally as a mitogen receptor

Thus, viral infection of B lymphocytes leading to the expression of gP70 in the surface membrane has been found to render these B cells susceptible to stimulation by anti-gP70 antibodies. This suggests that products of endogenous viruses may become parts of mitogen receptor complexes of the host. Episomal genes introduced through infection may, therefore, influence B-cell growth and development.

On the other hand, the structures of mitogen receptors, encoded for by germlike genes of the mouse, are at present unknown. However, it has recently been suggested (16) that they may carry determinants cross-reactive with known antibody idiotypes. An extension of this speculation suggests that, in fact, a given germline mitogen receptor is recognized by at least one of the V_H–V_L genes carried in the germ line.

The stimulatory 7 S Ig molecules present in normal serum could either be induced by external influence (i.e., virus infection) in which case the likely targets on B-cell membranes are viral products, or they could be naturally occurring during the development of the immune system, a likely possibility if they have a germline origin.

Along these lines, it would follow that some germline V_H and V_L genes could code for antibodies with binding sites specific for viral (and bacterial) products introduced through symbiosis in an episomal way. In this case, these germline V_H and V_L genes may as well be expressed as "natural" antibodies and thereby constitute the normal serum 7 S Ig molecules, which we find to be mitogenic.

Alternatively, the original specificities of V_H and V_L germline-encoded gene products could be directed to growth-regulating molecules (mitogen receptors) expressed on B cells, also germline encoded. Since the latter are endogenous to the organism and would necessarily be expressed on the cell surface membrane at a given point in development, those postulated germline antibody specificities would ensure the conditions necessary to drive precursor cells into proliferation, allowing thereby for accumulation of mutatnts which could be selected for in a number of ways. This postulate for a set of germ line antibody specificities would allow the regulation of B-cell development, and in a closed system which does not depend on external influence and would also offer an alternative explanation for the finding of natural mitogenic IgG molecules in normal mouse serum.

At the present time we have little knowledge of the cellular structures in the microenvironment where B lymphocytes develop and no information on which genes control the expression of these structures and, therefore, the development of B cells. It should be noted that the speculations of idiotype-bearing mitogen receptors as the genetic nature of such structures is only one of many possibilities and that other gene products *not* encoded for by V_H/V_L genes, but recognized by them, are equally likely.

From all these speculations, it appears clear that we need to know more of the structures, i.e., the receptors, which regulate growth and maturation of B cells and more of the genes which control the various components of them. It may also well be fruitful to have a new look into the interactions of the immune system with viruses and bacteria, which would appear to influence B cell function (and development) in a fashion paralleled by the MHC determination of T cell functions and development.

ACKNOWLEDGMENTS

The assistance of Deborrah Norman, Margaretha Tuneskog, and Luciana Forni is gratefully acknowledged. Jan Andersson was supported by the Swedish Cancer Society.

REFERENCES

1. Möller, G. (ed.) (1972) *Transplant. Rev.* **1**.
2. Andersson, J., Sjöberg, O., and Möller, G. (1972) *Eur. J. Immunol.* **2**, 349.
3. Melchers, F., Braun, V., and Galanos, C. (1975) *J. Exp. Med.* **142**, 473.
4. Coutinho, A., and Möller, G. (1973) *Nature (London), New Biol.* **245**, 12.
5. Rietschel, E. R., Gottert, H., Lüderitz, O., and Westphal, O. (1972) *Eur. J. Biochem.* **28**, 166.
6. Braun, V., and Rehn, K. (1974) *Eur. J. Biochem.* **30**, 426.
7. Watson, J., and Riblet, R. (1974) *J. Exp. Med.* **140**, 1147.
8. Coutinho, A., Möller, G., and Gronowicz, E. (1975) *J. Exp. Med.* **142**, 253.
9. Watson, J., Largen, M., and McAdam, K. P. W. J. (1978) *J. Exp. Med.* **147**, 39.
10. Coutinho, A., and Meo, T. (1978) *Immunogenetics* **7**, 17.
11. Andersson, J., Bullock, W. W., and Melchers, F. (1974) *Eur. J. Immunol.* **4**, 715.
12. Kearney, J. E. M., Cooper, M. D., and Lawton, A. R. (1976) *J. Immunol.* **116**, 1664.
13. Andersson, J., and Melchers, F. (1977) In "Dynamic Aspects of Cell Surface Organization" (G. Poste and G. L. Nicholson, eds.), pp. 601–618. Elsevier, Amsterdam.
14. Forni, L., and Coutinho, A. (1978) *Eur. J. Immunol.* **8**, 56.
15. Coutinho, A., Forni, L., and Watanabe, T. (1978) *Eur. J. Immunol.* **8**, 63.
16. Coutinho, A., Forni, L., and Blomberg, B. (1978) *J. Exp. Med.* **148**, 862.
17. Melchers, F., Coutinho, A., Heinrich, G., and Andersson, J. (1975) *Scand. J. Immunol.* **4**, 853.
18. Andersson, J., Coutinho, A., Lernhardt, W., and Melchers, F. (1977) *Cell* **10**, 27.
19. Andersson, J., Coutinho, A., and Melchers, F. (1977) *J. Exp. Med.* **145**, 1511.
20. Gronowicz, E., Coutinho, A., and Melchers, F. (1976) *Eur. J. Immunol.* **6**, 588.

Role of the Fc Portion of Antibody in Immune Regulation

WILLIAM O. WEIGLE AND MONIQUE A. BERMAN

Department of Immunopathology
Scripps Clinic and Research Foundation
La Jolla, California

INTRODUCTION

INHIBITION OF THE ANTIBODY RESPONSE WITH PASSIVE ANTIBODY

Complexes formed between antigen and antibody clearly have biological activity in that they initiate pharmacological reactions resulting in tissue injury (reviewed in Weigle *et al.*, 1–3). Furthermore, detection of antigen–antibody complexes in the circulation is commonly used as an indication of autoimmune disorders (3). Such complexes have now been implicated as part of the intricate regulatory mechanisms involved in control of the immune response. Supportive evidence lies in the ability of passive antibody to suppress an immune response and the importance of the time interval between the administration of antibody and challenge with antigen in promoting such suppression (reviewed in Uhr *et al.*, 4,5). That the regulatory role involves the interaction of antibody with antigen is further evidenced by the fact that only passive antibody specific for the antigen in question induces suppression. The ability of passive antibody to suppress an immune response is also influenced by both the class (6) and affinity of antibody (5). It was first postulated that passive antibody functions by masking specific antigenic determinants, thus inhibiting their presentation to receptors on lymphocytes. Cerottini and co-workers (7,8) demonstrated that antibody directed to certain determinants on protein antigens inhibited the *in vivo* response to these determinants, but not to unrelated determinants on the same molecule. They also re-

ported that the F(ab)₂ fragment of antibody was as effective in inhibiting thymus-dependent immune responses as was intact IgG antibody
(8). Similarly, Feldmann and Diener (9) demonstrated that the F(ab)₂
fragment of IgG antibody inhibited the *in vitro* thymus-independent
response as well as the intact antibody did. On the other hand, others
reported that the Fc fragment was required for inhibition of both the *in
vivo* and *in vitro* immune responses by passive antibody (10–17). Kappler *et al.* (15) found that passive antibody to one determinant inhibited the immune response both to that determinant and to unrelated
determinants on the same molecule. Since neither the F(ab)₂ fragment
of rabbit antibody nor intact chicken antibody suppressed the response, the latter authors concluded that the Fc fragment was required. Of special interest was the point that a dose of antiserum
which severely suppressed the development of antibodies to sheep
red blood cells (SRBC) did not prevent the increase in specific helper
T cells (16). As a result of similar data, Chan and Sinclair (18) postulated that the F(ab)₂ fragment of antibody suppressed immune responses by simple masking of antigen, whereas intact IgG antibody
altered the immune responses through a further activity involving the
Fc region and occurring after the antigen and antibody interacted.
Along similar lines, Hoffmann and Kappler (19) postulated two mechanisms of antibody-mediated suppression of antibody production.
They suggested that one mechanism operates at low concentrations of
antibody and depends on the Fc portion of antibody, while the other
requires high concentrations of antibody and is independent of the Fc
portion. Suppression through the latter mechanism could be mediated
by intact rabbit antibody, the F(ab)₂ fragment of rabbit antibody or
chicken antibody while the former could be initiated only by intact
rabbit antibody (19). Furthermore, B cells are not directly affected
since inhibition with low concentrations of intact antibody to the carrier in a protein–hapten conjugate had no effect on the response to that
hapten combined with an unrelated carrier. Thus, since the mediator
of suppression does not directly affect either the T or B cells, passive
antibody apparently interferes with interactions between T and B
cells. One might therefore predict that interference with thymus-
independent responses would not be mediated by low doses of antibody requiring the Fc piece. Indeed, Feldmann and Diener (9) found
that the Fc piece in IgG antibody was not required for the inhibition of
the *in vitro* response to polymerized flagellin (thymus independent).
    It is of particular interest in characterizing immune regulation that
the Fc portion is required for allotypic suppression (20,21) and for the
suppression of specific immune responses by anti-idiotypic antibody

(22,23). More recently it was reported that guinea pig anti-idiotypic antibody could suppress (IgG_2) or amplify (IgG_1) the immune response in mice depending on the class of anti-idiotypic antibody (23). In view of the postulated role for anti-idiotypic suppression in the network theory (24–27), the interaction of the Fc portion of antibody complexed with antigen and lymphocytes may be a critical event in immune regulation.

ENHANCEMENT OF THE ANTIBODY RESPONSE WITH PASSIVE ANTIBODY

Although emphasis has been placed on the suppression of the immune response by passive antibody, enhancement has also been reported by a number of investigators. Such enhancement has been observed with isoantigens in the rabbit (28) and both particulate (29–33) and soluble antigens (34–40) in mice. Walker and Siskind (5) demonstrated that low concentrations of high affinity antibody to the dinitrophenyl (DNP) hapten enhanced antibody responses to DNP, and Pincus et al. (40) observed that relatively small doses of antiserum to bovine serum albumin (BSA) in mice injected with DNP–BSA resulted in enhanced responses to both the DNP hapten and BSA. In other experiments, passive antibody to the $F(ab)_2$ fragment of human gamma globulin (HGG) inhibited the anti-$F(ab)_2$ response, but enhanced the response to Fc (41). Murgita and Vas (6) observed suppression of the immune response in mice to SRBC at all concentrations of IgG_1 antibody, while suppression with IgG_2 antibody was observed only with high concentrations and enhancement was found at low concentrations. In contrast to the suppressive effect reported by others, Uyeki and Klassen (32) reported that passive antibody enhanced the production of antibody to SRBC. In monkeys, Houston et al. (42) used passive antibody to enhance the immune response to Venezuelan equine encephalomyelitis virus. That passive antibody suppressed the humoral response while enhancing delayed type hypersensitivity (43), suggests that antibody reacts at different sites.

REGULATION BY ANTIGEN–ANTIBODY COMPLEXES

Since the inhibition or enhancement of the immune response is dependent on the time intervening between administration of passive antibody and antigen, as mentioned above, it is not surprising that complexes of antigen and antibody are effective in both suppression (14) and enhancement (39). A series of experiments on antibody inhibition led Bystryn *et al.* (44) to propose that antibody production to both persisting and readily catabolized antigens is controlled via a dynamic equilibrium among circulating antibody, antigen, and antigen–antibody complexes throughout the extracellular compartment. Thus, one should expect that both suppression (45) and enhancement (37) depend on the antigen–antibody ratio of the complexes. Chan and Sinclair (18) postulated that antigen–antibody complexes destroy antibody forming cells as a mechanism of antibody-mediated suppression. Kontiainen (46) observed that antigen–antibody complexes formed *in vivo* and maintained for long periods of time were instrumental in blocking the antibody response. Similarly, the continued presence of circulating antigen–antibody complexes resulted in a tolerant state to the antigen (47). Certain antigen–antibody complexes can also enhance (48) or inhibit (48–51) *in vitro* lymphocyte transformation. Experiments by Sidman and Unanue (51) implicated the Fc piece of IgG in such complex induced inhibition. The latter workers observed that the Fc fragment was required in order for anti-immunoglobulin to inhibit the proliferative response of B cells to lipopolysaccharide. Activation of guinea pig B cells by anti-immunoglobulin also required the Fc piece (52). Studies on direct activation of normal, unsensitized lymphocytes by antigen–antibody complexes have produced conflicting results. Block–Shtacher *et al.* (53) and Möller (54) reported that antigen–antibody complexes could stimulate DNA synthesis in normal human peripheral blood lymphocytes. However, this finding could not be repeated with mouse lymphocytes (54–56), and it was concluded that lymphocytes were not directly activated via the Fc receptor. More recently, Soderberg and Coons (57) showed activation of rabbit lymphocytes by antigen–antibody complexes which required complement. A possible role for complement in the activation of T cells has been well documented (58–60), especially in thymus-dependent antibody responses (58–61).

Although the majority of the available data on regulation of the immune response by antigen–antibody complexes is concerned with the humoral response, cell-mediated immunity can also be modulated by such complexes (62–65). Mackaness and co-workers (64,65) have investigated a model in which immunization procedures favoring the induction of humoral immunity interfere with generation of delayed type hypersensitivity (DTH). It appears that a product of the interaction between antigen and antibody blocks activated T cells without interfering with helper T cells. This is somewhat expected, since passive antibody does not interfere with priming of helper T cells while suppressing the humoral response (16,19). The question in the studies of Mackaness *et al.* is whether suppression of cellular immunity is mediated by the interaction of the Fc site with T cells or by the interference with antigen presentation to specific receptors. Sinclair *et al.* (63) have more recently demonstrated that *in vitro* and *in vivo* sensitization of mouse T cells with allogeneic cells is suppressed by antibody specific for the sensitizing cells. Suppression of cell-mediated immunity generated in this model does not require the Fc fragment. Thus, it is not clear at the present time if complex-mediated suppression of cellular immunity involves the Fc piece, and if so, whether the mechanism of suppression is the same as that involved in humoral immunity.

Fc RECEPTORS ON LYMPHOCYTES

The necessity of the Fc piece for modulation of the immune response by antigen and antibody complexes implicated an interaction between this fragment and receptor sites on appropriate cells. That lymphocytes have a strong affinity for these complexes was first demonstrated by Uhr and Phillips (66,67). Antigen–antibody complexes, aggregated IgG, and at times IgG itself were shown to bind to lymphocytes by rosette formation with antibody-coated erythrocytes, autoradiography, and immunofluorescence. Since a requirement for binding was an intact immunoglobulin containing the Fc piece, it was assumed that the binding lymphocytes contained Fc receptors (67–73). Although it is clear that most lymphocytes with Ig receptors (67,70,72,74–86) are much more active in binding than those without, the distribution of Fc receptors on B cells, T cells, and thymus cells varies from one report to another (reviewed in Dickler, 87). Basten and co-workers (69) observed that 25% of mouse peripheral lymphocytes with T cell markers contained Fc receptors (FcR+) as detected by aggregated immunoglobulin and antigen–antibody complexes, whereas FcR+ T cells in the thymus could be detected only with aggregates and no FcR+ cells were present in the thoracic duct lymphocytes (69). It was concluded that the FcR+ T cells were a subpopulation of noncirculating T cells. Kramer *et al.* (81) were also unable to find FcR+ cells in the thoracic duct lymphocytes. Anderson and Grey (88), using aggregated myelomas, reported that 80% of B cells, 30% of T cells, and 60% of null cells were FcR+ while Stout and Herzenberg (89) detected 23% of spleen T cells and 10% of thymus cells as FcR+. Parish (90), using depletion of FcR+ cells by rosette formation, found lower numbers of FcR+ cells in T, B, and null cells. Other workers were either unable to detect FcR+ cells in peripheral T cells or in thymus cells or detected them at lower levels (reviewed in Dickler, 87).

It appears that the affinity of binding to B cells of immunoglobulin via the Fc portion is considerably greater than binding to T cells. This conclusion is reflected in the ability of ^{125}I-labeled aggregated immunoglobulin to cause suicide of B cells but not T cells (91) and the ability of large but not small aggregates of immunoglobulin to detect FcR+ T cells (88). In any event, it is well established that activated T cells show an increased level of FcR+ cells (73,81,92–94). In contrast, fully differentiated B cells (antibody-forming cells) lose their Fc receptors (67,72,95,96). Although the ontogeny of the development of FcR on T or B cells is not well documented, it has been reported that immature B cells contain Fc receptors (80). In the human, Hayward and Greaves (97) found a reduced level of FcR+ cells in fetal spleen cells in comparison to Ig+ cells, while neonatal spleens appear to have a normal complement of FcR+ cells, and only a few of these were Ig+ (98). On the other hand, Sidman and Unanue (99) reported that the percentage of lymphocytes binding Ig was low in neonatal mouse spleens and approximately equal to that which bore surface Ig. Others have reported that the Fc receptor on mice does not appear on B cells until birth, although cells bearing Fc receptors are present in fetal liver at all stages (100).

Binding via the Fc receptor of lymphocytes is dependent on the immunoglobulin class as shown by Basten et al. (67), who observed that mouse IgG bound better to mouse B cells than IgM; IgG_1 bound better than IgG_2, and IgA failed to bind. Anderson and Grey (101), who also failed to observe binding with IgA in the mouse, reported that the affinity of binding to established T cell lines and spleen T and B cells was $IgG_1 > Ig_{2a} \geqslant IgG_{2b}$. The diverse functional effects of mouse IgG_1 and IgG_2 may reflect their differences in binding capacity since Murgita and Vas (6) reported that IgG_1 inhibited the in vitro response to SRBC better than IgG_2 did. A similar preferential binding to mouse lymphocytes was obtained with IgG subclass proteins aggregated with bis-diazotized benzidine (102). Although the cells have a considerably greater affinity for immunoglobulin when it is either aggregated or in the form of antigen–antibody complexes than for free immunoglobulin, the binding of monomeric preparations of Ig has been reported (reviewed in Dickler, 87). Klein et al. (93) reported comparable binding of human IgG_1, IgG_2, and IgG_3, but not IgG_4 to mouse T lymphocytes. Moretta et al. (103) reported that human peripheral blood T cells had Fc receptors for both IgG and IgM proteins, while Lamon et al. (104) found mouse T and B cells with receptors for

IgM antibody-coated erythrocytes. Lawrence *et al.* (105) examined human peripheral blood cells and observed that lymphocytes bound unaggregated human IgG_1 and IgG_3 proteins, but not IgG_2, or IgG_4 or immunoglobulins of the other classes. In contrast, after aggregation, IgG of all subclasses and IgE proteins bound to lymphocytes; aggregated immunoglobulins of the other classes did not bind. Ramasamy *et al.* (106) showed that although monomeric mouse IgG_1 and IgG_2 bound to lymphocytes, aggregated preparations bound more effectively. IgM bound either weakly or not at all.

An obvious question is where on the Fc portion of the IgG is the peptide sequence responsible for reaction with the Fc receptor. It is reasonably well established that the chains of IgG are folded into compact domains, each corresponding to one of the homology regions apparent in the primary structure (107). Although the Fc portion appears to be responsible for the nonspecific biological activities of the IgG molecules, the site involved in each of these activities may not be the same. The $C\gamma2$ domain of IgG has been implicated as the region in which the Cl_q reactive site (108) and site for catabolic regulation (109) are located, while the Fc site for the receptors on macrophages (109,110) and mast cells apparently resides in the $C\gamma3$ domain. Ramasamy *et al.* (106) presented evidence that the $C\gamma3$ region was required for reaction with lymphocyte Fc receptors and observed that an IgG_1 mutant protein lacking the $C\gamma3$ domain failed to bind. Klein *et al.* (93) observed that binding of the Fc fragment of human IgG_1 was not affected by mild reduction and that binding to T cells resided in the $C\gamma3$ domain between Gln_{342} and His_{433}. The monomeric $C\gamma2$ domain also showed binding, but it was tenfold less active than the $C\gamma3$ domain. It was suggested that the $C\gamma2$ and $C\gamma3$ domains may contribute to the formation of a cooperative binding site through quaternary interdomain interactions. It may be that the Fc site responsible for different functions of lymphocytes may also be different. Spiegelberg *et al.* (111), who investigated the reactivity of human IgG proteins with K cells in antibody-dependent cell cytotoxicity (ADCC), suggested two binding sites; one having triggering (enhancing) activity located on the $C\gamma2$ domain and one having high affinity binding located on the $C\gamma3$ domain. The complexity of the Fc regions expressing biological functions is further evidenced by the failure of either the $C\gamma2$ or $C\gamma3$ domains of IgG_1 to bind to the Fc placental receptor. MacLennan (112) presented evidence that the last 107 C-terminal amino acids of rabbit IgG were required to activate ADCC. Differential digestion of the antibody with pepsin and plasmin suggested two different sites were involved in Fc binding to complement and Fc receptors. Whatever the reactive site on IgG may be, it is apparently shared by other mammalian IgG molecules as evidenced by the absence of species-specific barriers in interactions with Fc receptors. On the other hand, it has been reported that aggregated fowl gamma globulin does not bind to receptors on mammalian lymphocytes (88), which is in accord with the failure of passive chicken antibody to inhibit the immune response in mice (17). Similarly, chicken lymphocytes do not bind to the Fc portion of mammalian immunoglobulins (113).

The physical conformation of aggregated IgG apparently dictates to some extent the degree of binding to the Fc receptors. Dickler and Kunkel (70) observed that aggregates of large sizes were optimal in binding to Fc receptors. Anderson and Grey (88) used aggregated myeloma IgG proteins and reported that aggregates of 100 molecules were optimal and that aggregates of 6–25 molecules could bind to splenocytes but not to thymocytes. Segal and Hurwitz (114), who used cross-linked rabbit IgG antibodies to determine affinity of binding to lymphocytes, observed that the binding affinity of trimers was stronger than that of dimers, and dimers bound more efficiently than monomers (115). However, as the size of the oligomers was increased, the binding affinity decreased. Thus, the size of antigen–antibody complexes is apparently critical for both suppression (116) and enhancement (38) of the humoral response.

Although antigen–antibody complexes in the presence of complement can bind to lymphocytes and macrophages through the C3 receptor (reviewed in Nussenzweig, 117), complement is not required for the binding of such complexes or aggregated IgG via the Fc receptor (68,70–72,88). However, complement has been shown to either amplify or inhibit binding via the Fc receptor (90), apparently because binding to C3 receptors occurs concomitantly. With this point in mind, it should be mentioned that 70% of spleen cells from normal and nude mice have receptors for both C3 and Fc sites. In view of the data implicating both complement and antibody in regulation of the humoral response, synergy in regulation via interaction of immunoglobulin with Fc and C3 receptors is not unlikely.

In addition to an association with the C3 receptor (CR), the Fc receptor has a close relationship to other surface markers, at least, on B lymphocytes. The majority of immunoglobulin positive B lymphocytes are FcR+. On the other hand, Fc and immunoglobulin receptors are distinct cell surface antigens (68,118,119), and each can be modulated independently of the other (119). Fc receptors on mouse B lymphocytes have also been related to antigens in the *H-2* complex. Antibodies directed against Ia antigens determined by I region genes inhibited the binding of immunoglobulin complexes to B lymphocytes (120–123). This inhibition was specific in that the Fc portion of the anti-Ia was not required, and antibodies against antigens determined by the K and D regions of the H-2 complex did not produce such inhibition. However, it was shown that capping of B lymphocyte-bound complexes did not lead to redistribution of Ia antigens and that binding of complexed immunoglobulin to B lymphocytes under non-capping conditions did not sterically hinder the detection of surface Ia by anti-Ia (124). Thus, it appears that Ia antigens do not lie in close physical proximity to B cell Fc receptors and that inhibition of Fc binding with anti-Ia results from a ligand-induced alteration of Ia antigens, which leads to interaction with the Fc receptors. However, there is evidence that the Fc receptor is linked to an antigen controlled by the M1s locus (125,126). The close association of Ia and FcR markers is not as apparent in certain non-B cells. Nelson *et al.* (127) presented data which indicated that the FcR+ cell (Ig−) involved in antibody-dependent cell cytotoxicity was Ia−.

IMMUNOLOGIC FUNCTION OF FcR+ LYMPHOCYTES

Although convincing evidence strongly implicates the Fc receptor as part of the regulatory mechanism that controls immune responses, the role of FcR+ cells in various parameters of the immune system has not been fully examined (128). Although it appears that helper T cells are FcR− cells (129,130), the status of antibody-precursor B cells is controversial. Parish (85,90) reported that depletion of Fc receptor bearing cells by rosette formation markedly diminished both primary and secondary PFC in mice. However, similar experiments in the rat (90) showed that depletion of FcR+ lymphocytes had no effect. Basten *et al.* (91) observed that when spleen cells from mice primed to several antigens were exposed to highly labeled radioactive aggregates, their capacity to transfer both a direct and indirect plaque-forming cell response to these antigens was abrogated. More recently, Miyama *et al.* (130) reported that the majority of precursor B cells in the primary response to a thymus-dependent and a thymus-independent antigen and a secondary thymus-dependent response were FcR−. On the other hand, it has been suggested that suppressor T cells are a sub-population of FcR+ T lymphocytes (16,19). It may be that antigen–antibody complexes that form *in vivo* and which persist for long periods of time interact with T cells resulting in the generation of suppressor activity (46,131–133). Moreover, alloantigen-activated suppressor cells were also shown to be FcR+ (134). Fridman and Golstein (135) demonstrated a receptor for IgG that is shed from activated mouse T cells and which they called immunoglobulin binding factor (IBF). IBF released from alloantigen-activated mouse T cells binds to the Fc portion of IgG and inhibits 19 and 7 S antibody responses (136). It was suggested that the IBF acts on differentiating B cells. Moretta *et al.* (137), who previously reported that human peripheral T cells bound erythrocytes coated with IgM antibody (EA-IgM), suggested that T cells with receptors for IgG (T_G) had suppressor activity while T cells with receptors for IgM (T_M) had helper activity (136). The model used by these investigators was pokeweed mitogen-induced differentiation of B lymphocytes. This finding contrasts with the results of others who failed to find FcR+ helper T cells in mice (129,130). A further association of suppressor and FcR+ T cells may be inferred by the differential response of FcR− and FcR+ cells to concanavalin A (Con A). Although both FcR+ and FcR− mouse T cells isolated on the fluorescence activated cell sorter respond to phytohemagglutinin, the response to Con A is characteristic of FcR+ lymphocytes (129).

The best documented association of FcR+ cells with an immunological event is that observed with ADCC. The Fc portion is required in ADCC since its removal from the antibody results in the loss of ADCC activity (113). Pape *et al.* (138,139) observed that effector cells (K) involved in ADCC are Ig− and FcR+ and that the Fc receptors on Ig+ cells were qualitatively different from those on K cells. Similarly, Kay *et al.* (140), working with human peripheral blood cells, reported that natural killer (NK) cells and effector (K) cells in ADCC are overlapping populations of FcR+ T lymphocytes. Hurwitz *et al.* (141) have also shown that FcR+ cells are effective in ADCC, whereas FcR− cells are ineffective. These observations are in agreement with those showing that heat (142,143) and chemically (111) aggregated preparations of IgG markedly inhibited ADCC. Larsson *et al.* (144) reported inhibition of ADCC with human IgG subclasses. More recently, Spiegelberg *et al.* (111) reported that preparations of IgG_1 and IgG_3 markedly inhibited ADCC, while IgG_2 and IgG_4 were less effective. Likewise, IgG_1 and IgG_3 coated columns were capable of removing ADCC activity from lymphocyte preparations. Although aggregated preparations of IgG_2 and IgG_4 showed increased inhibition of ADCC, small amounts of unaggregated IgG_2 and IgG_4 enhanced ADCC and their Fc fragments caused lysis of target cells in the absence of antibody. These observations suggested that two active sites were present on the Fc portion (possibly involving two receptors); one having a triggering action and the other having high affinity binding activity.

The presence of two Fc receptors involved in ADCC was previously suggested by Dickler (118).

Alloantigen-activated T cells possessing cytotoxic activity were also reported to be FcR+ (145,146), but modulation of the Fc receptors from the surface of the cells did not reverse the cytotoxic activity (146). FcR+ cells appear not to be involved in the mixed lymphocyte culture (MLC) since no distinction in the MLC-stimulated T cell population could be made on the basis of Fc receptors (147).

Macrophages also contain surface receptors for the Fc portion of immunoglobulin. Boyden and Sorkin (148,149) were the first to demonstrate cytophilic antibody for macrophages. Berken and Benacerraf (150) characterized this antibody as IgG and showed that binding occurred by the Fc fragment. Uhr and Phillips (66) and Rabinovitch (151) also demonstrated that the Fc portion of IgG was a requisite for binding of antigen–antibody complexes to macrophages. LoBuglio et $al.$ (152) reported an Fc requirement for fixation of human anti-red blood cell antibody to human monocytes and Hay et $al.$ (153) showed this binding to be a property of IgG_1 and IgG_3 subclasses of human IgG. Walker (154,155) presented data which suggested that macrophages possess two different Fc receptors; one that binds single IgG molecules and one which only binds aggregated IgG. Similarly, Unkeless (156) presented data that implicated two receptors for IgG on macrophages. One receptor was reactive with mouse IgG_2, while the other bound rabbit antigen–antibody complexes. These two receptors differ in their sensitivity to trypsin. Additional evidence for two distinct Fc receptors on macrophages was presented by Heusser et $al.$ (102), who suggested that one receptor was specific for monomeric IgG_{2a}, and also bound aggregated IgG_{2a}, and another receptor was reactive with aggregated preparations of all three IgG subclasses as well as monomeric IgG_{2b}. The presence of two Fc receptors on macrophages, one capable of binding monomeric IgG_{2a}, was also proposed by Segal and Titus (115). In a comprehensive study, Unkeless and Eisen (157), using mouse myelomas and peritoneal exudate cells, demonstrated that IgG_{2a} bound strongly to macrophages while IgG_{2b} bound weakly and IgM, IgA, and IgG_1 did not bind. As shown by others, in these latter studies the Fc fragment was required for macrophage binding. Reaction of macrophages with antibody (complexed with antigen) has been shown to cause specific suppression of the immune response (158,159), suggesting a role for Fc receptors on macrophages as part of the regulatory system of humoral immunity.

In addition to the possible role of Fc in the regulation of the immune response by macrophages, the Fc site and its reaction with Fc receptors is associated with phagocytosis and cytolysis by mononuclear cells. Huber and co-workers (160,161) showed that phagocytosis and cytolysis of isologous red blood cells coated with antibody by human monocytes was the result of IgG rather than IgM antibody and did not require complement. In this study, IgG_1 and IgG_3 proteins, but not IgG_2 and IgG_4, bound to the human monocytes. Larsson *et al.* (144) observed that initiation of phagocytosis of chicken erythrocytes coated with antibody also occurred with human IgG_1 and IgG_3 proteins but not with either IgG_2 or IgG_4 proteins.

ACTIVATION OF B LYMPHOCYTES BY THE Fc PORTION OF IMMUNOGLOBULIN

PROLIFERATIVE RESPONSE TO ANTIGEN–ANTIBODY COMPLEXES

As evidenced by the uptake of ^{3}H-thymidine *in vitro,* mouse spleen cells undergo a proliferative response in the presence of antigen–

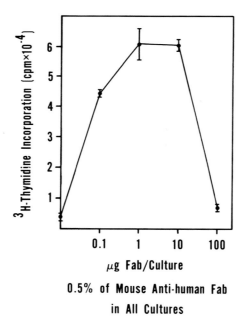

0.5% of Mouse Anti-human Fab

in All Cultures

Fig. 1. Stimulation of DNA synthesis in normal mouse spleen cells by antigen–antibody complexes. 5×10^5 A/J spleen cells were cultured in triplicate in 0.2 ml RPMI medium supplemented with fresh L-glutamine, vitamins, and 5×10^{-5} *M* 2-ME and pulsed with 1 μCi ^{3}H-thymidine on day 4 and harvested on day 5.

antibody complexes formed after the separate addition of antigen and antibody to the cultures (Fig. 1). These complexes were formed between the Fab fragment of human IgG and mouse anti-Fab. No stimulation occurred with Fab fragments added with normal mouse serum. Although complexes in both antibody and antigen excess were effective, the complexes in antigen excess appear to be more stimulatory. On the other hand, complexes formed in large antigen excess (2000×) caused no significant stimulation. These observations contrast with the fact that others failed to observe a proliferative effect of antigen–antibody complexes on mouse B cells (54,55), although Block–Shtacher *et al.* (53) and Möller (54) have reported that complexes did stimulate DNA synthesis in human peripheral blood cells. The effect of antigen dose and, in all likelihood, complex size on the proliferative response to antigen–antibody complexes again emphasizes the importance of complex size in both suppression (116) and enhancement (38) of the humoral response. Aggregate size is also critical in the binding of aggregated mouse IgG myeloma proteins to T and B cells (88). In addition, Segal and Hurwitz (114), working with cross-linked rabbit IgG, reported that trimers fixed to lymphocytes better than dimers or monomers; however, with an increase in the oligomer size, inhibition was observed.

PROLIFERATIVE RESPONSE TO Fc FRAGMENTS

Not only can immunoglobulin complexed to specific antigen stimulate proliferative responses in mouse spleen cells, but the Fc fragment isolated from human IgG is effective in stimulation (162). Fc fragments obtained by digestion of human IgG with papain cause a proliferative response when added to mouse spleen cells *in vitro*. The kinetics of the response is such that maximal uptake of ^{3}H-thymidine occurs between days 4 and 5 (Fig. 2). The peak response is quite pronounced in that it is five times as high as the response that occurs between days 3 and 4. After day 5, the proliferative response is diminished. The kinetics of the proliferative response to Fc is quite different from that observed with lipopolysaccharide (LPS), which reaches a peak between days 1 and 2 and thereafter slowly declines.

As in binding experiments of others with aggregated IgG and antigen–antibody complexes, the Fab and F(ab)$_2$ fragments of human IgG are inactive in mouse spleen cell cultures, while aggregated IgG induces proliferative activity but of considerably lower intensity than that of the Fc fragment (Fig. 3). The small amount of activity observed with human gamma globulin (HGG) alone is probably insignificant

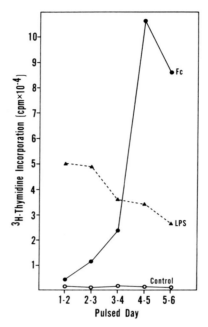

Fig. 2. Kinetics of the proliferative response induced by Fc fragments. Cultures were pulsed with 1 μCi ^{3}H-thymidine for 18 hr following 1, 2, 3, 4, or 5 days of incubation. Spleen cells were cultured alone (O——O), with 10 μg Fc per culture (5 × 10^5 cells in 0.2 ml) (●——●), or with 10 μg lipopolysaccharide (LPS) per culture (▲——▲). From Berman and Weigle (162).

and results from the presence of trace amounts of aggregates, since deaggregated (ultracentrifuge) preparations (DHGG) induce no proliferative activity.

In addition to inducing an *in vitro* proliferative response, Fc fragments cause an *in vitro* polyclonal activation (Table I). Fc added to normal mouse spleen cells results in induction of plaque-forming cells (PFC) to goat red blood cells and the trinitrophenyl (TNP) hapten. This observation is of particular interest since it suggests that the precursor B lymphocytes are FcR+. This observation is in agreement with that of Sidman and Unanue (51) who reported that inhibition of the LPS proliferative response of mouse B cells required the intact anti-Ig molecule, suggesting that the combining (anti-Ig) site and the Fc site react with the respective receptors on the same cells. Although some authors reported that precursor B cells are FcR+ (85,91), others found these precursor B cells to be FcR− (90,130). At the present, it is not

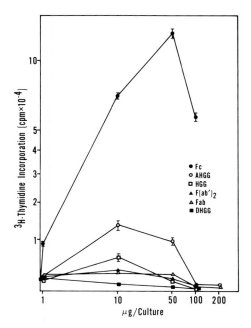

Fig. 3. Stimulation of normal mouse spleen cells with human gamma globulin (HGG) and HGG fragments. Spleen cells were cultured with Fc fragments of HGG (●——●), heat-aggregated HGG (AHGG) (○——○), HGG (□——□), F(ab')₂ fragments of HGG (▲——▲), Fab fragment of HGG (△——△), or deaggregated (by ultracentrifugation) HGG (DHGG) (■——■). Triplicate cultures were pulsed after 4 days of culture and harvested on the fifth day. From Berman and Weigle (162).

clear whether activation of cells by Fc fragments occurs through an Fc receptor or through some other surface interaction. An alternative possibility is that B cells stimulated by polyclonal activators are FcR+ while precursor B cells triggered by antigen may be either FcR− or FcR+. Furthermore, Fc fragments may be able to activate cells which have only few Fc receptors and which are not detected with rosetting reagents.

The addition of Fc fragments to normal spleen cells does not result in an anti-HGG response, which suggests that the proliferative response to the Fc fragment of HGG is nonspecific. This latter point is further emphasized by the ability of human Fc fragments to cause comparable proliferative responses in spleen cells from normal mice and spleen cells from mice in which both the T and B cells were tolerant to HGG. Further evidence that mouse spleen cells respond nonspecifically to the Fc fragment is the observation that the Fc frag-

TABLE I
Antibody Response Induced by Fc Fragments[a]

	Direct PFC/10⁷ cells cultured			Indirect PFC/10⁷
	Anti-HGG[b]	Anti-GRBC	Anti-TNP[c]	Anti-HGG
EXP. 1				
Normal spleen cells control	<1	<1	—	<1
Normal spleen cells + 50 μg Fc/ml	<1	153	—	<1
EXP. 2				
Normal spleen cells control	<1	<1	<1	<1
Normal spleen cells + 150 μg Fc/ml	<1	260	204	<1

[a] A/J spleen cells were cultured with or without Fc in RPMI containing 0.5% mouse serum and harvested for plaquing on day 5.

[b] Plaques against unconjugated GRBC were subtracted from the number of plaques obtained against HGG-conjugated GRBC.

[c] The anti-TNP response was determined against burro red blood cells (BRBC) heavily conjugated with TNP. No plaques to BRBC were detectable.

ment obtained from mouse IgG caused a proliferative response comparable to that observed with Fc from human IgG (Table II). In addition, a proliferative response is seen with Fc fragment obtained from goat IgG but not from turkey IgG. It was previously shown that there was either little or no species restriction in the binding of mammalian immunoglobulin to Fc receptors (cited in Dickler, 87), whereas mammalian lymphocytes were unable to bind fowl immunoglobulin via the Fc receptor (88). Likewise, fowl lymphocytes lack binding receptors for mammalian IgG (113). An exception to the above observation is the failure of the Fc receptor from rabbit IgG to cause a proliferative response with mouse spleen cells. The failure of rabbit Fc fragment to stimulate may be the result of the crystalline state of rabbit Fc when obtained by papain digestion.

EFFECT OF CLASS AND SUBCLASS OF Fc FRAGMENTS

Since the biological activity and lymphocyte binding properties of antigen–antibody complexes are dependent on both the class and subclass of the antibody, similar dependency may be expected for lymphocyte activation by the Fc fragment. In studies using human

TABLE II
Stimulation with Fc Fragments of IgG from Different
Species

	cpm ^{3}H-thymidine uptake (day 4–5)
	Fc (10 μg/culture)^a
Medium (control)	1,737
Human Fc	53,224
Mouse Fc	51,786
Goat Fc	64,028
Turkey Fc	1,802

^{a} 5 × 10^5 A/J spleen cells were cultured in 0.2 ml RPMI (L-glutamine, vitamins, 5 × 10^{-5} M 2-ME, and 0.5% A/J serum added). ^{3}H-thymidine was added on day 4 and harvested on day 5 of culture.

myeloma immunoglobulin, the results of stimulating mouse spleen cells *in vitro* with Fab and Fc fragments were compared. These results were expressed as the ratio of Fc/Fab proliferative responses (uptake of ^{3}H-thymidine). Only background stimulation was observed with soluble IgG, Fab, and F(ab)$_2$ fragments (Table III). If the comparison is made in terms of Fc/Fab ratios, it appears that the Fc fragments of IgG and IgA are equally potent and gave the highest stimulation, while the Fc fragment of IgD is intermediate, Fc of IgM is very weak, and the Fc fragment of IgE did not promote proliferation (163). These observations, however, are not in complete agreement with binding studies. In sharp contrast is the ability of the Fc fragment of IgA to promote ^{3}H-thymidine uptake and the failure of mouse (67,101) or human (105) IgA to bind to lymphocytes even when aggregated. IgD also shows little binding (105) to human lymphocytes but it does cause a proliferative response in mouse spleen lymphocytes. Such discrepancies may result from differences in the sensitivity of the techniques for detecting direct binding and binding as a secondary phenomenon of cell proliferation.

The ability of Fc fragments from different subclasses of IgG to cause proliferation of mouse spleen cells correlates with the ability of aggregated IgG subclasses to bind to human peripheral blood lymphocytes. Although human lymphocytes bind only IgG$_1$ and IgG$_3$ preparations, when the IgG proteins are aggregated all four subclasses bind (105). Likewise, the Fc fragments of all four subclasses cause proliferation of mouse spleen cells (Table IV) (163). As suggested by the differential

TABLE III
Stimulation of DNA Synthesis by Human IgG Fragments and
Different Ig Classes[a]

Ig Class	Fragment (50 μg/ml)	cpm ^{3}H-thymidine per culture	Stimulation ratio Fc/Fab
IgG soluble	Whole	3,541	—
IgG aggregated		23,835	7.5
	F (ab')$_2$	3,209	1.0
	Fab	3,178	—
	Fc	102,432	32.2
aggregated	Fc	102,866	32.4
IgM	Fab	11,811	—
	Fc	51,828	4.4
IgA	Fab	2,458	—
	Fc	80,929	32.9
IgD	Fab	6,141	—
	Fc	123,436	20.1
IgE	Fab	3,163	—
	Fc	3,140	1.0

[a] A/J spleen cell cultures as described in Table II and Berman *et al.* (163).

binding of unaggregated and aggregated preparations of IgG sub-classes to bind to lymphocytes, the affinity of binding of IgG$_1$ and IgG$_3$ may be greater than that of IgG$_2$ and IgG$_4$. The proliferative response of the various subclasses of mouse spleen cells appears to be consistent with the preferential binding of IgG$_1$ and IgG$_3$ proteins; however, the differences in the proliferative responses are not large and only one myeloma representing each subclass was studied.

As pointed out above, preparations of immunoglobulins bind better when aggregated than when unaggregated (67,70,71,74,77,88,105, 118,143,144). The increased binding affinity of antibody either com-plexed to antigen or in aggregated form over that of free immuno-globulin molecules may result from the arrangement of the molecules or from a conformational change or a combination of both. The stimu-latory property of the Fc fragment is compatible with a conformational change in the Fc fragment which permits a more favorable interaction between the Fc sites and their cell receptors. Although this change is not brought about in the same manner *in vivo*, the use of such Fc preparations should permit an easier and more quantitative appraisal of cell activation through the Fc receptor. Aggregation does not ap-pear to be a requisite for the proliferative response of mouse spleen cells to the Fc fragment of human IgG. Evidence for an association

TABLE IV

Stimulation of DNA Synthesis in Mouse Spleen Cell
Cultures by Fc and Fab Fragments of Human IgG Subclasses
(Myelomas)[a]

IgG subclass (myeloma)	Papain fragment (10 μg/culture)	cpm ^{3}H-thymidine uptake day 4–5 of culture ($\pm$SE)
—	—	5,422 ($\pm$ 196)
IgG$_1$	Fab	5,093 ($\pm$ 374)
(Eri)	Fc	94,237 ($\pm$2,257)
IgG$_2$	Fab	5,945 ($\pm$ 270)
(Kel)	Fc	76,471 ($\pm$2,829)
IgG$_3$	Fab	5,500 ($\pm$ 285)
(Cal)	Fc	98,866 ($\pm$6,090)
IgG$_4$	Fab	5,944 ($\pm$ 427)
(Heb)	Fc	73,620 ($\pm$1,460)

[a] Cultures as in Table II.

of mitogenesis with monomeric Fc, a protein with a sedimentation rate of 3.5 S, rather than with aggregated Fc fragments of higher sedimentation rates, was obtained by sucrose density centrifugation (162). The maximal activity was found in the pooled fractions having the highest protein concentration and migrating between 3 and 5 S (Fig. 4). Moreover, aggregation of the Fc fragment by bis-diazotized benzidine did not further increase its mitogenic properties (Table III). The mechanisms by which monomeric preparations of Fc fragment can modulate surface receptors in a significant manner so as to cause intracellular communication that results in cellular proliferation are not obvious.

Whatever the mechanism of stimulation, the binding site appears to be associated with the pFc' (Cγ3 domain) portion of the Fc fragment (163). The pFc' portion of the Fc fragment was obtained by 24-hr pepsin digestion and separation on a Sephadex G 150 column. Aliquots of the material in the fractions from the F(ab)$_2$, pFc' and peptide peaks were tested for their proliferative effect on mouse spleen cells (Table V). Only the pFc' fraction caused uptake of ^{3}H-thymidine when added to mouse spleen cells. These results are in agreement with others who previously implicated the Cγ3 domain in the binding of immunoglobulin to lymphocytes (93,106) and in ADCC (111).

The cell type activated to undergo a proliferative response to the Fc fragment in the mouse spleen is an Ig+, FcR+, Cr+, Ia+ B lymphocyte. In contrast to the binding of immune complexes and aggregated

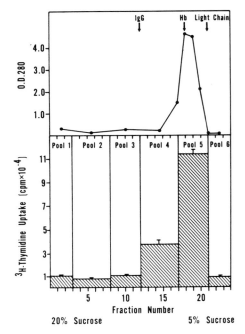

Fig. 4. Sucrose density gradient centrifugation of Fc preparation (from human gamma globulin). The protein concentration of pool 5 was adjusted to 10 μg/0.1 ml for addition to cultures. The same dilution as for pool 5 was performed on each pool. Triplicate cultures were pulsed with ^{3}H-thymidine between days 4 and 5 (hatched bar). ●——● Fc protein concentration. From Berman and Weigle (162).

TABLE V
Stimulation with pFc' Fragments

		cpm ^{3}H-thymidine uptake (day 4–5) ($\pm$SE)
Medium (control)		2,048 ($\pm$109)
IgG fragments[a]:	F(ab')$_2$	2,501 ($\pm$212)
	Peptides	2,387 ($\pm$186)
	pFc'	35,466 ($\pm$137)
	Fc	87,901 ($\pm$844)

[a] 50 μg protein/culture; cultures as in Table II.

immunoglobulins by B cells and subpopulations of T cells, proliferative responses to the Fc fragment of human IgG occurred only in B lymphocytes (162). Deletion of T lymphocytes from mouse spleen cell populations had no effect on stimulation by the Fc fragment, whereas an enriched preparation of T cells obtained by passage through nylon wool or after removal of Ig+ cells by rosetting was unresponsive (Table VI). The affinity of the Fc fragments for T cells may be too weak to trigger proliferation. Alternatively, Fc could trigger a different function in T cells which may be regulatory, but not manifested by increased DNA synthesis.

The Fc receptors on lymphocytes are associated with the presence of other surface markers (87). Although Fc receptors are clearly different from Ig receptors for antigen (68,118,119), and modulation of surface FcR has no effect on the distribution of surface Ig receptors (119), there seems to be a close association between the two receptors. This association is evident in the present studies, since deletion of Ig+ cells by rosetting with erythrocytes coated with anti-Ig abrogates the proliferative response with Fc fragments (Table VI). Furthermore, rosetting of spleen cells with erythrocytes coated with anti-μ also eliminates the proliferative response to the Fc fragment, suggesting that IgM+ cells are responsive to Fc fragments.

The presence of lymphocytes containing both Ia and FcR proteins is apparent because the Fc-induced proliferative response in mouse spleen cells is markedly reduced by depletion of Ia+ lymphocytes (Table VI). A close association between Ia proteins and FcR was suggested previously by several workers who demonstrated that anti-Ia antibodies inhibited the ability of lymphocytes to bind Ig (120–123). As would be expected, deletion of FcR+ cells resulted in elimination of the proliferative response of the Fc fragment. Capping of B cell-bound immune complexes did not result in a redistribution of Ia antigens (124). Thus, it appears that although some B cells express both Ia and FcR, these two surface antigens are not linked on the membrane of B cells.

Complement has been implicated in the immune response to thymus-dependent antigens (58), and it has been suggested that interaction between C3 and the C3 receptor on B cells may supply an effective signal to these cells (59). Moreover, Hartmann and Bokisch (164) have demonstrated stimulation of DNA synthesis and blast transformation in mouse lymphocyte cultures by isolated C3b. It is unlikely that complement plays any role in the stimulation of B cells by the Fc fragment since heat-inactivated or aged mouse serum was as effective

TABLE VI
Effect of Depletion of Various Spleen Cell Populations on the Proliferative Response

Exp. No.	Pretreatment	cpm ³H-thymidine uptake (day 4–5) (±SE)	
		Medium	Fc[a]
1	Normal rabbit serum + C	1,508(±251)	122,974(± 929)
	Anti-T cell serum + C[b]	3,429(±232)	124,060(±3,334)
2	None	1,740(± 48)	118,920(±7,093)
	Anti-Ig rosette depletion[b]	745(± 83)	5,276(± 160)
3	None	2,287(±108)	88,344(±5,222)
	Anti-μ rosette depletion[c]	1,503(± 17)	1,878(± 756)
4	Normal BALB/c (nu/+)[b]	957(±101)	98,208(±5,402)
	Athymic BALB/c (nu/nu)	2,348(± 72)	100,542(±3,263)
5	Normal mouse serum + C	1,782(± 65)	78,981(±2,307)
	Anti/Ia serum + C[d]	6,842(±202)	12,264(±2,833)
6	None	1,283(±116)	41,061(±4,525)
	Macrophage depletion[e]	217(± 9)	39,266(±4,620)
7	None	1,001(± 54)	46,027(±1,634)
	Nylon wool nonadherent[b]	280(± 10)	1,514(± 46)
8	Unseparated[b]	2,422(±128)	150,743(±4,595)
	FcR − spleen cells	803(± 65)	32,608(±1,901)
	FcR + spleen cells	11,044(± 95)	153,787(±3,806)
9	Unseparated[f]	4,112(±186)	40,188(± 668)
	CR − spleen cells	2,347(±202)	7,237(± 360)
	CR + spleen cells	4,408(± 64)	132,246(±3,586)

[a] Results shown for 10 μg Fc/culture in Exp. 3, 4, 5, 6, 7, and 50 μg Fc/culture in Exp. 1, 2.

[b] As in Berman and Weigle (162).

[c] Anti-$\lambda\mu$ serum, immunoabsorbent-purified on Kμ, was coupled to SRBC for rosetting.

[d] A.TH anti-A.TL serum was kindly provided by D. Shreffler.

[e] Spleen cells were cultured in plastic petri dishes at 37°C for 1 hr, then the nonadherent cells were recultured twice for 1 hr for further removal of adherent cells.

[f] Ficoll-Isopaque purified spleen cells were rosetted with EAC (sheep erythrocytes treated with rabbit anti-sheep IgM, then incubated in fresh A/J mouse serum for 30 min at 37° C). Rosette-forming cells (CR + cells, 45–75%) were separated from CR − cells on Ficoll-Isopaque.

as fresh serum in supporting the stimulation. On the other hand, B cells responding to Fc fragments bear complement receptors (CR). Cr+ cells obtained by rosette formation with erythrocytes coated with IgM antibody and complement showed a marked increase over unseparated cells in the proliferative response to Fc fragment, while spleen cells depleted of CR+ cells (CR− cells) responded only minimally to the Fc fragment (Table VI). Although the proliferative response to the Fc fragment appears to be associated with an FcR+ and CR+ population of B cells, the binding of complement is probably not required. Complement is also not required for the binding of either antigen–antibody complexes or aggregated IgG to lymphocytes; however, some evidence suggests that complement may either amplify or interfere with binding via the Fc receptor (90).

MODULATION OF THE *in Vitro* SECONDARY RESPONSE

Similar to antigen–antibody complexes, the Fc fragment was found to both suppress and enhance the antibody response. The addition of human Fc fragment to cultures of mouse spleen cells from primed mice along with the specific antigen resulted in either a suppressed or enhanced antibody response depending on the immune status of the donor mice. Spleen cells taken from mice 6 weeks after immunization with alum-precipitated turkey gamma globulin (TGG) incorporated in complete Freund's adjuvant (CFA) showed a suppressed antibody response to TGG in the presence of Fc fragment (Table VII). On the other hand, spleen cells taken from mice 6 weeks after immunization with bovine serum albumin (BSA) in CFA showed an enhanced antibody response to BSA in the presence of Fc fragment. It should be noted that the normal *in vitro* secondary response to TGG was strong (suppressed by Fc fragment) while the normal *in vitro* secondary response to BSA was weak (enhanced by Fc fragment). The importance of the immune status of primed mice for the subsequent effect of Fc on the *in vitro* secondary response is emphasized by using two different immunization schedules with the same antigen. In such experiments, the effect of Fc fragment on the *in vitro* secondary response to the Fab fragment of human IgG was examined. When donor mice were primed once with Fab in CFA and their cells cultured and stimulated with antigen 6 weeks later, the response was weak and the addition of Fc fragments resulted in a markedly enhanced response. On the other hand, when donor mice were immunized with Fab in CFA and subsequently boosted intraperitoneally (i.p.) with Fab 7 days before their cells were cultured and stimulated with antigen, the response was strong and the addition of Fc fragment resulted in a 72% suppression of the response (Table VII). Thus, it appears that the Fc fragment is capable of either a positive or negative effect on the immune response and that the direction of regulation is dictated by the immune status of the cells.

The mechanism for this suppression and enhancement of the *in vitro*

TABLE VII
Modulation of the Secondary Antibody Response by Fc Fragments

Priming of donor mice (A/J)	Antigen added in vitro[a]	Fc fragments added	Indirect PFC/10^7 cells cultured	Suppression (%)
100 μg	—	—	65	
alum TGG	TGG	—	17,007	
in CFA i.p.	TGG	50 μg/ml	1,548	91
(at 6 weeks)	TGG	5 μg/ml	2,436	86
50 μg human Fab (from IgG) in CFA s.c.	—	—	3,700	
(at 6 weeks)	Fab	—	32,000	
+ boosted with 10 μg Fab i.p. (on day 7)	Fab	50 μg/ml	9,000	72
50 μg Fab in CFA s.c.	—	—	16	
(at 6 weeks)	Fab	—	250	
	Fab	50 μg/ml	5,100	
50 μg BSA in CFA s.c.	—	—	5	
(at 6 weeks)	BSA	—	100	
	BSA	50 μg/ml	2,880	

[a] Spleen cells were treated with TGG (100 μg/ml) for 30 min at 4°C. Fab and BSA were added at 1 μg/ml. Cultures with TGG and FAB contained 7.5% fetal calf serum and 0.5% mouse serum; to cultures with BSA only 0.5% mouse serum was added.

immune response is under study. At the present, it is not known whether the effect of the Fc fragment on the *in vitro* secondary response is the result of a direct interaction of Fc with precursor B cells or whether the effect is mediated by other cells. There appears to be some question whether the Fc sites on antigen–antibody complexes can react directly with lymphocytes involved in thymus-independent responses. It has been reported that primed and secondary precursor B cells are both FcR+ (85,90,91) and FcR− (90,130). Moreover, Hoffmann and Kappler (19) have presented convincing data which suggest that in the suppression of the *in vitro* response with passive antibody, neither helper T cells or precursor B cells were affected, but that the effect was on T and B cell cooperation. Since considerable data has been accumulated showing that suppressor T cells contain Fc receptors and since their participation in control of the immune response is well documented (133,135,137), their role in Fc-mediated suppression should be considered as a likely possibility.

SUMMARY

An *in vitro* proliferative response was induced in mouse spleens with both antigen–antibody complexes and Fc fragments of IgG. Although complexes in antibody excess were stimulatory, complexes formed in antigen excess were somewhat more efficient.

Addition of human Fc fragments (50 μg) to the spleen cells resulted in uptake of ^{3}H-thymidine which was optimal between the fourth and fifth days of culture. Fc fragments from homologous IgG or goat IgG (but not from turkey gamma globulin) were also effective. In studies with Fc fragments from various classes and subclasses of human Ig (myelomas), IgG and IgA stimulated equally well, whereas IgM showed only a weak proliferative response and IgD was intermediate. Fc from human IgE did not stimulate mouse spleen cells. All of the IgG subclasses caused a good proliferative response. Stimulation with fragments obtained by pepsin degradation showed the activity to be in the pFc' (third domain) fraction.

The cell type stimulated to proliferate by Fc fragments was an Ig+, Ia+, FcR+, CR+ B cell. Splenic T cells showed no proliferative response to Fc fragment. Although the stimulated cells bear complement receptors, complement was not required for the proliferative response. Spleen cells with and without macrophages were equally affected by Fc fragments.

Fc fragments of human IgG can cause both suppression and enhancement of the *in vitro* secondary response to several protein (thymus-dependent) antigens. Whether suppression or enhancement occurred was dependent on the immune status of the spleen cell donor. Fc fragment, when added alone (without antigens) to normal spleen cells, caused a polyclonal activation of the B cells.

ACKNOWLEDGMENTS

This is publication no. 1568 from the Department of Immunopathology, Scripps Clinic and Research Foundation, La Jolla, California. Supported by U.S. Public Health Service Grant AI-07007, National Institutes of Health Grant AI-12449, and American Cancer Society Grant IM-42G. Monique A. Berman is a recipient of National Institute of Health Fellowship Award AI-05345.

The authors wish to acknowledge the technical assistance of Ms. Elysa Waltzer and the secretarial assistance of Ms. Chris VanLeeuwen.

REFERENCES

1. Weigle, W. O. (1961) *Adv. Immunol.* **1**, 283.
2. Cochrane, C. G., and Koffler, D. (1973) *Adv. Immunol.* **16**, 185.
3. Haakenstad, A. O., and Mannik, M. (1977) *In* "Autoimmunity" (N. Talal, ed.) p. 277. Academic Press, New York.
4. Uhr, J. W., and Möller, G. (1968) *Adv. Immunol.* **8**, 81.
5. Walker, J. G., and Siskind, G. W. (1968) *Immunology* **14**, 21.
6. Murgita, R. A., and Vas, S. I. (1972) *Immunology* **22**, 319.
7. Cerottini, J.-C., McConahey, P. J., and Dixon, F. J. (1969) *J. Immunol.* **103**, 268.
8. Cerottini, J.-C., McConahey, P. J., and Dixon, F. J. (1969) *J. Immunol.* **102**, 1008.
9. Feldmann, M., and Diener, E. (1972) *J. Immunol.* **108**, 93.
10. Sinclair, N. R. St.C. (1969) *J. Exp. Med.* **129**, 1183.
11. Kappler, J. W., Hoffmann, M., and Dutton, R. W. (1971) *J. Exp. Med.* **134**, 577.
12. Lees, R. K., and Sinclair, N. R. St.C. (1973) *Immunology* **24**, 735.
13. Sinclair, N. R. St.C., and Chan, P. L. (1971) *In* "Morphological and Functional Aspects of Immunity" (K. Lindahl-Kiessling, G. Alm, and M. G. Hanna, eds.), p. 609. Plenum, New York.
14. Sinclair, N. R. St.C., Lees, R. K., Abrahams, S., Chan, P. L., Fagan, G., and Stiller, C. R. (1974) *J. Immunol.* **113**, 1493.
15. Kappler, J. W., van der Hoven, A., Dharmarajan, U., and Hoffmann, M. (1973) *J. Immunol.* **111**, 1228.
16. Hoffmann, M. K., Kappler, J. W., Hirst, J. A., and Oettgen, H. F. (1974) *Eur. J. Immunol.* **4**, 282.
17. Wason, W. M., and Fitch, F. W. (1973) *J. Immunol.* **110**, 1427.
18. Chan, P. L., and Sinclair, N. R. St.C. (1971) *Immunology* **21**, 967.
19. Hoffmann, M., and Kappler, J. W. (1978) *Nature (London)* **272**, 64.
20. Dubiski, S., and Swierczynska, Z. (1971) *Int. Arch. Allergy Appl. Immunol.* **40**, 1.
21. Shek, P., and Dubiski, S. (1975) *J. Immunol.* **114**, 621.
22. Eichmann, K. (1975) *Eur. J. Immunol.* **5**, 511.
23. Pawlak, L. Y., Hart, D. A., and Nisonoff, A. (1973) *J. Exp. Med.* **137**, 1442.
24. Jerne, N. K. (1974) *Ann. Immunol. (Paris)* **125c**, 373.
25. Rodkey, L. S. (1974) *J. Exp. Med.* **139**, 712.
26. Köhler, H. (1975) *Transplant. Rev.* **27**, 24.
27. Pierce, S., and Klinman, N. R. (1977) *J. Exp. Med.* **146**, 509.
28. Cohn, C., and Allton, W. H. (1962) *Nature (London)* **193**, 990.
29. Ryder, R. J. W., and Schwartz, R. S. (1969) *J. Immunol.* **103**, 970.
30. Playfair, J. H. L. (1974) *Clin. Exp. Immunol.* **17**, 1.
31. Dennert, G. (1971) *J. Immunol.* **106**, 951.
32. Uyeki, E. M., and Klassen, R. S. (1968) *J. Immunol.* **101**, 271.
33. Wason, W. M. (1973) *J. Immunol.* **110**, 1245.
34. Stoner, R. D., and Terres, G. (1963) *J. Immunol.* **91**, 761.
35. Terres, G., and Wolins, W. (1959) *Proc. Soc. Exp. Biol. Med.* **102**, 632.
36. Weigle, W. O. (1964) *J. Immunol.* **92**, 113.
37. Morrison, S. L., and Terres, G. (1966) *J. Immunol.* **96**, 901.
38. Terres, G., Morrison, S. L., Habicht, G. S., and Stoner, R. D. (1972) *J. Immunol.* **108**, 1473.
39. Terres, G., Habicht, G. S., and Stoner, R. D. (1974) *J. Immunol.* **112**, 804.
40. Pincus, C., Miller, G., and Nussenzweig, V. (1973) *J. Immunol.* **110**, 301.
41. Pincus, C. S., Lamm, M. E., and Nussenzweig, V. (1971) *J. Exp. Med.* **133**, 987.

42. Houston, W. E., Pederson, C. E., Jr., Cole, F. E., Jr., and Spertzel, R. O. (1974) *Infect. Immun.* **10**, 437.
43. Liew, F. Y., and Parish, C. R. (1972) *Cell. Immunol.* **4**, 66.
44. Bystryn, J.-C., Schenkein, J., and Uhr, J. W. (1971) *Prog. Immunol., Int. Congr. Immunol., 1st, 1971*, p. 627.
45. Rowley, D. A., Fitch, F. W., Axelrad, M. A., and Pierce, C. W. (1969) *Immunology* **16**, 549.
46. Kontiainen, S. (1975) *Immunology* **28**, 535.
47. Boyns, A. R., and Hardwicke, J. (1968) *Immunology* **15**, 263.
48. Oppenheim, J. J. (1972) *Cell. Immunol.* **3**, 341.
49. Ryan, J. L., Arbeit, R. D., Dickler, H. B., and Henkart, P. A. (1975) *J. Exp. Med.* **142**, 814.
50. Ryan, J. L., and Henkart, P. A. (1976) *J. Exp. Med.* **144**, 768.
51. Sidman, C. L., and Unanue, E. R. (1976) *J. Exp. Med.* **144**, 882.
52. Wahl, S. M., Iverson, G. M., and Oppenheim, J. J. (1974) *J. Exp. Med.* **140**, 1631.
53. Bloch-Shtacher, N., Hirschhorn, K., and Uhr, J. W. (1968) *Clin. Exp. Immunol.* **3**, 889.
54. Möller, G. (1969) *Clin. Exp. Immunol.* **4**, 65.
55. Möller, G., and Coutinho, A. (1975) *J. Exp. Med.* **141**, 647.
56. Ramasamy, R. (1976) *Immunology* **30**, 559.
57. Soderberg, L. F., and Coons, A. H. (1978) *J. Immunol.* **120**, 806.
58. Pepys, M. B. (1974) *J. Exp. Med.* **140**, 126.
59. Dukor, P., and Hartmann, K. U. (1973) *Cell. Immunol.* **7**, 349.
60. Dukor, P., Schumann, G., Giesler, R. H., Dierich, M., Konig, W., Hadding, U., and Bitter-Suermann, D. (1974) *J. Exp. Med.* **139**, 337.
61. Pepys, M. B., Mirjah, D. D., Dash, A. C., and Wansbrough-Jones, M. H. (1976) *Cell. Immunol.* **21**, 327.
62. Axelrad, M. A. (1968) *Immunology* **15**, 159.
63. Sinclair, N. R. St.C., Lees, R. K., Fagen, G., and Birnbaum, A. (1975) *Cell. Immunol.* **16**, 330.
64. Mackaness, G. B., Lagrange, P. H., Miller, T. E., and Ishibashi, T. (1974) *J. Exp. Med.* **139**, 543.
65. Lagrange, P. H., Mackaness, G. B., and Miller, T. E. (1974) *J. Exp. Med.* **139**, 528.
66. Uhr, J. W., and Phillips, J. M. (1966) *Ann. N.Y. Acad. Sci.* **129**, 793.
67. Basten, A., Miller, J. F. A. P., Sprent, J., and Pye, J. (1972) *J. Exp. Med.* **135**, 610.
68. Basten, A., Warner, N. L., and Mandel, T. (1972) *J. Exp. Med.* **135**, 627.
69. Basten, A., Miller, J. F. A. P., Warner, N. L., Abraham, R., Chia, E., and Gamble, J. (1975) *J. Immunol.* **115**, 1159.
70. Dickler, H. B., and Kunkel, H. G. (1972) *J. Exp. Med.* **136**, 191.
71. Paraskevas, F., Lee, S.-T., and Orr, K. B. (1972) *J. Immunol.* **108**, 1319.
72. Cline, M. J., Sprent, J., Warner, M. L., and Harris, A. W. (1972) *J. Immunol.* **108**, 1126.
73. Grey, H. M., Kubo, R. T., and Cerottini, J.-C. (1972) *J. Exp. Med.* **136**, 1323.
74. Yoshida, T. O., and Andersson, B. (1972) *Scand. J. Immunol.* **1**, 401.
75. Dickler, H. B., Adkinson, N. F., and Terry, W. D. (1974) *Nature (London)* **247**, 213.
76. Ferrarini, M., Tonda, G. P., Risso, A., and Vial, G. (1975) *Eur. J. Immunol.* **5**, 89.
77. Dickler, H. B., and Sachs, D. H. (1974) *J. Exp. Med.* **140**, 779.
78. Abbas, A. K., and Unanue, E. R. (1975) *J. Immunol.* **115**, 1665.
79. Rask, L., Klareskog, L., Östberg, L., and Peterson, P. A. (1975) *Nature (London)* **257**, 231.

80. Möller, G. (1974) *J. Exp. Med.* **139**, 969.
81. Kramer, P. H., Hudson, L., and Sprent, J. (1975) *J. Exp. Med.* **142**, 1403.
82. Dickler, H. B., Siegal, F. P., Bentwich, Z. H., and Kunkel, H. G. (1973) *Clin. Exp. Immunol.* **14**, 97.
83. Hallberg, T., Gurner, B. W., and Coombs, R. R. A. (1973) *Int. Arch. Allergy Appl. Immunol.* **44**, 500.
84. Frøland, S. S., Natvig, J. B., and Michaelsen, T. E. (1974) *Scand. J. Immunol.* **3**, 375.
85. Parish, C. R., and Hayward, J. A. (1974) *Proc. R. Soc. London, Ser. B* **187**, 65.
86. Brown, G., and Greaves, M. F. (1974) *Eur. J. Immunol.* **4**, 302.
87. Dickler, H. B. (1976) *Adv. Immunol.* **24**, 167.
88. Anderson, C. L., and Grey, H. M. (1974) *J. Exp. Med.* **139**, 1175.
89. Stout, R. D., and Herzenberg, L. A. (1975) *J. Exp. Med.* **142**, 611.
90. Parish, C. R. (1975) *Transplant. Rev.* **25**, 98.
91. Basten, A., Miller, J. F. A. P., and Abraham, R. (1975) *J. Exp. Med.* **141**, 547.
92. Van Boxel, J. A., and Rosenstreich, D. L. (1974) *J. Exp. Med.* **139**, 1002.
93. Klein, M., Neauport-Sautes, C., Ellerson, J. R., and Fridman, W. H. (1977) *J. Immunol.* **119**, 1077.
94. Smeraldi, R. S., Villa, M. G. S., Perussia, B., Fabio, G., Casali, P., and Rugarli, C. (1977) *Immunology* **32**, 827.
95. Ramasamy, R., Munro, A., and Milstein, C. (1974) *Nature (London)* **249**, 573.
96. Warner, N. L., Harris, A. W., and Gutman, G. A. (1975) *In* "Membrane Receptors of Lymphocytes" (M. Seligmann, J. L. Preud'homme, and F. M. Kourilsky, eds.), p. 203. North-Holland Publ., Amsterdam.
97. Hayward, A. R., and Greaves, M. F. (1975) *Clin. Immunol. Immunopathol.* **3**, 461.
98. Forni, L., and Pernis, B. (1975) *In* "Membrane Receptors of Lymphocytes" (M. Seligmann, J. L. Preud'homme, and F. M. Kourilsky, eds.), p. 193. North-Holland Publ., Amsterdam.
99. Sidman, C. L., and Unanue, E. R. (1975) *J. Immunol.* **114**, 1730.
100. Rosenberg, Y. J., and Parish, C. R. (1977) *J. Immunol.* **118**, 612.
101. Anderson, C. L., and Grey, H. M. (1977) *J. Immunol.* **118**, 7.
102. Heusser, C. H., Anderson, C. L., and Grey, M. H. (1977) *J. Exp. Med.* **145**, 1316.
103. Moretta, L., Ferrarini, M., Mingari, M. C., Moretta, A., and Webb, S. R. (1976) *J. Immunol.* **117**, 2171.
104. Lamon, E. W., Andersson, B., Whitten, H. D., Hurst, M. M., and Ghanta, V. (1976) *J. Immunol.* **116**, 1199.
105. Lawrence, D. A., Weigle, W. O., and Spiegelberg, H. L. (1975) *J. Clin. Invest.* **55**, 368.
106. Ramasamy, R., Richardson, N. E., and Feinstein, A. (1976) *Immunology* **30**, 851.
107. Cathou, R., and Dorrington, K. J. (1975) *In* "Biological Macromolecules, Subunits in Biological Systems" (G. D. Fasman and S. N. Timasheff, eds.) p. 91. Marcel Dekker, New York.
108. Ellerson, J. R., Yasmeen, D., Painter, R. H., and Dorrington, K. J. (1976) *J. Immunol.* **116**, 510.
109. Yasmeen, D., Ellerson, J. R., Dorrington, K. J., and Painter, R. H. (1976) *J. Immunol.* **116**, 518.
110. Yasmeen, D., Ellerson, J. R., Dorrington, K. J., and Painter, R. H. (1973) *J. Immunol.* **110**, 1706.
111. Spiegelberg, H. L., Perlmann, H., and Perlmann, P. (1976) *J. Immunol.* **117**, 1464.
112. MacLennan, J.-C. M. (1972) *Transplant. Rev.* **13**, 67.

113. Ewald, S., Freedman, L., and Sanders, B. G. (1976) *Immunology* **31**, 847.
114. Segal, D. M., and Hurwitz, E. (1977) *J. Immunol.* **118**, 1338.
115. Segal, D. M., and Titus, J. A. (1978) *J. Immunol.* **120**, 1395.
116. Rowley, D. A., Fitch, F. W., Axelrad, M. A., and Pierce, C. W. (1969) *Immunology* **16**, 549.
117. Nussenzweig, V. (1974) *Adv. Immunol.* **19**, 217.
118. Dickler, H. B. (1974) *J. Exp. Med.* **140**, 508.
119. Unanue, E. R., Dorf, M. C., David, C. S., and Benacerraf, B. (1974) *Proc. Natl. Acad. Sci. U.S.A.* **71**, 5014.
120. Dickler, H. B., Cone, J. L., Kubicek, M. T., and Sachs, D. H. (1975) *J. Exp. Med.* **142**, 796.
121. Schirrmacher, V., Halloran, P., and David, C. S. (1975) *J. Exp. Med.* **141**, 1201.
122. Samarut, C., Gebuhrer, L. Brochier, J., Betuel, H., and Revillard, J.-P. (1977) *Eur. J. Immunol.* **7**, 908.
123. Stout, R. D., Murphy, D. B., McDevitt, H. O., and Herzenberg, L. A. (1977) *J. Exp. Med.* **145**, 187.
124. Dickler, H. B., Kubicek, M. T., Arbeit, R. D., and Sharrow, S. O. (1977) *J. Immunol.* **119**, 348.
125. Dickler, H. B., Ahmed, A., and Sachs, D. H. (1977) *J. Exp. Med.* **146**, 1678.
126. Kuribayashi, K., and Masuda, T. (1978) *Cell. Immunol.* **35**, 279.
127. Nelson, D. L., Sachs, D. H., and Dickler, H. B. (1977) *J. Immunol.* **119**, 1034.
128. Kerbel, R. S., and Davies, A. J. S. (1974) *Cell* **3**, 105.
129. Stout, R. D., and Herzenberg, L. A. (1975) *J. Exp. Med.* **142**, 1041.
130. Miyama, M., Kuribayashi, K., Yodoi, J., Takabayashi, A., and Masuda, T. (1978) *Cell. Immunol.* **35**, 253.
131. Kontiainen, S., and Mitchison, N. A. (1975) *Immunology* **28**, 523.
132. Taylor, R. B., and Basten, A. (1976) *Br. Med. Bull.* **32**, 152.
133. Gorczynski, R., Kontiainen, S., Mitchison, N. A., and Tigelaar, R. E. (1974) In "Cellular Selection and Regulation in the Immune Response" (G. M. Edelman, ed.), p. 143. Raven, New York.
134. Fridman, W. H., Fradelizi, D., Guimezanes, A., Plater, C., and Leclerc, J. C. (1977) *Eur. J. Immunol.* **7**, 549.
135. Fridman, W. H., and Golstein, P. (1974) *Cell. Immunol.* **11**, 442.
136. Gisler, R. H., and Fridman, W. H. (1976) *Cell. Immunol.* **23**, 99.
137. Moretta, L., Webb, S. R., Grossi, C. E., Lydyard, P. M., and Cooper, M. D. (1977) *J. Exp. Med.* **146**, 184.
138. Pape, G. R., Troye, M., and Perlmann, P. (1977) *J. Immunol.* **118**, 1919.
139. Pape, G. R., Troye, M., and Perlmann, P. (1977) *J. Immunol.* **118**, 1925.
140. Kay, H. D., Bonnard, G. D., West, W. H., and Herberman, R. B. (1977) *J. Immunol.* **118**, 2058.
141. Hurwitz, E., Zatz, M. M., and Segal, D. M. (1977) *J. Immunol.* **118**, 1348.
142. MacLennan, I. C. M. (1972) *Clin. Exp. Immunol.* **10**, 275.
143. Wisloff, F., Michaelsen, T. E., and Frøland, S. S. (1974) *Scand. J. Immunol.* **3**, 29.
144. Larsson, A., Perlmann, P., and Natvig, J. B. (1973) *Immunology* **25**, 675.
145. Stout, R. D., Waksal, S. D., and Herzenberg, L. A. (1976) *J. Exp. Med.* **144**, 54.
146. Leclerc, J. C., Plater, C., and Fridman, W. H. (1977) *Eur. J. Immunol.* **7**, 543.
147. Häyry, P., and Andersson, L. C. (1976) *Cell. Immunol.* **25**, 237.
148. Boyden, S. V., and Sorkin, E. (1960) *Immunology* **3**, 272.
149. Boyden, S. V., and Sorkin, E. (1961) *Immunology* **4**, 244.
150. Berken, A., and Benacerraf, B. (1966) *J. Exp. Med.* **123**, 119.

151. Rabinovitch, M. (1967) *J. Immunol.* **99**, 1115.
152. LoBuglio, A. F., Cotran, R. S., and Jandl, J. H. (1967) *Science* **158**, 1582.
153. Hay, F. C., Torrigiani, G., and Roitt, I. M. (1972) *Eur. J. Immunol.* **2**, 257.
154. Walker, W. S. (1976) *J. Immunol.* **116**, 911.
155. Walker, W. S. (1977) *J. Immunol.* **119**, 367.
156. Unkeless, J. C. (1977) *J. Exp. Med.* **145**, 931.
157. Unkeless, J. C., and Eisen, H. N. (1975) *J. Exp. Med.* **142**, 1520.
158. Ivanyi, J. (1970) *Nature (London)* **226**, 550.
159. Ptak, W., and Pryjma, J. (1971) *Eur. J. Immunol.* **1**, 408.
160. Huber, H., and Fudenberg, H. H. (1968) *Int. Arch. Allergy Appl. Immunol.* **34**, 18.
161. Huber, H., Douglas, S. D., Musbacher, J., Kochwa, S., and Rosenfield, R. E. (1971) *Nature (London)* **229**, 419.
162. Berman, M. A., and Weigle, W. O. (1972) *J. Exp. Med.* **146**, 241.
163. Berman, M. A., Spiegelberg, H. L., and Weigle, W. O. (1979) *J. Immunol.* **122**, 89.
164. Hartmann, K.-U., and Bokisch, V. A. (1975) *J. Exp. Med.* **142**, 600.

Factors Affecting the Triggering of the B-Cell Repertoire

SUSAN K. PIERCE

Department of Biochemistry and Molecular Biology
Northwestern University, Evanston, Illinois

ELEANOR S. METCALF

Department of Microbiology, Uniformed Services
University of the Health Sciences. Bethesda, Maryland

NORMAN R. KLINMAN

Department of Pathology, University of Pennsylvania
School of Medicine, Philadelphia, Pennsylvania

INTRODUCTION

The specificity of the humoral immune response depends upon the generation of a vast array of B-cell clonotypes and an exquisitely specific stimulatory mechanism which permits antigen to select from among this array (1–4). Antigen selection may, on the one extreme, stimulate B cells to yield clones of antibody-forming cells and lead to the generation of immunologic memory (1,5). On the other extreme, antigen may serve to dampen antibody responses or to eliminate a B-cell clonotype from the repertoire (6–9). In addition, the stimulatory mechanism appears to have the inherent potential to modulate or regulate the response of individual B cells to an antigen. Thus, the ultimate humoral response to any antigenic challenge may be viewed as a composite of a multitude of factors both stimulatory and inhibitory.

Over the past 10 years this laboratory has examined a variety of B-cell responses at the single cell level by the use of an *in vitro* cloning procedure (1,3). In addition to defining large segments of the murine B-cell repertoire, these techniques have also enabled us to study, at a well defined level, factors which may ultimately affect the antigenic stimulation of the B-cell repertoire. In this manuscript we will present an overview of the factors which we believe determine the outcome of any antigen challenge of the humoral immune system. These factors appear to include the functional characteristics of the individual B cells, the form in which antigenic determinants are presented to the B cells, and the individual's previous antigenic history.

THE CLONOTYPE REPERTOIRE

Studies from several laboratories now indicate that the B-cell repertoire in mature mice is composed of greater than 2×10^7 unique antibody specificities (clonotypes) (1–4). In general this estimate was reached by determining the frequency in which identifiable B-cell clonotypes reoccur within the B-cell repertoire. We have carried out several such analyses in this laboratory using an *in vitro* B-cell cloning technique in which individual B cells are isolated and antigenically stimulated in spleen fragment cultures (1,3). Employing this system one has the ability to examine and identify individual monoclonal B-cell antibody responses.

In summary, our results indicate that for a variety of antigens, which include: 2,4-dintrophenyl (DNP), 2,4,6-trinitrophenyl (TNP), phosphorylcholine (PC), and the hemagglutinin of the PR8 strain of influenza virus (PR8-HA), the identifiable clonotypes are present in the primary B-cell repertoire at a frequency lower than 1 in 2×10^7 B cells (1,3,4,10,11). It is important to note that in spite of so diverse a B-cell repertoire which is responsive to a given antigen, the stimulation of B cells by antigenic determinants appears to be exquisitely specific. The specificity of the stimulatory mechanism is most clearly evident in antibody responses to very similar antigenic determinants. Although a large number of different B-cell clonotypes respond to determinants such as DNP and TNP, it has been demonstrated that there is very little overlap stimulation of the primary nonimmune B cells responsive to either DNP or TNP (1,12).

For the purposes of this discussion one can envisage the B-cell repertoire as depicted in Fig. 1. Here it can be seen that an individual animal may express a vast array of unique antibody specificities. At any particular point in time, this array, although extensive, may not represent the entire repertoire of the strain (13,14). It should also be noted that this number has been demonstrated to vary during an individual's lifetime. Thus, the B-cell clonotype repertoire of an individ-

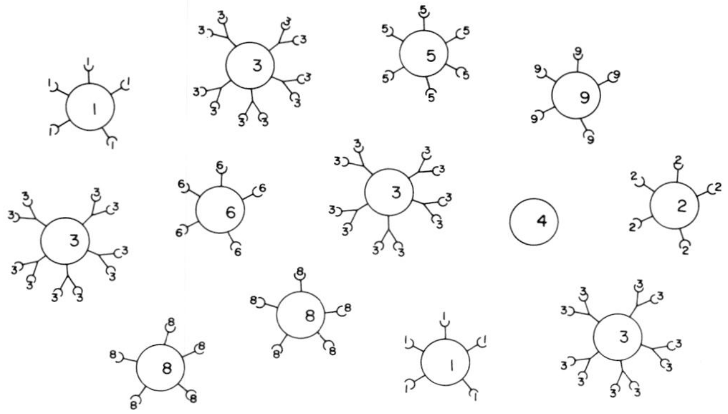

Fig. 1.   The B-cell repertoire is depicted as a heterogeneous population of cells each bearing immunoglobulin receptors of a single specificity.

ual appears to be in a state of dynamic equilibrium in which the expression of any given clonotype waxes and wanes with time.

It is this vast B-cell repertoire which antigen confronts upon entering an individual's immune system. In terms of the clonal selection theory, antigen entering the system serves to either turn B cells of a given clonotype on or off. Thus, each antigen has the potential to stimulate or tolerize more than 10^7 clonotypes. Moreover, the system can potentially express 2×10^7 different antibody populations in response to the antigenic universe. In this context, considering the possible repercussions of antigenic stimulation, it is not surprising that a number of regulatory mechanisms govern the response of each individual B cell to antigen at many different stages of the cells response. In the following sections we will discuss various elements of the regulation of the humoral immune response which are mediated both through the characteristics of B-cell subpopulations and the presentation of the antigenic determinant.

B-CELL SUBPOPULATIONS

Several years ago an analysis of B-cell antibody responses in the splenic focus culture system demonstrated that B cells are not homogeneous in their response to antigen (15). B cells derived from mice at different developmental stages and at various times following immunization were found to differ in their responses in a characteristic manner. These differences appeared to define three distinct B-cell subpopulations. Although many investigators have subsequently sub-divided the B-cell population by a variety of criteria (16–18), for simplicity we will consider only three subpopulations. It is important to stress that these subpopulations are defined by the functional differences between the B cell's response to antigen and are not dependent on the specificity of the B cells. In fact, at any point in time a clonotype may be represented by B cells in any functional subpopulation.

The first subpopulation of B cells we will refer to as the mature primary B-cell population. This subpopulation represents the majority of B cells in a mature nonimmune animal. The second subpopulation of interest is that population which is generated in an animal after immunization. These are termed secondary B cells. In conventional animals, several studies now indicate that these cells represent less than 2% of the B cells in the spleen responsive to any given antigen (1,15,19). After immunization this subpopulation appears to be greatly expanded in the B-cell repertoire specific for the immunizing antigen. When examined, the specificity repertoire of secondary B cells appears to be somewhat less extensive than the primary B-cell clonotypes responsive to a given antigen. The most extensive analysis of this phenomenon has recently been reported from our laboratory in the analysis of the response to PR8-HA (4). The third B-cell subpopulation is that of immature developing B cells. This population predominates in the neonatal and fetal liver and spleen. By the end of the first week of life, developing B cells represent a minority population in these organs and are represented primarily in the bone marrow of mature mice (20,21). Recent studies from this laboratory suggest that approximately 25% of the B cells in adult bone marrow are immature developing B cells (22). In this context, a mutant strain of mice (CBA/N), which carries a recessive X-linked immunodeficiency, is of interest. The defective phenotype of this strain is expressed in the B lymphocyte's inability to respond to certain "T-independent antigens" (23,24). This immunodeficiency may reflect a developmental defect in B-cell maturation (25). As will be discussed in the following sections, when analyzed in the fragment culture system, B cells from the CBA/N mouse strain appear to respond to antigen in a fashion very similar to immature neonatal B cells of other mouse strains.

In the following sections we will present a detailed discussion of the responses of these three subpopulations to antigenic determinants presented in various forms. At this time it would be useful to briefly describe the response pattern of these subpopulations. The primary adult B cells can be characterized as cells which are readily stimulated and not readily tolerized. The secondary B cells can be distinguished from primary B cells by several behavioral characteristics which include their recirculation patterns and relative longevity (26,27). In response to antigen they appear to be more readily stimulated and less susceptible to the specific immunoregulatory phenomena which will be discussed in a later section. The distinguishing characteristic of immature B cells is their susceptibility to *in vitro* tolerance induction (6,7). While the population of neonatal developing B cells may differ somewhat from that developing population found in bone marrow, they also share this unique susceptibility to tolerance induction (22). The parameters of the *in vitro* tolerance susceptibility will be discussed in subsequent sections. Suffice it to say that it is likely that the availability of this tolerance mechanism may be crucial to the process of self-discrimination.

ANTIGEN FORM

If one is to consider the interaction of antigen with the B-cell subpopulations of the clonotype repertoire, it is important to note that antigens vary markedly from one another and can be classified in a rather artificial way according to their ability to interact with B cells. For this discussion we will divide antigens into five categories which describe the context in which the antigenic haptenic determinants are presented to the B cell. Although this classification may be rather artificial, to some extent it is in these differences which one might best understand the mechanisms of B-cell triggering. In the following sections, where possible, we will attempt to relate the responsiveness of the three subpopulations of B cells to their possible molecular requisites of stimulation.

The first most simplistic form in which an antigen may be presented to a B cell is as a monovalent determinant. The best example of such an antigen is a simple haptenic determinant although multideterminant antigens which express only a single copy of any given determinant would also be included in this category, as these antigens would be functionally monovalent with respect to any given determinant. Many protein antigens and monosubstituted hapten–antigen complexes such as DNP_1-S-papain would fall into this category.

The second category of antigens are those which may be considered multivalent antigens. These include all antigens which present multiple copies of the same determinant on a single molecule. The best example of such antigens is a hapten–protein complex in which multiple haptenic determinants are substituted on a protein, DNP_{10}-HSA would be an example of such an antigen. Included in this group would also be a variety of other antigens whose determinants are naturally expressed in multiple copies. Viruses and bacteria which repeatedly express identical surface determinants and many proteins and carbohydrates certainly fulfill this criterion. We will consider the interactions of this class of antigens with the B-cell subpopulations in the absence of antigen-specific T cells.

The third category is that set of multivalent antigens which themselves act as B-cell mitogens. This set of antigens has been best described by Coutinho and Möller (28) and is the subject of one of the papers in this volume. It is important to note that the mitogenicity of such antigens need not be related to the antigenic determinant which presumably binds the immunoglobulin receptors of B cells.

The fourth and fifth categories of antigens which will be described are those which are presented to the B cell in the presence of primed T cells which also recognize the antigen. These antigens can then be recognized by both T and B lymphocytes through one or more antigenic determinants on the molecule and are presented to B cells in the presence of antigen-specific T cells. Within this group of antigens there are two definable modes in which T cells, B cells, and antigen interact. These different modes of interaction describe the fourth and fifth "antigen" categories. The fourth category of antigens are those which are recognized by T cells which are not maximally suited for interaction with the antigen-specific B cells. This type of interaction is best exemplified by antigen-specific collaborating T cells which are allogeneic to the B cells in the *I* region of the major histocompatibility complex (29,30). Although this mode of antigen may not represent a physiological means of antigenic stimulation, it has been included in this list as it represents a novel mode of antigenic stimulation from which it may be possible to gain insights to the role of T cells in B-cell stimulation. In addition, it remains to be seen if this type of antigenic stimulation is akin to a stage of *in vivo* stimulation when T and B lymphocytes within an individual have not had adequate time for appropriate associative recognition or matching.

The fifth and final category of antigens are those for which a non-limiting number of syngeneic antigen-specific helper T-cells are available. These antigens obviously represent any antigen for which T-cell recognition is possible and, in the system to be discussed, for which the recipient has been carrier primed (1,3).

MODES OF ANTIGENIC STIMULATION

The process of B-cell triggering by antigen may have a number of consequences which depend both on the form of the antigen and the B-cell subpopulation stimulated. Antigen may trigger B cells to proliferate and differentiate to a clone of antibody-forming cells. The size of this clone and the heavy chain class of antibody synthesized appears to be dictated by the interaction of antigen with the B cell. It is also possible under appropriate circumstances for the antigen–B cell interaction to yield secondary B cells and under still different circumstances to tolerize B cells. One can therefore evaluate any triggering mechanism by not only determining if B cells are triggered but more pointedly by determining the precise outcome of the triggering event. Table I summarizes the findings of this laboratory in carrying out such an analysis. We have investigated the response of each B-cell subpopulation following interaction with antigens of each of the five defined categories. We have described whether a given interaction resulted in antibody synthesis, tolerance, or secondary B-cell generation. In addition we have also described each stimulatory interaction in terms of the amount and heavy chain isotype of the antibody synthesized.

TABLE I
The Interplay of Antigen and B-Cell Subpopulations

	Immature B cell	Mature B cell	Secondary B-cell generation	Secondary B cell
Monovalent antigen	—[a]	—	—	—
Multivalent antigen	Tolerance	—	—	10% +(IgG)
Mitogenic "antigen"	Tolerance	+(IgM)[b]	—[b]	+(IgM or IgG)[b]
Antigen + antigen-specific allogeneic T cells[c]	+(IgM)?	+(IgM)	—?	+(IgG)
Antigen + antigen-specific syngeneic T cells[c]	++(IgM) (IgG)	(IgM) +++(IgG) (IgA)	+++	(IgM) ++++(IgG) (IgA)

[a] Dash represents no demonstrable effect.
[b] These findings were abstracted from other systems.
[c] Syngeneic T cells share genes with responding B cells in the I region of the H-2 gene complex, allogeneic T cells do not.

It can be seen in Table I that the interaction of the simple monovalent antigen with B cells of each subpopulation has no apparent effect (1,6). It can be shown that the B cells of each subpopulation do in fact bind monovalent antigens such as simple haptens since the presence of the hapten in large excess can inhibit the interaction of these cells with antigen presented in a stimulatory form (1,6,31). There are a few reports which suggest that when B cells are nonspecifically stimulated by mitogens at high doses, monovalent antigenic determinants may trigger a small subset of B cells specific for that antigen (32,33).

The second subset of antigens, multivalent antigens, appears to have a more profound effect on the B cells which it encounters. These antigens are more competent than simple monovalent haptens in inhibiting B cell triggering by more complex antigenic forms which can perhaps be related to the multivalent presentation of the antigenic determinants (1,31,34). In the absence of antigen-specific T cells, a multivalent antigen can trigger approximately 10% of the secondary B cells specific for the antigen (1,15,35). This stimulation results in rather small IgG-producing B-cell clones. These antigens do not, however, have any measurable effect on the vast majority of secondary B cells or on primary B cells. In contrast, antigens presented in this form in the absence of T cells are potent tolerogens for developing B cells (6,7). One might imagine that a neonatal tolerance mechanism of this type normally operates in individuals to eliminate emerging self-reacting B-cell clonotypes within the B-cell repertoire during development and throughout the lifetime of the individual. The parameters of this simple form of antigenic triggering of immature B cells to nonresponsiveness has been further investigated with a view toward elucidating the molecular requisites of B-cell triggering.

If neonatal tolerance does indeed serve to eliminate self-reacting B-cell clonotypes there are certain predictions one would make concerning such a mechanism. First it would be anticipated that a tolerance mechanism designed to eliminate self-reactivity would be exquisitely specific, since one would like to remove only the self-reactive specificities in the B-cell repertoire and not reactivity to closely related nonself antigens. The tolerance induction of neonatal cells *in vitro* which we have described, appears to be exquisitely specific (6). Not only is it possible to readily demonstrate that tolerance induced with DNP does not affect the repertoire to other unrelated antigens, but also that it has no demonstrable affect on the developing B cells responsive to the very closely related hapten TNP. Since the neonatal repertoire for DNP and TNP are well defined (36), it is possible to state with great certainty that DNP_{10}-HSA, at a DNP concentration high enough to not only saturate the neonatal anti-DNP clonotypes but also the neonatal anti-TNP clonotypes, is capable of tolerizing only those cells specific for DNP. It may be assumed, therefore, that, in spite of the fact that the TNP-specific cells bind this antigen, they do not bind it with sufficient affinity to be triggered. This then introduces the first criterion of antigenic stimulation, that the antigen-cell receptor interaction be of a sufficient affinity to permit triggering.

Affinity requisites for the triggering of B cells may be envisaged as depending on either of two mechanisms. One could postulate that the binding of antigen to the B-cell receptor must have a sufficient energy to permit any energy-dependent conformational change in the receptor molecule. Since haptenic determinants or monovalent antigens are not adequate for inducing tolerance, it is not likely that such an affinity-dependent conformational change is the sole explanation for the affinity dependence of the triggering phenomenon. A more likely possibility is that the affinity must be sufficiently high to enable the stable tethering of receptors in the membrane with respect to one another. This mechanism accommodates both the affinity requisite and the fact that the antigen must be present in a multivalent form. Tethering of receptors in cell membranes has been suggested as a possible mechanism of triggering in other immunological and biological systems (37,38). Since the duration of the receptor tethering would be directly related to the dissociation rate of the antigen receptor complex, one could imagine that affinity requisites of B-cells triggering reflect a requirement to stabilize immunoglobulin receptors in complexes in the membrane.

It is of interest that the tolerance triggering phenomenon of immune B cells requires only rather small multivalent molecules such as DNP_{10}-HSA (6). Previous studies on the hapten inhibition of primary and secondary B-cell triggering had led us to postulate that the immunoglobulin receptors of primary B cells were functionally monovalent, whereas the receptors of secondary B cells were at least bivalent (1). This postulate was derived from the observation that the triggering of secondary B cells was somewhat less specific than that of primary B cells (1,12). It was demonstrated that secondary B cells specific for the hapten TNP could be triggered by DNP whereas TNP-specific primary B cells were not. This phenomenon could reflect the greater avidity of cross-reacting antigens to a multivalent receptor. Indeed, primary B cells do not appear to display bivalent interactions in binding large multivalent antigens. If the primary and developing B-cell immunoglobulin receptors are actually monovalent, then the evidence presented here, that small hapten protein complexes are adequate for the tolerance trigger in developing B cells, indicates that stabilization of very few receptors into membrane complexes may be adequate for the tolerance trigger.

Referring back to Table I, it can be seen that the third category of antigens, antigens which are mitogenic, also appears to have profound effects on the B-cell repertoire. It should be noted at this point that many of the results reported in this table for mitogenic antigens are abstracted from the work of other laboratories. Mitogenic antigens do not appear adequate for stimulation of monoclonal B-cell responses in the spleen fragment culture assays employed in this laboratory. However, even though these antigens do not stimulate antibody synthesis in spleen fragment cultures, such antigen serve as specific tolerogens of neonatal B cells (39). While, as stated, such antigens stimulate neither primary nor secondary B cells in our culture system, other laboratories do report that such antigens are adequate for the direct stimulation of both primary and secondary B cells to antibody production (28,40). Since the antigens in this category are able to stimulate primary and secondary B cells to antibody production in the absence of any available T cells, they are commonly referred to as "T-independent antigens." In general, B-cell responses to these antigens result in small antibody-producing clones synthesizing antibody of primarily the IgM heavy chain class (28,40). Findings in several laboratories indicate that B-cell stimulation with a high concentration of nonspecific mitogen results in the synthesis of antibody of multiple heavy chain isotypes (41). In general, however, low concentrations of haptenated mitogens trigger hapten-specific primary B cells to synthesize only antibody of the IgM heavy chain isotype. Some reports have indicated that stimulation of secondary B cells under these conditions leads to IgG antibody production (42).

One could imagine that such stimulation with hapten-coupled mitogens involves the concentration of the mitogen on the cell surface by virtue of the specific receptor–hapten interaction. Since the triggering of B cells via mitogenic antigen probably occurs through a mitogen receptor as opposed to the immunoglobulin receptor per se, it remains problematic whether such triggering would have an affinity requisite similar to that observed when the immunoglobulin receptor alone is involved in the triggering event. Affinity dependence of such triggering could be evidenced in the ability of cells of higher affinity for the haptenic determinant to trap such antigens. It is also conceivable that the mitogen receptor serves to tether immunoglobulin receptors which are simultaneously specifically binding the antigenic determinant in an affinity-dependent manner. However, it is perhaps less likely that such an exquisitely specific triggering process would be observed if the triggering event were mediated solely through the mitogen receptor. This prediction is borne out by the results from laboratories using such mitogenic antigens for the stimulation of anti-hapten responses (28,43).

The fourth mode of antigenic stimulation presented in Table I is that of antigens which are presented to B cells in the presence of antigen-specific T cells which are not maximally suited for interaction with the B cells. Most experiments done in this context have utilized T and B lymphocytes which differ in the *I* region of the *H-2* gene complex (29,30). Although such use of allogeneic T and B lymphocytes may appear to represent a rather nonphysiological interaction, it is important to note that interactions between *I* region mismatched T and B lymphocytes may constitute the majority of T cell–B cell interactions within an individual at certain stages of the immune response. One could imagine that early in an immune response the majority of T and B cell interactions might be between T and B lymphocytes which were not appropriately matched or maximally suited to interact if the expression of *I* region gene products were clonally distributed among the T and B lymphocytes.

Preliminary results from this laboratory indicate that antigenic challenge in the presence of allogeneic antigen-specific T cells is stimulatory to immature B cells unlike antigens of the first two categories which tolerize these cells. Thus, it appears that allogeneic T cells are capable of preventing the induction of tolerance in neonatal cells.

Mature primary B cells are invariably stimulated by antigen in collaboration with allogeneic carrier specific T lymphocytes to yield IgM antibody-producing cell clones (30). This response of mature nonimmune B cells is very reminiscent of the response of these cells to mitogenic antigens. It is possible to discriminate between these two responses by examining the response of the CBA/N male mice which as mentioned earlier are unable to respond to many "T-independent" antigens. B cells from CBA/N male mice synthesize small amounts of IgM antibody when stimulated by antigen in the presence of antigen-specific allogeneic T lymphocytes. Thus, it appears that allogeneic T cells are presenting antigenic determinants to B cells in a form distinct from mitogenic antigens.

The response of mature B cells in the presence of allogeneic T cells is in marked contrast to the response of the B cells stimulated by the fifth category of antigens, antigens presented in an excess of syngeneic antigen-specific T cells. B cells stimulated with these antigens yield antibody-producing cell clones which synthesize IgG, IgA, or IgM antibody (30). This finding has several implications for the mechanism of antigenic stimulation. First, it appears that the same B cells triggered under different circumstances may give qualitatively different antibody responses; in this case IgM responses when stimulated in collaboration with allogeneic T cells and antibody of several heavy chain classes when stimulated in collaboration with syngeneic T cells. Second, it would appear that for the more sophisticated triggering of primary B cells syngeny in the *I* region between collaborating T and B cells is a necessary requisite. This finding is consistent with a role for *I* region gene products in regulating cell–cell interactions (29). An interesting parallel finding from this lab indicates that a small subpopulation of small B lymphocytes which expresses little or. no *I* region-associated antigens are triggered in collaboration with syngeneic antigen specific T cells to synthesize only IgM antibody (44). Thus, syngeny in the *I* region between individual T and B lymphocytes may play a crucial role in the generation of maximum B-cell antibody responses, multiple heavy chain isotype production, and perhaps the generation of secondary B cells although little evidence is yet available for the latter.

In the splenic focus system secondary B cells are stimulated to synthesize IgG antibody in collaboration with allogeneic antigen-specific T cells as shown in Table I (19). This response is somewhat less efficient than antibody responses resulting from antigenic stimulation in the presence of syngeneic T cells in that only approximately 50% of the secondary B cells available for stimulation are stimulated. The IgG antibody response of secondary B cells is, however, in sharp contrast to the primary B cells' IgM antibody responses and may be used as a means of discriminating between primary and secondary B lymphocytes. It is perhaps important to note that these findings are not in agreement with those of other laboratories (29). The results summarized in Table I were obtained by a limiting dilution of secondary B cells into a lethally irradiated carrier-primed recipient which might provide a more enhancing and less inhibitory environment for B cells than those used by other investigators. Thus, if one postulates a small population of carrier-specific T cells within an "allogeneic" recipient which are not in fact restricted to interacting with B cells which share genes in the *I* region, such IgG antibody responses might be expected. In this context one would have to assume that primary B cells were not as efficient in seeking out these recipient T cells.

The final mode of stimulation to be discussed is that in which the antigen is recognized by an excess of antigen-specific T cells which are syngeneic in the *I* region to the B cells being stimulated. Under these conditions all subpopulations of B cells appear to be maximally stimulated. Developing cells are stimulated to antibody synthesis rather than tolerized. In general, stimulation of developing neonatal B cells yields IgM antibody-forming cell clones although these cells at times may give rise to IgG or IgA antibody responses in the presence of maximum syngeneic T-cell help (6,45). In contrast, developing B cells in the adult bone marrow invariably yield IgM antibody responses, while mature primary B cells in the adult bone marrow and in the adult spleen may give rise to antibodies of multiple isotypes when stimulated in this mode (22). Furthermore, as shown in Table I, it is probable that antigen presented in this form *in vivo* maximizes the generation of secondary B cells (46). Secondary B cells themselves are stimulated by antigen presented in this form to synthesize relatively large quantities of antibody of the isotype the secondary B cell was precommitted to synthesize.

One might best review the requisites of B-cell triggering in the context of this maximal stimulation. It appears that for triggering to occur, the antigenic determinant must be presented in a multivalent fashion to the B cell. However, monovalent antigens can serve as triggers if the antigenic determinants are recognized by both T and B lymphocytes. From this finding one may presume that part of the function of the antigen-specific T cell is to polymerize the antigenic determinants. This function for antigen-specific T cells is highly reminiscent of the antigen focusing mechanism initially postulated by Mitchison as the role for T cells in B cell stimulation (47). In this context, the collaborative interaction between T and B lymphocytes would be important in providing the cells with multivalent antigens through which to interact. Such multivalent interactions between the cell receptors and antigenic determinant would be of greater affinity. If receptor interlinkage on the cells' surface is essential for triggering, this cell–cell interaction would prove most beneficial to both the T and B cells involved. As discussed earlier, primary B-cell triggering appears to require rather large antigen–cell receptor complexes to form at the cell surface while immature B cells appear to require fewer receptors to be bound in antigen–receptor complexes for tolerization. This has been incorporated into the immunon theory of Dintzis in which he postulates that at least ten to twelve receptors must be interlinked in order to obtain stimulation of primary B cells (48). Along this line, secondary B cells, which appear to have multivalent antigen receptors, can be triggered by multivalent antigens in the absence of ancillary antigen-specific T cells. The stimulation appears to be rather inefficient as only 10% of the secondary cells available for stimulation are actually stimulated. It is possible that the multivalent secondary B-cell receptors polymerize antigen sufficiently on the cell surface to promote triggering in the absence of T cells.

It would appear that allogeneic T cells like syngeneic T cells are capable of fulfilling this antigen presentation requisite of stimulation. However, more pertinent to this discussion is the marked differences in the B-cell responses to antigens presented in these two different modes. The differences in the B-cell responses is most likely due to cell–cell interactions which occur during B-cell triggering. It seems clear that maximum B-cell stimulation requires syngeneic T-cell interactions which implies a very powerful regulatory mechanism for cell–cell interactions in B-cell triggering. Finally, this finding implies that B-cell triggering is not a simple on–off switch but a far more sophisticated event which has the potential to modulate B-cell responses. The triggering events which have the potential to modulate antibody isotype expression will surely be one of the more interesting questions to be asked in future years.

SUPPRESSION

Thus far we have discussed various factors, inherent in the B-cell subpopulation and antigen form, which affect the ultimate outcome of any antigen–B cell interaction. We would like to turn to a discussion of the effect on B-cell stimulation of an immunoregulatory phenomenon we have recently described which is generated following or concomitant with a primary humoral immune response (8). In recent years several studies have indicated that individuals possess the ability to recognize their antibody idiotypes and that such recognition mediated either through T or B lymphocytes may either enhance or suppress responses (49–51). It was of interest to determine if such recognition plays a role in regulating primary B-cell antibody responses during the course of a humoral immune response to an antigenic determinant. To this end we have carried out an investigation which utilizes the transfer of mature nonimmune and secondary B cells to recipients which have been primed either to the carrier alone or to the carrier plus the relevant hapten carrier complex. It was reasoned that if a suppressive mechanism developed which was specific for hapten-responsive B cells, then recipients primed to a hapten as well as the carrier would suppress responses of hapten-specific B cells whereas recipients primed to the carrier alone would not. Table II presents the results of

TABLE II
Antibody Specific Immunoregulation

| | | | In vitro stimulating antigen | | | |
| | | | DNP-HY | | FL-HY | |
Donor cells[a]	Recipient	Recipient priming	No. anti-DNP[b] positive foci per 10⁶ spleen cells transferred	Response in HY-primed recipients (%)	No. anti-FL positive foci per 10⁶ spleen cells transferred	Response in HY-primed recipients (%)
BALB/c	BALB/c	HY	1.83	—	1.4	—
BALB/c	BALB/c	DNP-HY + HY	0.54	29.5	1.5	107.1
CB20	BALB/c	HY	1.87	—		
CB20	BALB/c	DNP-HY + HY	2.00	106.9		
DNP-HY BALB/c	BALB/c	HY	6.97	—		
DNP-HY BALB/c	BALB/c	DNP-HY + HY	6.78	97.3		

[a] 4×10^6 donor spleen cells were transferred to irradiated recipient mice which had been previously primed to either HY alone or DNP-HY plus HY. Fragments of the recipient spleens were cultured individually in media containing either DNP-HY or FL-HY at a hapten concentration of $10^{-6} M$ as described in detail elsewhere (1, 3, 8).

[b] Positive foci were determined by a radioimmunoassay detecting either DNP or FL specific antibody using I^{125}-labeled rabbit anti-mouse Fab as a detecting reagent as described previously (30).

such an analysis. It can be seen from this table that primary BALB/c B cells transferred to irradiated BALB/c recipients primed to hemocyanin give three times the response of the same cells transferred to recipients primed to DNP-hemocyanin as well. It can also be seen that this suppression is specific since primary B-cell responses to a second hapten fluorescein (FL) coupled to the same carrier, are not suppressed. This suppression does not appear to be due to trivial effects of immunization or the presence of DNP-specific antibody as evidenced by two results presented in Table II.

First, it can be seen that secondary B cells from BALB/c donors are not suppressed in DNP-primed recipients. This finding demonstrates another characteristic difference between primary and secondary B cells which is their relative susceptibility to suppression. This difference would not appear to be related to the specificity of the B cells since, as mentioned earlier, studies from this laboratory investigating the anti-PR8-HA response of primary and secondary B cells indicates that the two subpopulations share much of the same specificity repertoire. Perhaps of greater interest is the finding that primary B cells of a CB20 donor are not suppressed in the DNP immunized BALB/c recipient. These two murine strains are genetically identical except for genes which control the expression of both antibody heavy chain isotype and idiotype (52). Considering the specificity of the regulation for the antibody response to the immunizing hapten it may be argued that the pertinent difference between these two strains is the expression of antibody idiotypes. Thus, following a normal primary immune response it appears that an immunoregulatory phenomenon develops which is capable of suppressing the B cells reactive to that antigen and bearing the idiotypes of the B cells which presumably responded in the immunized animal itself. To what extent such an immunoregulatory phenomenon pertains in a conventional animal faced with a novel antigenic determinant has yet to be determined.

CONCLUSION

In this paper we have reviewed many of the elements which have an influence in determining how an individual will respond to antigenic confrontation. First it is crucial to an understanding of the immune response to realize that the B-cell repertoire is composed of a vast array of clonotypes which is potentially sufficient to discriminate between 2×10^7 different antigenic determinants providing that the antigen's interactions with the B-cell repertoire is random. Antigen plays upon this repertoire in a highly selective way. The outcome of any antigenic stimulation is dependent first on the fact that antigen interacts with a given B cell with a sufficient affinity to enable triggering to occur. Since there also seems to be a necessity for antigen multivalence and presumably receptor interlinkage, it would seem most likely that the requisite for triggering is the stable interaction of receptors tethered with respect to one another within the membrane. The size of such antigen–receptor complexes may be different for different triggering modes, in that tolerance induction may require smaller complexes. However, it is crucial for the specificity of the antigen dependent triggering processes that the antigen receptors of primary B cells interact with antigen in a monovalent way. This is consistent with the antigen binding capabilities known for monomer subunits of IgM antibody. It remains to be seen if other immunoglobulins which are reported to be present on the surface of mature primary lymphocytes such as IgD interact with antigen in a similar fashion. It is interesting to speculate that if IgD can bind antigen in a multivalent fashion, its role in the immune mechanism may be to serve as a focus for antigen such that the monovalent triggering probe, IgM, can interact with antigen and decide for or against stimulation, depending on the stability of that interaction.

It is possible that the triggering mechanism which operates through immunoglobulin receptors may, to some extent, be bypassed by mitogens or specific and nonspecific "factors" synthesized by T cells. However, in general, such modes of stimulation can be clearly discriminated from stimulation by antigen presented in the context of antigen-specific T cells.

The use of allogeneic T cells to dissect the antigen triggering event has enabled an understanding of some important factors governing B-cell antibody responses. First, it appears that antigen presentation in the presence of antigen-specific T cells is a more sophisticated mode of antigen presentation than antigen presentation in the absence of T cells. This is evidenced by the ability of antigen presented in the presence of either allogeneic of syngeneic T cells to stimulate CBA/N male B cells which would not respond otherwise. It may be that T cells are actually serving to prevent the tolerization of these B cells. One could imagine that the ability of allogeneic T cells to carry out this function may reflect an important feature of primary immune responses. If the expression of *I* region gene products were expressed clonally within the T and B cell population of an individual, the majority of T–B cell interactions early in an immune response may be allogeneic in nature and it would become crucial that allogeneic T cells were capable of interacting with primary B cells. Thus, the first B-cell antibody response one sees may be the result of T–B cell interactions which are allogeneiclike in nature; such interactions serve to prevent tolerance in developing B cells and promote IgM antibody synthesis in mature B cells.

The final point to be made from these analyses is that much of what occurs subsequent to antigenic stimulation is dependent not only on the antigen used and its mode of presentation, but also on the B cell that is being acted upon. Thus an immature B cell is likely to be tolerized under conditions which would not affect a mature B cell and similarly secondary B cells may be triggered by a process which would not affect a mature primary B cell. Inherent in this concept is the fact that definable stages of B cells may be crucial for an individual's well being. Thus, it is probably essential that B cells pass through a stage in which self antigens, if present, would induce tolerance. It is possibly equally as important that secondary B cells are generated as a consequence of primary immunization and are able to be stimulated in the suppressive milieu which prohibits the stimulation of primary B cells.

Thus, the immune system would appear to be an extraordinarily specific system which may be stimulated in an exquisitely specific and sophisticated manner and may have built within itself its own regulation.

REFERENCES

1. Klinman, N. (1972) *J. Exp. Med.* **135**, 241.
2. Kreth, H. W., and Williamson, A. H. (1973) *Eur. J. Immunol.* **3**, 141.
3. Klinman, N. R., and Press, J. L. (1975) *Transplant. Rev.* **24**, 41.
4. Cancro, M. P., Gerhard, W., and Klinman, N. R. (1978) *J. Exp. Med.* **147**, 776.
5. Klinman, N. R., and Taylor, R. B. (1969) *Clin. Exp. Immunol.* **4**, 473.
6. Metcalf, E. S., and Klinman, N. R. (1976) *J. Exp. Med.* **143**, 1327.
7. Cambier, J. C., Kettman, J. R., Vitetta, E. S., and Uhr, J. W. (1976) *J. Exp. Med.* **144**, 293.
8. Pierce, S. K., and Klinman, N. R. (1977) *J. Exp. Med.* **146**, 509.
9. Gershon, R. K. (1976) *Transplant. Rev.* **26**, 170.
10. Gearhart, P. J., Sigal, N. H., and Klinman, N. R. (1975) *J. Exp. Med.* **141**, 56.
11. Klinman, N. R., Sigal, N. H., Metcalf, E. S., Pierce, S. K., and Gearhart, P. J. (1976) *Cold Spring Harbor Symp. Quant. Biol.* **41**, 165.
12. Klinman, N. R., Press, J. L., and Segal, G. (1973) *J. Exp. Med.* **138**, 1276.
13. Klinman, N. R., Press, J. L., Sigal, N. H., and Gearhart, P. J. (1976) *In* "The Generation of Diversity: A New Look" (A. J. Cunningham, ed.), p. 127. Academic Press, New York.
14. Kohler, G. (1976) *Eur. J. Immunol.* **6**, 340.
15. Klinman, N. R., Press, J. L., Pickard, A. K., Woodland, R. T., and Dewey, A. F. (1974)

In "The Immune System: Genes, Receptors, Signals" (E. E. Sercarz, A. R. Williamson, and C. F. Fox, eds.), p. 357. Academic Press, New York.

16. Basten, A., Miller, J., Sprent, J., and Pye, J. (1972) *J. Exp. Med.* **135**, 160.
17. Bianco, C., Patrick, R., and Nussenzweig, V. (1970) *J. Exp. Med.* **132**, 702.
18. Hammerling, J., Deak, B., Mauve, G., Hammerling, V., and McDevitt, H. O. (1974) *Immunogenetics* **1**, 69.
19. Pierce, S. K., and Klinman, N. R. (1976) *J. Exp. Med.* **144**, 1254.
20. LaFleur, L., Underdown, B. J., Miller, R. G., and Phillips, R. A. (1972) *Ser. Haematol.* **5**, 58.
21. Nossal, G. J. V., and Pike, B. L. (1975) *J. Exp. Med.* **141**, 904.
22. Metcalf, E. S., and Klinman, N. R. (1977) *J. Immunol.* **118**, 2111.
23. Amsbaugh, D., Hansen, C., Prescott, B., Stashak, P., Barthold, D., and Baker, P. (1972) *J. Exp. Med.* **136**, 931.
24. Scher, I., Steinberg, A., Berning, A. K., and Paul, W. E. (1975) *J. Exp. Med.* **142**, 637.
25. Metcalf, E. S. (1978) *Fed. Proc., Fed. Am. Soc. Exp. Biol.* **37**, 674.
26. Strober, S. (1975) *Transplant. Rev.* **24**, 84.
27. Gowans, J. L., and Manson, D. W. (1976) *Ann. Immunol. (Paris)* **127**, 74.
28. Coutinho, A., and Möller, G. (1975) *Adv. Immunol.* **21**, 113.
29. Katz, D. H., and Benacerraf, B. (1976) *In* "The Role of Products of the Histocompatibility Gene Complex in Immune Responses" (D. H. Katz and B. Benacerraf, eds.), p. 355. Academic Press, New York.
30. Pierce, S. K., and Klinman, N. R. (1975) *J. Exp. Med.* **142**, 1165.
31. Feldman, M. (1972) *J. Exp. Med.* **136**, 532.
32. Watson, J., Trenker, E., and Cohn, M. (1973) *J. Exp. Med.* **138**, 699.
33. Anderson, J., Sjöberg, O., and Möller, G. (1972) *Transplant. Rev.* **11**, 131.
34. Feldman, M., Howard, J., and Desaymord, C. (1975) *Transplant. Rev.* **23**, 78.
35. Klinman, N. R., and Doughty, R. A. (1973) *J. Exp. Med.* **138**, 473.
36. Klinman, N. R., and Press, J. L. (1975) *J. Exp. Med.* **141**, 1133.
37. Metgzer, H. (1977) *In* "Regulatory Genetics of the Immune System" (E. E. Sercarz, L. A. Herzenberg, and C. F. Fox, eds.), p. 679. Academic Press, New York.
38. Anderson, M. J., and Cohen, M. W. (1977) *J. Physiol. (London)* **268**, 757.
39. Metcalf, E. S., Sigal, N. H., Pickard, A., and Klinman, N. R. (1977) *Prog. Immunol., Int. Congr. Immunol., 3rd, 1977* p. 162.
40. Möller, G. (1976) *Cold Spring Harbor Symp. Quant. Biol.* **41**, 217.
41. Kearney, J., and Lawton, A. (1975) *J. Immunol.* **115**, 671.
42. Klaus, G., and Humphrey, J. H. (1975) *Transplant. Rev.* **23**, 105.
43. Anderson, J., Sjöberg, O., and Möller, G. (1972) *Eur. J. Immunol.* **2**, 349.
44. Press, J., Klinman, N., Henry, C., Wofsy, L., Delovitch, T., and McDevitt, H. (1975) *In* "Membrane Receptors of Lymphocytes" (M. Seligmann, J. L. Preud'homme, and F. M. Kourlsky, eds.), p. 247. Elsevier, Amsterdam.
45. Owen, J. A. (1978) Ph.D. Thesis, University of Pennsylvania, Philadelphia.
46. Schrader, J. W. (1975) *J. Immunol.* **114**, 665.
47. Mitchinson, N. A. (1967) *Cold Spring Harbor Symp. Quant. Biol.* **32**, 431.
48. Dintzis, H. N., Dintzis, R. C., and Vogelstein, B. (1976) *Proc. Natl. Acad. Sci. U.S.A.* **73**, 3671.
49. Rodkey, L. (1974) *J. Exp. Med.* **139**, 712.
50. Köhler, H. (1975) *Transplant. Rev.* **27**, 24.
51. Jerne, N. (1974) *Ann. Immunol. (Paris)* **125c**, 373.
52. Leiberman, R., Potter, M., Mushinski, B., Humphrey, W., and Rudikoff, S. (1974) *J. Exp. Med.* **139**, 983.

PART V

LYMPHOCYTE HYBRIDS

Fusion of Immunoglobulin Secreting Cells

MARC SHULMAN AND GEORGES KÖHLER

Basel Institute for Immunology
Basel, Switzerland

INTRODUCTION

Immunoglobulins (Ig) have been intensively studied with two goals in mind. On the one hand, immunoglobulins are a reagent whose specificity in antigen binding is used to distinguish different biochemical entities. On the other hand, antibodies themselves represent a very interesting phenomenon, and challenge our ingenuity to understand cellular and molecular control mechanisms through which the organism generates antibodies that react with foreign substances of great variety, yet not with the organism itself. This review will consider the ways in which hybridomas, the hybrid cells derived from the fusion of tumor and normal Ig producing cells, aid the attainment of these two goals: First, hybridomas synthesize monoclonal antibody, and thus provide an unlimited supply of monospecific antibody which is used to define antigenic determinants. Second, hybridomas are material for the study of the molecular biology of immunoglobulin synthesis.

IMPORTANCE OF MONOCLONAL ANTIBODY

An antibody producing cell and its progeny make antibody of only one specificity, i.e., in any cell, only one light (L) chain variable (V) region and one heavy (H) chain variable region are expressed. There-

275

fore, the population of antibody producing cells is as heterogeneous as the antibody population.

Estimates of the antibody repertoire in the mouse strain range between 1 and 5×10^7 (1–3). By transfer of limiting amounts of spleen cells into irradiated hosts, a single mouse has been shown to make at least 138 different anti-NIP antibodies (2) and at least 43 different anti-β-galactosidase antibodies against one determinant of the enzyme (3). The total potential repertoire of a single mouse might be comparable to the repertoire of the mouse strain (3) which for the two antigens mentioned above has been determined to be around 8100 antiNIP and 1200 anti-β-galactosidase antibodies. Nevertheless when a conventional mouse response to these antigens is analyzed, only 5–10 different antibody species are seen, representing probably a random sample of the total repertoire. These considerations indicate that it is very difficult or even impossible to make reproducible reagents against a given antigenic determinant. Figure 1 demonstrates the situation encountered when, for example, mice are immunized with xenogeneic cells. The mouse recognizes perhaps between 10 and 100 different antigens on the cell surface which might have 5 different major antigenic determinants. Against each determinant one mouse might produce 5 distinct antibodies which will in general differ from the antibodies made by a second mouse against the same determinant. By employing appropriate adsorptions and allogeneic immunizations, one can reduce the heterogeneity. However, even under these conditions the sera obtained have four major disadvantages: (1) the titers are low, (2) the antibodies, while specific for a single determinant, are nevertheless heterogeneous, (3) the supply is limited, and (4) the same combination of specific antibodies is impossible to reproduce in a new animal.

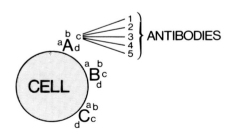

Fig. 1.   Heterogeneous antibody response to xenogeneic immunization.

HYBRIDOMAS

The goal of an unlimited supply of monoclonal antibody of predetermined specificity is achieved by making a hybridoma, a hybrid cell
derived from the fusion of a myeloma tumor cell and a specific antibody producing spleen cell from an immunized animal (4). From the
myeloma tumor cell parent comes the capacity for unlimited growth in
culture and from the spleen cell, the capacity for synthesizing the
specific antibody.

Although other techniques are available to generate monoclonal antibodies they all suffer from some disadvantages not encountered in
the lymphocyte fusion technique (Table I).

SELECTION OF HYBRIDOMAS

Hybridomas are made by fusing the parental cells and selecting the
rare viable hybrid cells with the "HAT" selection medium (12). The
basis for this selection is the following. Aminopterin (A) inhibits the *de
novo* pathways of purine and pyridine synthesis. Normal tumor cells
can, however, grow in aminopterin-containing medium if such medium also contains hypoxanthine (H) and thymidine (T) which by
alternative "scavenger" pathways can be used as nucleotide precur-

TABLE I
Methods of Preparation of Monoclonal Antibodies

Technique		Limitation	Reference
Monoclonal antibodies from normal cells			
Transfer of limiting	a. Whole animal	Concentration of	3,5
amount of lymphocytes.	b. Spleen focus	Ig is low and	1,6
Clone expansion in	c. Microculture	supply is limited.	6,7
Monoclonal antibodies from tumor cells			
Myeloma induction		Specificity cannot be predetermined. Some species are refractory to myeloma induction.	8
SV40 transformation of lymphocyte		Concentration of Ig is low. Transformation is rare.	9
Epstein–Barr virus transformation of lymphocytes		Only primate lympho-cytes are transformable.	10,11

sors. The myeloma tumor cell lines such as X63-Ag8 used for making such hybridomas are defective in the enzyme hypoxanthine guanine phosphoribosyltransferase (HGPRT), necessary for making purine nucleotides from hypoxanthine, and therefore these cells cannot grow in HAT medium. Normal spleen cells are capable of only limited growth in tissue culture, but are able to supply the enzyme HGPRT. Therefore, only hybrid cells gaining HGPRT from the normal spleen cell partner and the capacity for growth in tissue culture from the myeloma can grow in HAT medium. Myeloma cells are fused with spleen cells from immunized animals using inactivated Sendai virus or polyethylene glycol to "glue" the cells together. The mixture of

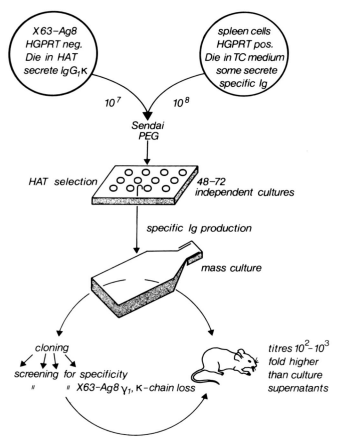

Fig. 2.   Hybridoma production, screening, and propagation.

cells is then distributed to many wells containing HAT medium so that each well yields approximately one viable hybrid cell line. Such hybrids are then grown to mass culture and recloned or grown in mice (Fig. 2). (An extensive description of methods for making hybridomas and of the Ig specificity of those hybridomas generated to date is presented in Melchers *et al.*, 13).

ANTIBODY SPECIFICITIES AVAILABLE FROM HYBRIDOMAS

Over the last years, cell lines making monoclonal antibodies of many different specificities have been generated. Table II summarizes the types of antibody producing cell lines available. This library of monoclonal reagents will continue to grow rapidly.

Table II
Hybridoma Antibody Specificities[a]

Specificity	Types of H and L chains
Haptens	
Trinitrophenyl	$\mu,\gamma1,\gamma2a,\gamma2b,\gamma3,\lambda,\kappa$
Phosphoryl choline	
Ig allotype	
Ig-1 (mouse $\gamma2a$)	
Ig-5 (mouse δ)	$\gamma1,\gamma2a$
Virus	
SV40	
Rabies	
Herpes Zoster	Human Ig
Influenza	
Cell surface antigens	
Mouse H-2K	$\gamma2a$
Mouse I-A	$\gamma2a,\gamma2b,\gamma3$
Rat H-IA	
Forssman	
Thy 1	
Chick brain	
Sheep red cells	$\mu,\gamma1,\gamma2b,\kappa$
Miscellaneous	
Ovalbumin	ϵ
MOPC 460 idiotype	γ
Hen egg lysozyme	

[a] See Melchers *et al.* (13) for detailed description of the origin of such hybridomas.

CELLULAR RESTRICTIONS ON HYBRIDOMA FUSION

The choice of tumor cell line is important for the successful generation of hybridomas, because for some types of normal and tumor cells
fusion might be impossible. Furthermore, as will be discussed below,
the tumor cell parent can enhance or extinguish Ig expression of the
normal parent. Some of these effects work to the advantage of the
experimenter, and some to his disadvantage. Some will provide a fruitful area for research.

Often the tumor and normal cells differ in genetic markers. The
ontogenetic state of the cell can be characterized by the expression of
specific products. For example, T cells but not B cells express the Thy
1 antigen, for which two allelic forms, Thy 1.1 and Thy 1.2, are known;
liver cells are characterized by the synthesis of albumin. In some cases
the ontogenetic state of the normal cell parent of a hybrid has been
inferred by the expression of ontogenetically specific products (14).
However, cases exist where the expression of a silent gene of one
partner was induced in the hybrid. In a hybrid derived from a rat
hepatoma and mouse fibroblasts or lymphoblasts, expression of mouse
albumin (15,16) and another mouse serum protein (17) was activated.
Fusion of the thymoma BW5147 (Thy 1.1) with different Thy 1 expressing and nonexpressing cell populations of a genetically Thy 1.2 animal produced in both cases hybrids expressing Thy 1.2, arguing that
the tumor cell parent can activate Thy 1 expression of the normal cell
parent (18).

By contrast Ig *specificity* is likely to be a reliable marker. Because
an Ig producing cell makes only one of the thousands of different
possible specificities, it is correspondingly unlikely that a cell could be
"induced" to express the specificity looked for, i.e., the Ig specificity
expressed in the hybridoma is the same as the specificity of the Ig
made by the normal parent spleen cell. However, the quantity or class
of antibody expressed might behave as a phenotypic marker, subject to
induction and repression.

SELECTIVE FUSION TO Ig SECRETING SPLEEN CELLS

With the above cautions in mind, we wish to review the evidence
that myeloma cells yield viable hybrids preferentially from the fusions
with the Ig secreting cells of the spleen.

Among hybridomas, the frequency of specific and nonspecific antibody producing cells is the same as in the fraction of the Ig secreting
spleen cells, which in turn is different from that observed for the frac-

tion of small spleen B cells. For example, the number of sheep red cell (SRC) precursor spleen B cells in unimmunized or hyperimmunized mice is 0.1% (19) or 0.5% (A. Coutinho, personal communication) respectively. At the time of fusion SRC-specific Ig secreting (plaque forming) cells comprised 0.0005 and 0.05% of the total spleen cells of unimmunized and immunized animals, respectively (Table III). If we assume random fusion of the myeloma cells with the spleen cells we would expect at most 0.5% of the hybrids to be SRC specific. By contrast we observed that 20% of the hybrids were SRC specific. It was found that specific hybridomas were most frequently obtained in fusions with spleen cells having the highest frequency of specific plaque forming cells (21), suggesting that fusions of myeloma and plaque forming cell preferentially yielded hybrids. In the spleen, plaque forming cells comprise 1% of the total cells (19) so that if there is preferential fusion with Ig secreting cells, one would expect that among hybridomas derived from spleen cells of an unimmunized animal 0.05% would be SRC specific, whereas fusion with spleen cells of an immunized animal would yield hybridomas of which 5% would have SRC specificity. These figures are in approximate agreement with our finding that in fusions with spleen cells of unimmunized and immunized mice, the frequency of specific hybrids was <0.2 and 20%, respectively. Furthermore, the IgG/IgM class distribution of specific and nonspecific hybrids corresponds to that seen for plaque forming spleen cells. An additional argument for this hypothesis that Ig secreting cells are the preferred parent are the fusion results using lipopolysaccharide (LPS) stimulated cells as fusion partners. Addition of LPS to spleen B cells stimulates the cells to divide and secrete Ig. LPS-stimulated cells fused more efficiently than unstimulated cells and blast cells more efficiently than small lymphocytes (22). These results argue that the dividing Ig secreting cells as opposed to the nondividing surface Ig positive small B cells of the spleen are the major fusion partners of the myeloma cell. Therefore the successful generation of hybrid cells secreting antigen-specific antibodies is very dependent on the frequency of antigen-specific plaque forming cells.

PHYLOGENETIC RESTRICTIONS

The mouse myeloma line X63-Ag8 [derived from MOPC 21 (8)] has been fused to syngeneic (21) and allogeneic (23) mouse spleen cells and with similar high fusion and success rates to rat spleen cells (24). In collaboration with A. Kelus we have fused X63-Ag8 to rabbit splenocytes. The derivation of hybrids was about tenfold lower than

TABLE III

Comparison of Ig Secreting Spleen Cells to Hybridoma Cells Obtained in Myeloma × Spleen Cell Fusions[a]

	Ig secretors			4 Days after 2nd stim. SRC-specific secretors			Fraction of total Ig secreting cells that are SRC specific	
	Total	IgM	IgG	Total	IgM	IgG	After Imm.	Before Imm.
Spleen	1	90	10	0.05	50	50	5	0.05
Hybrids	50[b] (49/95)	93 (91/98)	7 (7/98)	10 (5/54)	40 (2/54)	60 (3/54)	20	<0.2

[a] Results expressed as percentages.

[b] In these hybrids the myeloma IgG and additional new immunoglobulin could be detected.

[c] The results for nonspecific Ig secreting cells are taken from Andersson et al. (19). Other data are from Köhler and Shulman (20).

with mouse splenocytes and only occasionally a hybrid secreted a rabbit light chain, but never a complete rabbit Ig. Peripheral blood lymphocytes grown in the presence of Epstein–Barr virus and antigen (SRC) were fused with X63-Ag8. Only a few of the hybrids secreted normal amounts of human Ig, and reclones of these hybrids secreted no human Ig and showed loss of almost all human chromosomes (25). Fusions to frog lymphocytes resulted in even fewer hybrids, and they exhibited no stable Ig secretion (25). However, exceptions emerge showing the feasibility of generating functional hybrids by fusing mouse myeloma with rabbit spleen cells (J. Andersson, personal communication) or with human cells (26,27). Nevertheless the results so far suggest a phylogenetic restriction of the lymphocyte fusion: greater phylogenetic separation between the normal lymphocyte and the tumor cell parents makes it more difficult to generate functional (specific antibody secreting) hybrids. To obtain hybridomas from other species, a myeloma cell line from that species will probably be a better fusion partner.

ONTOGENETIC RESTRICTIONS

Tumor cells of various kinds have been fused with Ig producing cells, and the resulting hybrids have been examined for Ig production and other markers. Fusion of myeloma cells to spleen cells rescues spleen cell Ig production but not the T-cell marker Thy 1 (23).

Fusion of thymoma cells to spleen cells rescues the spleen cell Thy 1 marker but not Ig production (14,28). Fibroblasts, ontogenetically less related to the lymphoid cell lineage, have been fused to thymoma cells or myeloma cells. The hybrids showed extinction of Thy 1 (29) and Ig production (30,31), respectively. These results suggest a simple rule for function rescue fusions. Only tumor lines ontogenetically closely related to the normal cell fusion partner yield hybrids expressing the specialized function of normal cells.

HYBRID ANTIBODY MOLECULES

The first hybrids were obtained by fusing the BALB/c myeloma cell X63-Ag8, which makes an IgG_1 (κ) of unknown specificity. The resulting hybrid cells expressed not only the specific heavy and light chains of the spleen cell fusion partner but also the nonspecific myeloma Ig chains. We have observed that some such hybrid cells synthesize hybrid antibody molecules (32). The test for hybrid heavy chain molecules took advantage of conditions in which $\gamma 2b$ chains bind strongly to the protein A of *Staphylococcus aureus* whereas μ and $\gamma 1$ do not (33). When a mixture of IgG_1 and IgG_{2b} molecules was mixed with *S. aureus* we found that only IgG_{2b} could be eluted from the bacteria, whereas IgG_1 remained in the supernatant. However, from the supernatant of a hybrid line secreting both IgG_1 and IgG_{2b} molecules, about half of the $\gamma 1$ chains could be eluted together with IgG_{2b}. This indicates that $\gamma 1$–$\gamma 2b$ hybrid molecules were secreted and that the association of these chains is about random. There was, however, no hybrid molecule formation between μ and $\gamma 2b$. The light chains L_1 (μ origin) and L_2 ($\gamma 2b$ origin) were evenly distributed in the IgM molecules but there was a preferential association of L_2 with $\gamma 2b$. No hybrid molecule formation for μ and δ chains has been reported (34,35). It is interesting to note that the formation of hybrid heavy chains (e.g., $\gamma 1$–$\gamma 2b$) molecules seems to be correlated with the nonexistence of normal cells which coexpress these chains (36), and that the nonformation of hybrid heavy chains (e.g., no μ–δ or μ–$\gamma 2b$) is found in those cases where coexpression has been demonstrated in normal lymphocytes. The formation of heavy chain hybrid molecules may, therefore, be indicative of a forbidden combination of heavy chain classes in normal cells.

A hybrid cell making distinct γ heavy chains and two distinct light chains which are randomly associated produces ten different IgG molecules, one of which is the antigen binding monospecific IgG which represents only one-sixteenth of the total amount of IgG secreted. Even after purification with antigen columns, (assuming that one antigen binding site per IgG molecule is sufficient for binding), there are four different antibodies, only one of which is monospecific and represents one-seventh of the total amount.

For some applications the heterogeneous antibody production poses no problem. In fact, hybrid antibody molecules would be useful in cases where antibodies with two different binding activities are needed. However, if the hybridoma antibodies are to be used, for example, to derive anti-idiotype antibodies, truly monospecific preparations are required. One way to overcome this problem is to isolate a reclone that has lost expression of the nonspecific chains. Generally we found that among hybridoma reclones, about one reclone in 50 had lost expression of the nonspecific H chain. From this clone, at a similar frequency could be isolated clones which no longer expressed the remaining nonspecific L chain (see the next Section). However, although clones which have ceased to make a nonspecific chain are not rare (one in 50), such recloning is very time consuming.

Another possibility is to use a myeloma line which does not synthesize Ig chains but supports synthesis of the spleen cell-derived Ig chains. A subclone (NSI-Ag4/1) of the MOPC 21 myeloma which synthesizes only the myeloma κ but not the γ1 chain has been successfully used (see Melchers *et al.*, 13).

Recently we have generated hybridomas using as the tumor cell parent, the cell line Sp2/0-Ag, which itself synthesizes neither an H nor an L chain. Sp2/0-Ag is derived from Sp2/HLGK (21), a hybrid between a BALB/c spleen cell contributing a γ2b (H) and κ (L) chain with anti-SRC activity and X63-Ag8 (γ1 (G) and κ (K)). The line Sp2/0-Ag is 8-azaguanine resistant, dies in HAT supplemented medium, and synthesizes no Ig chains. It was isolated by D. Wilde (MRC, Cambridge) as a reclone from Sp2/HL-Ag. It has about 73 chromosomes which is only 8 more than the chromosome number of X63-Ag8.

In our first experiments, the efficiency of fusion of mouse spleen cells with Sp2/0-Ag was about twentyfold lower than with X63-Ag8. More recently, fusion with Sp2/0-Ag has been as efficient as has been reported for X63-Ag8 and other myeloma-derived tumor cells. In a particular experiment we fused Sp2/0-Ag cells with spleen cells of BALB/c immunized against TNP-KLH. We derived eight hybrid lines each synthesizing a monoclonal antibody as judged by polyacrylamide gel electrophoressis of [^{14}C]leucine-labeled culture supernatants. Four of them synthesizing IgG were found to be specific for the TNP hapten. All four lines were recloned and showed continued synthesis of antiTNP antibodies over several months. Such hybrids can be grown as tumors in BALB/c mice yielding ascites with anti-TNP titers much higher than those obtained from cell culture supernatants. Since no reexpression of the Sp2/0-Ag parental Ig chains was observed, this line is indeed suitable for producing hybrid lines secreting truly monospecific antibodies.

MOLECULAR BIOLOGY OF IMMUNOGLOBULINS

Immunoglobulin structure and synthesis present several interesting problems. We would like to outline the ways in which such problems have been or can be studied by applying biochemical analysis and somatic cell genetics to Ig producing cell lines. While many of the studies cited have used myeloma cell lines, future experiments will probably exploit the greater variety of Ig that hybridomas make available.

NONRANDOM LOSS OF H AND L CHAIN EXPRESSION IN HYBRIDOMAS

Hybridomas can express more than one immunoglobulin, thus overcoming the restriction in normal lymphocytes which show isotypic, allotypic, and idiotypic exclusion. But another restriction seems to be imposed on the lymphocyte hybrids. Although Ig chain expression was lost quite frequently, the light and heavy chain expression was lost in a nonrandom way (Table IV). Cells where the number of different L chains expressed is the same as the number of different H chains yielded reclones that had lost expression of an H chain, but none that had lost only L chain expression. By contrast, cells making a greater number of different L chains than the number of different H chains yielded reclones among which loss of L chain expression was as frequent as loss of H chain expression. Reexpression of the lost chain did not occur in any of 10^7 cells, nor in hybrids derived from the fusion of such cells with an Ig secreting tumor (37). This result taken together with the observation that chain loss was more frequent when the analyzed hybrid had more chromosomes (Table IV) suggests that chain loss is due to chromosome loss. Since chain loss is random in those cases where the number of light chains exceeds the number of heavy chains, chromosome loss presumably also occurs at random. In explanation for this pattern we suggest that the free heavy chain (i.e., not bound to light chain) which accumulates in a cell that has lost a light chain encoding chromosome is toxic, and such cells therefore escape our analysis.

IMMUNOGLOBULIN BIOCHEMISTRY

Hybridoma technology permits the rapid accumulation of specific antibodies, permitting comparative studies. For a series of similar an-

TABLE IV
Loss of H or L Chain Expression in Hybridomas

Number of chromosomes	Chains	Frequency of loss of H chain	L chain
130–150	2H + 3L	0.23	0.23
90–100	2H + 2L	0.04	<0.003
	1H + 2L	0.01	0.02
70–90	1H + 1L	0.007	<0.0003
	0H + 1L		[a]

[a] Such variants have been reported by Coffino and Scharff (36a).

tibodies one could examine such parameters as antigen binding, amino acid sequence, or contribution of light and heavy chains, and thus better define the basis of antibody–antigen reactions. One such study has been reported by Imanishi–Kari *et al.* (38) for nitrophenyl-binding antibodies. From such a comparison these authors concluded that heteroclitic binding was associated with the occurrence of the λ chain, homoclitic with the occurrence of the κ chain.

Unusual antibody properties which are masked by their low concentration in sera might be revealed as more monoclonal preparations are studied. For example, we have found that about 10% of the IgM producing hybridomas secrete a μ chain that is 5000 daltons larger than the usual μ (32). High molecular μ secreting hybridomas were found in all the mouse strains tested (BALB/c, AKR/J, and C57B1/6). The molecule is secreted as a pentamer and cross-reacts with a specific sheep antiMOPC104E μ-sera. Intracellularly, where only a small fraction of core sugars have been added to the μ chain, the same apparent molecular weight difference of about 5000 daltons is observed, arguing against the hypothesis that the additional molecular weight reflects sugar attachment. Furthermore, we have fused a high molecular weight IgM secreting hybridoma with a low (normal) molecular weight IgM secreting line. The hybrid expressed μ chains of both parental types, arguing against postsynthetic regulatory differences being the cause of the molecular weight difference. This high molecular weight μ might therefore represent a new subclass.

GENERATION OF DIVERSITY

For many years it was argued whether all antibodies that were observed were encoded in the germ line DNA, or whether the variety reflected events such as mutation, or recombination that occurred somatically (39). Mouse lambda light chain genes have been counted by several methods (40–44) and the number of genes is less than number of amino acid sequences observed, implying that the diversity is for the most part generated somatically.

The origin of antibody diversity is a difficult problem to analyze, because it is not evident whether there is a special mechanism or special stage of development for altering Ig genes. Nevertheless, over the last years, mutant cell lines making an altered Ig have been isolated from different myelomas. Milstein *et al.* (45) screened 7000 clones of the MOPC 21 cell line for the appearance of Ig with altered electrophoretic properties. From this screening were isolated seven mutants, of which four were characterized for their amino acid sequence. One of these mutants was apparently an A–G transition, another a frameshift, the third caused a deletion of the CH1 domain, the fourth a terminal deletion, perhaps resulting from a nonsense triplet created by mutation. The frequency with which such mutants are found suggests a mutation frequency of 3×10^{-6}/cell per generation. Scharff and his colleagues have isolated variant clones making Ig with altered tryptic peptides. The first such variants were recognized by screening clones for the loss of H chain antigenic determinants (46) and more recently for the loss of hapten binding (47). The frequency of such hapten nonbinding variants is in the range 0.1–0.6%, and the variants are remarkable for their instability, that is, the high frequency with which they revert to the original or near original state.

Using a hybridoma cell line secreting IgM with trinitrophenyl (TNP) binding activity, we have recently developed methods for selecting mutants that have lost this activity (Fig. 3). To obtain this selection we couple TNP to the cell membrane. Wild-type cells secrete IgM that binds to the TNP on their own membrane which in the presence of complement kills the cell. On the other hand, mutant cells secreting, for example, IgM which does not bind TNP or that does not fix complement (C') will survive this treatment. Along with this selection we have developed a plaque assay that is specific for mutants that

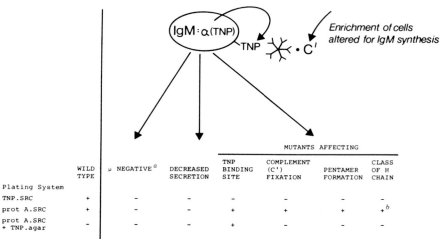

	WILD TYPE	μ NEGATIVE[a]	DECREASED SECRETION	TNP BINDING SITE	COMPLEMENT (C') FIXATION	PENTAMER FORMATION	CLASS OF H CHAIN
Plating System							
TNP.SRC	+	-	-	-	-	-	-
prot A.SRC	+	-	-	+	+	+	+[b]
prot A.SRC + TNP.agar	-	-	-	+	-	-	-

[a] Loss of light chain expression is observed only for cells which have already lost heavy chain expression.

[b] Other heavy chain classes can be detected with appropriate developing sera.

Fig. 3. Isolation of mutants making altered immunoglobulin.

have lost the TNP binding activity (Fig. 3). For this assay we use the protein A plaque method in which protein A is coupled to sheep red cells (SRC) on which any Ig-secreting cell makes a plaque, regardless of its specificity (48). By including TNP-coupled agar in the assay system we are able to suppress plaques from the wild-type cells whose antibody binds to the TNP agar instead of protein A–SRC. By contrast the mutants whose IgM does not bind TNP make a plaque. From this system we have isolated a mutant making a μ chain that is about 10,000 daltons smaller than the parent chain. Another mutant appears to have altered the regulation of L chain synthesis.

The results obtained to date are consistent with the conjecture that significant variability is generated in plasma cells, the normal cells analogous to myeloma tumor cells used in these studies. On the other hand, it is premature to conclude that these observations reflect events analogous to those underlying somatic diversification. However, the plaque assay for mutants offers a simple test for the occurrence of mutations affecting the variable region, and therefore can be used to test whether in a cell one can achieve conditions increasing the frequency of diversification.

IMMUNOGLOBULIN SYNTHESIS

Immunoglobulin synthesis presents several peculiar problems. First, the variable (V) and constant (C) parts of the Ig chains appear to be encoded by physically separate genes. Nevertheless, the RNA transcript of these genes contains the V and C nucleotide sequences in tandem (49). A second problem is that there appear to be more V genes than C genes. Third, the variable region of the heavy chain, V_H, can apparently be expressed in conjunction with different C_H genes (heavy chain class switch) (36,50–52).

As a solution to these problems, Dreyer and Bennett (53) suggested that the separate V and C genes of the germ line were translocated to be in tandem in the Ig producing cell, thus generating a continuous template. An alternative model that V and C were transcribed into separate RNA molecules which were subsequently joined was made unlikely by the finding that hybridomas derived by fusing parents making two distinct heavy chains, here denoted V_1C_1 and V_2C_2 did not make the "scrambled" molecules V_1C_2 and V_2C_1 (4,45,54).

Direct evidence of translocation for mouse light chain V and C regions was found by Hozumi and Tonegawa (41) and Rabbits and Forster (42) by comparing the restriction maps of DNA from Ig producing and other cells: they found that in the germ line DNA arrangement, V and C are on separate restriction fragments whereas in Ig producing myeloma cells, V and C are closer together on the same fragment.

The heavy chain switch might also involve DNA translocation. According to such a model, in a cell making IgM, the V_H region would be adjacent to the μ constant ($C\mu$) region. Switching to IgG production would require apposing the V_H and $C\gamma$ regions.

Recently, several examples involving viral and mammalian genes have been found where nucleotide sequences which are separate on the DNA template are in tandem in the RNA transcript [see Gilbert (55), for a summary of these results]. This phenomenon, called "RNA splicing," has suggested an alternative model for the activation of heavy chain constant genes (44,55). First, translocation would bring together the cluster of C_H genes and a particular V_H gene. An RNA for this V_H–C_H region would be transcribed. For an IgM producer this primary transcript would be processed to yield an RNA in which the V_H region would be in tandem with C_μ, whereas for an IgG producer the RNA would be processed so that V_H and C_γ would be in tandem. The fusion of an IgG producing cell (making V_1C_γ) with an IgM producing cell (making V_2C_μ) yields a hybrid producing both IgG and IgM. The RNA processing model predicts that such a hybrid should have both γ and μ processing enzymes and that these enzymes should act on the primary transcripts of both the V_1 and the V_2 expressing chromosomes, thus predicting that the hybrid should make the scrambled chains V_1C_μ and V_2C_γ as well as the parental V_1C_γ and V_2C_γ chains.

Using more sensitive techniques than were employed earlier, we have again tested for scrambled molecules. In this case we used a hybridoma Sp2/HLML′ derived from the fusion of the hybridoma Sp2/HL-Ag-14, which makes an IgG_{2b} specific for SRC, with a spleen cell making an IgM of unknown specificity. We have looked, on the one hand, for IgM with SRC specificity, and on the other, for direct SRC plaques, and have found no evidence of scrambled molecules: in the hybrid, less than 0.15% of the μ molecules bear the SRC-specific region contributed by the IgG parent, and fewer than 1 among 5×10^6 cells have switched to making SRC-specific IgM.

We conclude from these experiments that for the pair IgG and IgM (a) V–C expression is stable, (b) the RNA processing model in its simplest form is incorrect, and (c) the regulation of class expression might be determined by some mechanism such as class-specific translocation which exerts its effect prior to RNA transcription.

While we have shown that regulation of the IgM to IgG switch is probably not due to a change in RNA splicing of the same transcript, the RNA splicing model might be valid for the regulation of the expression of other classes. For example, the membrane of some normal B cells contains both μ and δ bearing the same V region (51). Hybridomas derived from the fusion of transformed hamster cells with a mouse spleen cell making both mouse μ and δ have been isolated (35), suggesting that normal cells might synthesize these two heavy chains simultaneously. As described above for the fusion of IgG and IgM producing cells, the fusion of these μ and δ producing cells with cells making an IgM with a distinct specificity would provide the material to answer this question.

BASIS OF DIFFERENTIATION

Higher organisms contain cells of very many different types. At the present time, normal cells cannot be grown indefinitely outside the organism, and it has not been possible to assess the importance of the internal as opposed to the external environment of the cell in determining the differentiated state. For many tumor cell lines the differentiated state is stable and inherited by the progeny cells over many generations, and therefore we might use these cells to investigate the mechanisms that maintain and transmit the differentiated state.

Hybridomas provide several advantages in the study of the basis of differentiation. First, assays exist for the Ig, its RNA, and its DNA, and therefore the state of these parameters can be examined. Analysis of the mechanism of differentiation requires the comparison of closely related states. If the number of determining factors distinguishing the different states is large, i.e., greater than one or two, then the analysis becomes very difficult. We might have already on hand appropriate cell lines to compare. Nonsecreting B lymphomas that bear IgM in their membrane might differ from Ig secreting hybridomas by only one factor, thus offering the possibility of simple analysis. A preliminary attempt at such an analysis was reported by Laskov et al. (56) who found that the fusion of B lymphoma cells making, but not secreting, IgM with an IgG secreting myeloma yielded hybrids secreting both IgG and IgM.

New closely related cell lines might be obtained when cells "mutate" to different states, e.g., from secretion to nonsecretion, or from IgM to IgG production. While attempts to achieve such transitions have failed in the past, the intervening years have provided a new technology which we can now apply.

REFERENCES

1. Klinman, N., and Press, J. (1975) *Transplant. Rev.* **24**, 41–83.
2. Kreth, H., and Williamson, A. (1973) *Eur. J. Immunol.* **3**, 141–147.
3. Köhler, G. (1976) *Eur. J. Immunol.* **6**, 340–347.
4. Köhler, G., and Milstein, C. (1975) *Nature (London)* **256**, 495–497.
5. Eichmann, K. (1972) *Eur. J. Immunol.* **2**, 301–307.
6. Levy, R., Dilley, J., Lampson, L. (1978) *Curr. Top. Microbiol. Immunol.* **81**, 164–169.
7. Andersson, J., Coutinho, A., Lernhardt, W., and Melchers, F. (1977) *Cell* **10**, 27–34.
8. Potter, M. (1972) *Physiol. Rev.* **52**, 631–719.
9. Strosberg, A., Collins, J., Black, P., Malamud, D., Wilbert, S., Bloch, K., and Haber, E. (1974) *Proc. Natl. Acad. Sci. U.S.A.* **71**, 263–264.
10. Zurawski, V., Spedden, S., Black, P., and Haber, E. (1978) *Curr. Top. Microbiol. Immunol.* **81**, 152–155.
11. Steinitz. M., Koskimies, S., Klein, G., and Mäkelä, O. (1978) *Curr. Top. Microbiol. Immunol.* **81**, 156–163.
12. Littlefield, J. (1964) *Science* **145**, 709–710.
13. Melchers, F., Potter, M., and Warner, N. (eds.) (1978) *Curr. Top. Microbiol. Immunol.* **81**.
14. Goldsby, R., Osborne, B., Simpson, E., and Herzenberg, L. (1977) *Nature (London)* **267**, 707–708.
15. Peterson, J., and Weiss, M. (1971) *Proc. Natl. Acad. Sci. U.S.A.* **69**, 571–575.
16. Malawista, S., and Weiss, M. (1974) *Proc. Natl. Acad. Sci. U.S.A.* **71**, 927–931.
17. Dannies, P., and Tashjian, A. (1974) *In* "Somatic Cell Hybridization" (R. Davidson and F. de la Cruz, eds.), pp. 163–172. Raven, New York.
18. Iverson, G., Goldsby, R., and Herzenberg, L. (1978) *Curr. Top. Microbiol. Immunol.* **81**, 192–194.
19. Andersson, J., Coutinho, A., and Melchers, F. (1977) *J. Exp. Med.* **145**, 1520–1530.
20. Köhler, G., and Shulman, M. (1978) *Curr. Top. Microbiol. Immunol.* **81**, 143–148.
21. Köhler, G., and Milstein, C. (1976) *Eur. J. Immunol.* **6**, 511–519.
22. Andersson, J., and Melchers, F. (1978) *Curr. Top. Microbiol. Immunol.* **81**, 130–139.
23. Köhler, G., Pearson, T., and Milstein, C. (1977) *Somatic Cell Genet.* **3**, 303–319.
24. Galfré, G., Howe, S., Milstein, C., Butcher, G., and Howard, J. (1977) *Nature (London)* **267**, 707–708.
25. Hengartner, H., Luzzati, A., and Schreier, M. (1978) *Curr. Top. Microbiol. Immunol.* **81**, 92–99.
26. Koprowski, H., Gerhard, W., Wiktor, T., Martins, J., Shander, M., and Croce, C. (1978) *Curr. Top. Microbiol. Immunol.* **81**, 8–19.
27. Levy, R., Dilley, J., Sikora, K., and Kucherlapati, R. (1978) *Curr. Top. Microbiol. Immunol.* **81**, 170–172.
28. Hämmerling, G. (1977) *Eur. J. Immunol.* **7**, 743–746.
29. Hyman, R., and Kelleher, T. (1975) *Somatic Cell Genet.* **1**, 335–343.
30. Periman, P. (1970) *Nature (London)* **228**, 1086–1087.
31. Coffino, P., Knowles, B., Nathenson, S., and Scharff, M. (1971) *Nature (London), New Biol.* **231**, 87–90.
32. Köhler, G., Hengartner, H., and Shulman, M. (1978) *Eur. J. Immunol.* **8**, 82–88.
33. Kronvall, G., Grey, H., and Williams, R. (1970) *J. Immunol.* **105**, 116–1123.
34. Melcher, U., Vitetta, E., McWilliams, M., Lamm, M., Philips-Quagliata, J., and Uhr, J. (1974) *J. Exp. Med.* **140**, 1427–1431.

35. Raschke, W. (1978) *Curr. Top. Microbiol. Immunol.* **81**, 70–76.
36. Pernis, B., Forni, L., and Luzzati, A. (1976) *Cold Spring Harbor Symp. Quant. Biol.* **41**, 175–183.
36a. Coffino, P., and Scharff, M. (1971) *Proc. Natl. Acad. Sci. U.S.A.* **68**, 219–223.
37. Köhler, G., Howe, S., and Milstein, C. (1976) *Eur. J. Immunol.* **6**, 292–295.
38. Imanishi-Kari, T., Reth, M., and Hammerling, G. (1978) *Curr. Top. Microbiol. Immunol.* **81**, 20–26.
39. Cunningham, A. (1976) "Generation of Antibody Diversity." Academic Press, New York.
40. Tonegawa, S., Hozumi, N., Matthyssens, G., and Schuller, R. (1976) *Cold Spring Harbor Symp. Quant. Biol.* **41**, 877–889.
41. Hozumi, N., and Tonegawa, S. (1976) *Proc. Natl. Acad. Sci. U.S.A.* **73**, 3628–3632.
42. Rabbits, T., and Forster, A. (1978) *Cell* **13**, 319–327.
43. Brack, C., and Tonegawa, S. (1977) *Proc. Natl. Acad. Sci. U.S.A.* **74**, 5652–5656.
44. Tonegawa, S., Maxam, A., Tizard, R., Bernard, O., and Gilbert, W. (1978) *Proc. Natl. Acad. Sci. U.S.A.* **75**, 1485–1489.
45. Milstein, C., Adetugbo, K., Cowan, N., Köhler, G., Secher, D., and Wilde, C. (1976) *Cold Spring Harbor Symp. Quant. Biol.* **41**, 793–803.
46. Birshstein, B., Preud'homme, J., and Scharff, M. (1974) *Proc. Natl. Acad. Sci. U.S.A.* **71**, 3478–3482.
47. Cook, W., and Scharff, M. (1977) *Proc. Natl. Acad. Sci. U.S.A.* **74**, 5687–5691.
48. Gronowitz, E., Coutinho, A., and Melchers, F. (1976) *Eur. J. Immunol.* **6**, 588–590.
49. Milstein, C., Brownlee, G., Cartwright, E., Jarvis, J., and Proudfoot, N. (1974) *Nature (London)* **252**, 354–362.
50. Kearney, J., and Lawton, A. (1975) *J. Immunol.* **115**, 671–676.
51. Goding, J., and Layton, J. (1976) *J. Exp. Med.* **144**, 852–857.
52. Wabl, M., Forni, L., and Loor, F. (1978) *Science* **199**, 1078–1079.
53. Dreyer, W., and Bennett, J. (1965) *Proc. Natl. Acad. Sci. U.S.A.* **54**, 864–869.
54. Cotton, R., and Milstein, C. (1973) *Nature (London)* **244**, 42–43.
55. Gilbert, W. (1978) *Nature (London)* **271**, 501.
56. Laskov, R., Kim, K., and Asofsky, R. (1978) *Curr. Top. Microbiol. Immunol.* **81**, 173–175.

Analysis of the Diversity of Murine Antibodies to α(1→3) Dextran

DANIEL HANSBURG, BRIAN CLEVINGER,
ROGER M. PERLMUTTER, ROGERS GRIFFITH,
DAVID E. BRILES, AND JOSEPH M. DAVIE

Department of Microbiology and Immunology
Washington University School of Medicine
St. Louis, Missouri

INTRODUCTION

A central issue in immunology is the mechanism by which the immune system generates the extraordinary diversity of immunoglobulins, a diversity which has fascinated several generations of immunologists. A variety of approaches has been taken to evaluate the problem of diversity, but as yet, few clear principles have emerged.

A major problem has been the estimation of how diverse antibodies really are. One approach has been to estimate the heterogeneity of antibodies produced to single antigenic determinants by techniques such as isoelectric focusing and binding site antigenicity, and extrapolating these results to all antigenic specificities. Estimates of the total diversity of antibodies extrapolated from the diversity seen to aromatic haptens (1,2) and proteins (3) have been very large, ranging from 10 to 80 million. However, similar studies using polysaccharide antigens have yielded estimates of total antibody diversity nearly three orders of magnitude lower (4,5). For more precise estimates of total antibody diversity to be generated, it is necessary that lymphocytes bearing different immunoglobulins be represented at equal frequencies and that techniques to identify different binding sites be extraordinarily discriminatory. Since neither of these requirements are presently available, estimates of total diversity can only be considered as approximations.

A different approach to the study of antibody diversity has been the study of amino acid sequences of random samples of the immunoglobulin repertoire, represented by myeloma proteins. Early estimates of the human repertoire of K light chains gave minimum estimates of several thousand (6). Similar estimates of mouse K chain diversity have been presented (7). The continued accumulation of sequence information of both heavy and light chains over the past decade has shown no tendency to demonstrate saturation of diverse sequences (8), so that again estimates of total diversity have not been possible.

Ideas concerning the mechanisms by which this vast array of different protein molecules might be generated have been distilled into four major types (8). The first is that for every immunoglobulin molecule, there is a V_H and a V_L gene encoded in the germ line. While everyone agrees that there must be several such genes in the germ line, the precise number is a matter of dispute. Invariant inheritance of variable region markers (9,10) and the demonstration of genetic recombination of variable region markers (11) provide strong evidence for a multiplicity of variable region genes. Nonetheless, attempts to enumerate variable region genes by nucleic acid hybridization have so far disclosed a paucity of such genes (12). This, and a variety of amino acid sequence studies (11), have led to the proposal that germ line genes may be further diversified in the soma through mutational means. This has taken the form of either insertional models in which different parts of germ line genes are redistributed to generate diversity (13), or through base changes within portions of germ line genes which encode for binding site structures during the development of immunocompetent cells (14). A potentially important mechanism of diversification is combinatorial diversity. Since each immunoglobulin molecule is the product of at least four separate genes, considerable diversity can be generated if the gene products can pair randomly. It has been clearly documented that V_H genes can pair with multiple C_H genes (15,16). In addition, it has been demonstrated that individual heavy chains can pair with multiple light chains (17) and vice versa (18,19). If, in fact, these processes are random, then several hundred V_H genes and V_L genes could pair with C_H and C_L genes to generate several hundred thousand distinct antibody molecules. Unknown in this formulation is the extent of randomness of these processes. Finally, further diversification has been proposed by means of each immunoglobulin molecule serving as recognition structures for more than one antigenic determinant. Multispecificity of binding sites has been documented clearly for several myeloma and normally induced antibodies (20).

It is possible, if not probable, that all of these mechanisms operate to generate antibody diversity to some degree. However, the precise contribution of each mechanism to antibody diversity and therefore the importance of each mechanism to the process remain unanswered.

For the past several years, our laboratory has been involved with an analysis of the diversity of antibodies raised to a variety of simple antigenic determinants, including phosphocholine, $\alpha(1 \to 3)$ dextran, and streptococcal group A carbohydrate. These antigenic determinants were chosen because of the knowledge that each population of antibodies was of limited heterogeneity. In each of these systems, our goal has been to determine both the extent of antibody diversity and to explore how diversity is generated in each system. What follows is a progress report of our studies of the murine response to $\alpha(1 \to 3)$ dextran.

EXTENT OF DIVERSITY OF ANTI-$\alpha(1 \to 3)$ DEXTRAN REPERTOIRE

Our study of anti-$\alpha(1 \to 3)$ antibodies was significantly simplified by a chance observation that *Escherichia coli* bacteria possess $\alpha(1 \to 3)$ determinants in their cell walls. An immunization protocol was devised in which mice were primed with 100 μg dextran B1355 in CFA and boosted 2 months later with several injections of 2×10^9 *E. coli;* this protocol in all strains tested of the IgCH^a allotype stimulated very large antibody responses, generally exceeding 10 mg/ml serum (21).

A second advantage for the study of anti-dextran antibodies is the existence of three myeloma proteins specific for $\alpha(1 \to 3)$ determinants which provide standards for comparison of induced antibodies. The idea here is that if the myeloma protein is the product of germ line genes, all animals may express an antibody identical to the myeloma protein; if the prototype is derived from somatically modified genes, only a rare animal will express it. In addition, if all animals express several "germ line" antibodies to the same determinant, it will be possible to determine whether the expression of the antibodies is equal or not, an important question for statistical estimates of total diversity.

The three myeloma proteins, M104, J558, and U102, have been shown to be structurally similar and all have the same λ light chain (22–24). We prepared antisera to variable regions (idiotypes) on the myelomas and demonstrated at least four distinct determinants (Table I): IdX, which is shared equally by all three myeloma proteins, and three determinants unique to each protein, IdI(M104), IdI(J558), and IdI(U102).

Earlier studies by Blomberg *et al.* (25) had demonstrated that induced antibodies to $\alpha(1 \rightarrow 3)$ dextran possessed λ chains predominantly and shared idiotypic determinants with M104 and J558, so that it was not unexpected that we would find similarities between myelomas and induced antibodies. What was not clear was whether the unique idiotypic determinants would be represented among the antibodies. We first demonstrated that the dextran/*E. coli* protocol stimulated antibodies primarily specific for $\alpha(1 \rightarrow 3)$ linkages. In addition, it was shown that these antibodies were found in both the 19 and 7 S serum fractions. Figure 1 shows the average serum concentration of total anti-dextran antibody and the four dextran-associated idiotypic determinants in two strains of mice. Several observations can be made from this figure: IdX is found on about half the antibody in both 19 and 7 S fractions; all three unique idiotypes are present; there is a hierarchy of expression of the unique antigenic determinants, IdI(M104) > IdI(J558) > IdI(U102); and the IdX-bearing population is much greater than the sum of the unique idiotype populations. These results imply that the myelomas are indeed samples of the anti-dextran repertoire, but that the repertoire is larger than three. In fact, at least five clonotypes must exist from these results: three clones each bearing a single myeloma-specific idiotype as well as the common idiotype; at least one clone expressing the common determinant, but lacking any

TABLE I
Idiotypic Characteristics of Myeloma Proteins

Protein	Class	Specificity	Idiotypic specificity			
			IdX	IdI(M104)	IdI(J558)	IdI(U102)
M104	IgMλ	Dextran	+	+	−	−
J558	IgAλ	Dextran	+	−	+	−
U102	IgAλ	Dextran	+	−	−	+
HOPC-1	$IgG_{2a}\lambda$	?	−	−	−	−
T183	IgMK	?	−	−	−	−

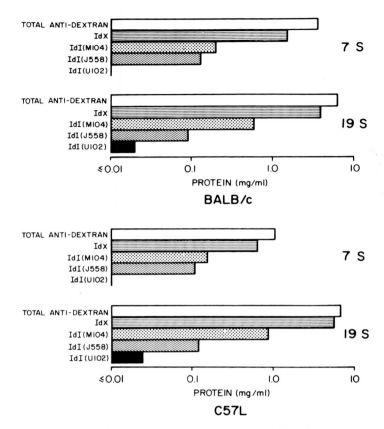

Fig. 1.   Anti-dextran and idiotype concentrations in sera from dextran immune mice (modified from Hansburg *et al.*, 26). Mice were immunized by the dextran/*E. coli* protocol, sera were separated into 19 and 7 S fractions by zonal centrifugation, and individual fractions were assayed for antibody and idiotype levels. Shown are the average values for eight BALB/c and nine C57L mice.

of the unique determinants; and at least one clone deficient in the cross-reactive determinants. It should be emphasized at this point, that anti-idiotypic reagents may be multispecific and that even the populations of antibodies which react with the "unique" idiotypes may be multiclonal.

A different approach to compare antibodies from different individuals for structural relatedness is isoelectric focusing (IEF). By this technique differences in as few as one charged amino acid between light chains are reflected in different pI. It is not yet clear that a similar degree of discrimination exists for intact immunoglobulin molecules.

Figure 2 shows the IEF pattern of 7 S anti-dextran antibodies. It is clear that the patterns are simple and repetitive with major bands appearing in most sera. While occasional disparate bands occur, one is struck more by the uniformity of focus patterns than by the differences. If an average protein produces three bands because of micro-heterogeneity, then the number of spectrotypes commonly present in the anti-dextran repertoire may be 10 or less.

Comparable studies of 19 S anti-dextran antibodies showed that IEF is probably not sufficiently discriminatory to be a useful measure of diversity (27). While clear differences could be detected between the focusing patterns of IgM monomers from different animals, the range of pI's was only about one pH unit. IgM antibodies of other specificities seemed limited as well to this range so that considerable overlap was encountered. While it was possible to detect IgM anti-dextran antibodies which cofocused with M104, the uncertainty of the technique does not allow one to conclude that the antibodies were identical to M104. Therefore, attempts to further characterize IEF diversity of anti-dextran antibodies have been concentrated on 7 S antibodies.

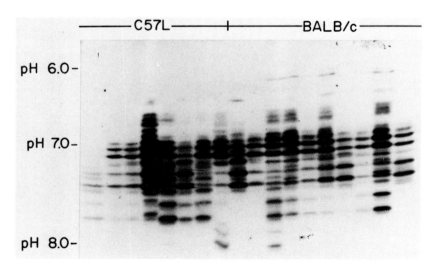

Fig. 2. Comparison of IEF spectrotypes of 7 S anti-dextran antibodies (21). Sera from eighteen individual, hyperimmune mice were focused in acrylamide gels; anti-dextran antibodies were detected by exposure to ^{125}I-dextran and radioautography.

CORRELATION BETWEEN SPECTROTYPE, IDIOTYPE, AND ISOTYPE

One means by which diversity can be generated is by variable regions pairing with more than one constant region. While this mechanism clearly has been implicated in the IgM to IgG switch, as demonstrated in Fig. 1, and other shifts in heavy chain class (15,16), the situation with regard to IgG subclass is less clear. In fact, a recent study from our laboratory has suggested that variable regions may not be shared by IgG subclasses, but rather are restricted to particular subclasses (28). This surprising conclusion was derived from the observation that the predominant isotype of a variety of purified anti-carbohydrate antibodies in the mouse, including anti-$\alpha(1 \rightarrow 3)$ dextran, groups A and C carbohydrate and phosphocholine, was IgG_3, a subclass which normally makes up only a few percent of serum immunoglobulin. Anti-protein antibodies were deficient in IgG_3.

Since IgG_3 represented a considerable fraction of total anti-dextran antibodies, it was expected that most bands of focused antibodies would be IgG_3. This was shown to be the case by separating immunoadsorbent purified IgG antibodies by preparative IEF and measuring IgG subclasses by radioimmune inhibition assays. The bulk of antibodies which focus from pH 7.0 to 8.0 were shown to be IgG_3 (27). Since this constitutes most 7 S anti-dextran antibodies, it is likely that little diversity is generated in this system by pairing of single V_H regions to multiple constant regions.

Similarly, in other systems, diversity has been shown to result from random pairing of heavy and light chains. Blomberg et al. (25) showed that IgM primary responses to $\alpha(1 \rightarrow 3)$ dextran were predominantly of the λ light chain class; we have confirmed this and shown that the massive responses elicited by the dextran/E. coli protocol are also almost entirely λ-bearing antibodies. IEF has been shown to be a useful and sensitive means to evaluate light chain heterogeneity. Figure 3 (left panel) shows that myeloma protein light chains typically focus as a distinctive triplet while light chains from normal pools of immunoglobulin are blurs of large numbers of bands. The IEF profiles of the light chains of M104, J558, and U102 are indistinguishable and cofocus with light chains from induced anti-dextran antibodies. Figure 3 (right panel) shows the comparison of light chains from two myelomas and antibodies from four individual animals. In extensive studies of antibodies from eleven strains of mice of the IgCH[a] allotype, no differences have been seen in light chain spectrotypes. We feel, therefore, that single λ light chains most likely are pairing with

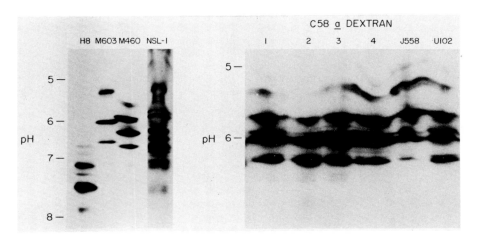

Fig. 3. L-chain isoelectric focusing patterns (modified from Perlmutter *et al.*, 29). Immunoglobulins were labeled with ^{125}I and separated into H and L chains by SDS acrylamide gel electrophoresis; L chains were focused in gels containing 0.5% Nonidet P-40. The left panel shows focusing patterns of ^{125}I-L chains derived from myeloma proteins and normal serum immunoglobulin. The right panel shows ^{125}I-L chains from dextran-binding myeloma proteins J558 and U102 and immunoadsorbent-purified anti-dextran antibodies from four C58 mice.

several different γ_3 heavy chains to generate both spectrotypic and idiotypic heterogeneity.

Having excluded a light chain or isotypic contribution to spectrotypic heterogeneity, we have attempted to correlate spectrotype with idiotype. These studies were performed by examining the spectrotypes of antibodies from animals with unusually elevated or depressed levels of particular idiotypes or by idiotypic analysis of antibodies isolated by preparative IEF. These approaches have allowed tentative assignments to be made for some of the IEF spectrotypes of 7 S anti-dextran antibodies (Fig. 4). The triplet of bands at pI 7.0 are the most prominent bands in sera from all dextran responder strains; these bands are IgG$_3\lambda$ antibodies which bear IdX alone or IdX and IdI(M104) and have been labeled CIAS to denote common idiotype-associated spectrotype. The region from pH 7.2 to 7.6 is complex both idiotypically and spectrotypically. While these antibodies are also IgG$_3\lambda$, it is likely that molecules bearing several different idiotypes will focus in this region. The most alkaline bands are IgG$_3\lambda$ which probably also contain IdI(J558) determinants (27). Even though tentative assignments can be made, it is probable that the relatively simple

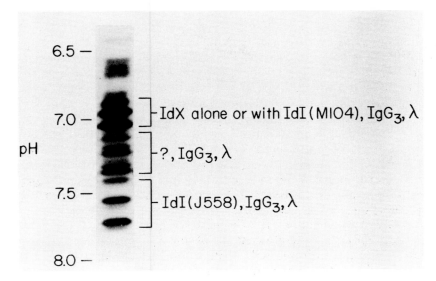

Fig. 4. Tentative assignment of idiotypes to spectrotypes (modified from Hansburg *et al.*, 27).

IEF patterns of 7 S anti-dextran antibodies may be composed of families of similar but not identical antibodies and possible that other molecules bearing idiotypes not presently known may be found to focus in positions indistinguishable from these. For these reasons, an approach to the enumeration of anti-dextran clonotypes was sought by means of somatic cell hybridization.

SOMATIC CELL HYBRIDS

Most antisera, even to simple determinants like $\alpha(1 \to 3)$ dextran, are generally complex, heterogeneous mixtures of antibodies. In addition, variability from animal to animal makes clonal analysis difficult. Thus, the desirability of continuous lines of cells producing homogeneous antibody of predetermined specificity is obvious. Several workers have recently documented the usefulness of somatic cell hybrids, resulting from the fusion of plasmacytomas with normal lymphoid cells, in the production of monoclonal antibodies to what is now an ever enlarging library of antigens (30–32).

Kohler, Milstein, and co-workers utilized Littlefield's methods (33) of hybrid selection and have developed methods with general applicability. Plasmacytoma mutants deficient in the enzyme hypoxanthine guanine phosphoribosyl transferase (HGPRT) were fused with polyethylene glycol to dextran-immune spleen cells. Hybrid cells were grown in a selective medium (HAT medium) which required HGPRT for cellular proliferation. Since spleen cells have only limited growth potential in this medium and since the reversion rate of HGPRT deficiency is low, only hybrid cells grow in the HAT medium. We have found, as have others, that about one hybrid line can be recovered for every 10^6 spleen cells in the initial fusion mixture (34). Even so, many of the hybrids express anti-dextran activity, presumably because of the preferential fusion of dividing B cells. Typically, the products of fusion of a single spleen are divided into 48 cultures; 2–3 weeks later, all cultures have growth and, if the spleen came from an animal making 10 mg of anti-dextran antibody per ml serum, then most cultures will contain anti-dextran antibody in the culture medium. Obviously, under these conditions many of the cultures will contain hybrids producing the same anti-dextran antibodies. We have found that a convenient screening assay for detecting hybrids producing different antibodies is IEF of culture media in acrylamide gels and exposure of the gels to ^{125}I-dextran. By this means it can be determined which cultures produce distinctive antibodies, whether the antibodies are IgM or IgG, and which cultures are producing the largest amounts of immunoglobulin. Since each culture probably contains more than one hybrid, cloning in soft agar is necessary. Finally, clones that demonstrated anti-dextran activity were grown as an ascites in histocompatible mice; within 7 to 10 days after injection of 10^7 hybrid cells secreting IgM anti-dextran antibody, the ascites fluid contained 7–16 mg/ml of dextran-precipitable protein.

Our experience with this technique over the last year has convinced us that the hybrids which are produced are representative idiotypically and isotypically of the antibodies secreted by the spleen cells at the time of fusion. Most of the hybrids are IgMλ producers; about 20% secrete IgGλ. The idiotypic makeup of several IgM clones is summarized in Table II.

These clones were all derived from the same mouse. It can be seen that all six clones have the same reactivity to anti-IdX as the myeloma proteins, none react with anti-IdI(M104), and four of six react only slightly with anti-IdI(J558). The other two, Dex-B1 and Dex-B2, have intermediate cross reaction with anti-IdI(J558). These hybrids represent the most frequent anti-dextran clonotypes, those which possess

TABLE II
Idiotypic Analysis of Anti-Dextran Hybrids

Clone	Class	IdX/λ	IdI(M104)/λ	IdI(J558)/λ
Dex-A	IgMλ	0.7	0.001	0.006
Dex-B1	IgMλ	1.2	0.001	0.056
Dex-B2	IgMλ	1.4	0.001	0.039
Dex-C1	IgMλ	0.8	0.001	0.003
Dex-C2	IgMλ	1.1	0.001	0.028
Dex-C3	IgMλ	1.0	0.001	0.008
M104	IgMλ	1.0	1.0	0.004
J558	IgAλ	0.9	0.001	1.0

IdX but little or no IdI. It is probable that each hybrid possesses different IdI determinants from the existing myeloma proteins and could provide additional serologic probes for enumerating the anti-dextran repertoire. Preparation of IdI reagents to hybrid products is underway. In fact, such serologic markers could allow us to determine whether the hybrids are derived from the same clonotype. Another means of comparing hybrid products is by IEF. The six clones shown in Table II were reduced to monomers with cysteine, desialidated with neuraminidase and focused in acrylamide gels (Fig. 5). It can be seen that none of the hybrids resemble M104 by this technique. Instead, the hybrids form two distinct focusing patterns which correspond with the idiotypic analysis: Dex-B1 and Dex-B2 cofocus and differ from the other hybrids which themselves cofocus. As was stated before, however, IEF of IgM proteins has limited resolving power so that additional differences could exist among the six hybrids.

A complication of the somatic hybrid technique is the opportunity it offers for the generation of artifactual molecules resulting from the pairing of myeloma and spleen cell immunoglobulin chains in combinations not seen normally. This process is seen in the anti-dextran hybrids where μ chains pair with both λ chains from the spleen cells and κ chains from the plasmacytoma; fortunately μ–γ mixtures do not take place. However, it is clear that $\mu\kappa$ pairs lose binding specificity for $\alpha(1 \rightarrow 3)$ dextran. It is probable that these mixed molecules are responsible for the existence in hybrids Dex-B1 and Dex-B2 of two IgM molecules, only one of which binds dextran. Therefore, many of these mixed molecules can be removed by immune adsorption. Another approach which we and others are taking to solve this problem is to fuse with plasmacytoma variants which have lost the ability to produce myeloma protein. These experiments are in progress.

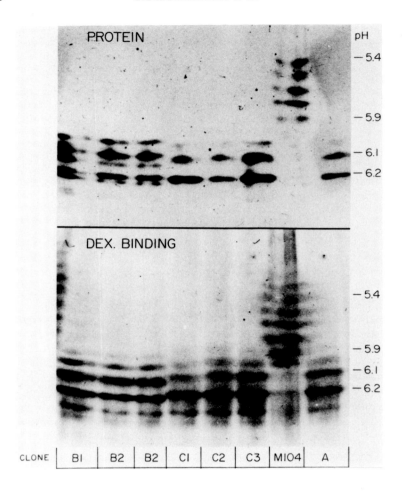

Fig. 5. IEF analysis of IgM anti-dextran antibodies from cloned hybrid cells (34). Cloned hybrid cells were grown as ascites tumors in syngeneic mice. The 19 S fractions of the ascites fluid were reduced to monomers by cysteine and desialidated by neuraminidase before focusing in acrylamide gels. Shown above is the negative image of the protein bands after salt precipitation; below is an autoradiograph of the same gel after exposure to ^{125}I-dextran.

SUMMARY

We have not reached our goal of characterizing the total repertoire of antibodies in the mouse directed to $\alpha(1 \rightarrow 3)$ dextran, but we have developed tools which will help us approach this goal. Using a combined approach of IEF and antigenic analysis of serum antibodies, a minimum estimate of eight clonotypes can be made. At this moment, it appears that these clonotypes are generated solely by differences in V_H structure. The new technology of somatic cell hybridization makes possible unambiguous enumeration of at least common clonotypes and ensures sufficient quantities of material for structural analysis. Major areas to be approached in the future are to determine the structural correlates of the different clonotypes, to determine whether each clonotype is derived from germ line genes, and to determine whether limits exist in the association of V_HDEX genes with particular C_H genes. We feel that continued exploration of phenotypic expression of families of antibody molecules will lead us to a better understanding of the means of the generation of antibody diversity.

ACKNOWLEDGMENTS

This research was supported by U.S. Public Health Service grant AI-11635, National Science Foundation grant PCM78-15318, by U.S. Public Health Service fellowships AI-05344, GM-02016, CA-09118 and HL-07081, and by Special Postdoctoral Fellowship (SPF-13) from the American Cancer Society.

REFERENCES

1. Kreth, H. W., and Williamson, A. R. (1973) *Eur. J. Immunol.* **3**, 141–147.
2. Klinman, N. R., and Press, J. L. (1975) *Transplant. Rev.* **24**, 41–83.
3. Kohler, G. (1976) *Eur. J. Immunol.* **6**, 340–347.
4. Sigal, N., Gearhart, P., and Klinman, N. R. (1975) *J. Immunol.* **114**, 1354–1358.
5. Cramer, M., and Braun, D. G. (1975) *Scand. J. Immunol.* **4**, 63–70.
6. Quattrochi, R., Cioli, R., and Baglioni, C. (1969) *J. Exp. Med.* **130**, 401–415.
7. Hood, L., McKean, D., Farnsworth, B., and Potter, M. (1973) *Biochemistry* **12**, 741–749.
8. Hood, L., Loh, E., Hubert, J., Barstad, P., Eaton, B., Early, P., Fuhrman, J., Johnson, N., Kronenberg, M., and Schilling, J. (1976) *Cold Spring Harbor Symp. Quant. Biol.* **51**, 817–836.
9. Pawlak, L. L., Mushinski, E. B., Nisonoff, A., and Potter, M. (1973) *J. Exp. Med.* **137**, 22–31.
10. Lieberman, R., Potter, M., Mushinski, E. B., Humphrey, W., and Rudikoff, S. (1974) *J. Exp. Med.* **139**, 983–1001.
11. Weigert, M., and Riblet, R. (1976) *Cold Spring Harbor Symp. Quant. Biol.* **51**, 837–846.
12. Tonegawa, S. (1976) *Proc. Natl. Acad. Sci. U.S.A.* **73**, 203–207.
13. Capra, J. D., and Kindt, T. J. (1975) *Immunogenetics* **1**, 417–427.

14. Cohn, M., Blomberg, B., Geckeler, W., Raschke, W., Riblet, R., and Weigert, M. (1974) *In* "The Immune System: Genes, Receptors, Signals" (E. E. Sercarz, A. R. Williamson, and C. F. Fox, eds.), pp. 89–117. Academic Press, New York.
15. Gearhart, P. J., Sigal, N. H., and Klinman, N. R. (1975) *Proc. Natl. Acad. Sci. U.S.A.* **72**, 1707–1711.
16. Wang, A. C., Wang. I. Y., and Fudenberg, H. H. (1977) *J. Biol. Chem.* **252**, 7192–7197.
17. Capra, J. D., Klapper, D. G., Tung, A. S., and Nisonoff, A. (1976). *Cold Spring Harbor Symp. Quant. Biol.* **51**, 847–853.
18. Braun, D. G., Huser, H., and Jaton, J. -C. (1975) *Nature (London)* **258**, 363–365.
19. Perlmutter, R. M., Briles, D. E., Greve, J. M., and Davie, J. M. (1978) *J. Immunol.* **121**, 149–158.
20. Richards, F. F., Konigsberg, W. H., Rosenstein, R. W., and Varga, J. M. (1975) *Science* **187**, 130–137.
21. Hansburg, D., Briles, D. E., and Davie, J. M. (1976) *J. Immunol.* **117**, 569–575.
22. Weigert, M., Cesari, I. M., Yonkovich, S. J., and Cohn, M. (1970) *Nature (London)* **228**, 1045–1047.
23. Barstad, P., Weigert, M., Cohn, M., and Hood, L. (1975) *Immunogenetics* **1**, 531–532.
24. Carson, D., and Weigert, M. (1973) *Proc. Natl. Acad. Sci. U.S.A.* **70**, 235–239.
25. Blomberg, B., Geckeler, W. R., and Weigert, M. (1972) *Science* **177**, 178–180.
26. Hansburg, D., Briles, D. E., and Davie, J. M. (1977) *J. Immunol.* **119**, 1406–1412.
27. Hansburg, D., Perlmutter, R. M., Briles, D. E., and Davie, J. M. (1978). *Eur. J. Immunol.* **8**, 352–359.
28. Perlmutter, R. M., Hansburg, D., Briles, D. E., Nicolotti, R. A., and Davie, J. M. (1978) *J. Immunol.* **121**, 566–572.
29. Perlmutter, R. M., Briles, D. E., and Davie, J. M. (1977) *J. Immunol.* **118**, 2161–2166.
30. Kohler, G., and Milstein, C. (1976) *Eur. J. Immunol.* **6**, 511–519.
31. Koprowski, H., Gerhard, W., and Croce, C. (1977) *Proc. Natl. Acad. Sci. U.S.A.* **74**, 2985–2988.
32. Margulies, D. H., Kuehl, W. M., and Scharff, M. D. (1976) *Cell* **8**, 405–415.
33. Littlefield, J. N. (1964) *Science* **145**, 709–710.
34. Clevinger, B., Hansburg, D., and Davie, J. M. (1978) *Curr. Top. Microbiol. Immunol.* **81**, 110–114.

Monoclonal Antibodies to Alloantigens and to Immunoglobulin Allotypes

JAMES W. GODING, VERNON T. OI,
PATRICIA P. JONES, LEONORE A. HERZENBERG,
AND LEONARD A. HERZENBERG

Department of Genetics
Stanford University School of Medicine
Stanford, California

INTRODUCTION

The specificity of the antigen–antibody bond provides an exquisitely precise probe for the identification and analysis of biological molecules. Until recently, though, the usefulness of antibodies has been limited by the variability of the immune response, the extreme heterogeneity of antibodies, and the presence of unwanted antibodies in many antisera. However, the demonstration by Köhler and Milstein (1) of the feasibility of the production of functional hybrids between myeloma cells and normal antibody-secreting cells has essentially solved these problems, and vastly increased the power of the serological approach. It is now possible to generate virtually unlimited quantities of homogeneous, monospecific antibodies to almost any desired antigenic determinant, even if the antigen is not pure. In this paper, we describe the production and properties of hybrid cell lines secreting antibodies to products of the major histocompatibility complex and to immunoglobulin allotypes of the mouse.

309

CELL HYBRIDS

The best known example of cell fusion is that of sperm and egg. In general, spontaneous fusion of somatic cells is rare, although the process does occur in myotubes, osteoclasts, and foreign body giant cells (2). However, the incidence of fusion of somatic cells can be greatly increased by certain agents, such as Sendai virus, lysolecithin and polyethylene glycol (PEG) (2). PEG is now the agent of choice. When the cytoplasmic membranes are fused by chemical treatment, bi- or multi-nucleated cells (heterokaryons) are produced. During the next division, the nuclei fuse, and cell hybrids are formed (2).

The hybrids are then isolated by growth on selective media. For example, normal cells may be fused with tumor cells that have been selected for resistance to thioguanine or azaguanine by virtue of loss of the X-linked "salvage" enzyme hypoxanthine guanine phosphoribosyl transferase (HGPRT). When the main biosynthetic pathways for purines and pyrimidines are blocked by aminopterin, cells must use HGPRT to convert hypoxanthine and guanine into ribonucleotides. Thus, if the cells are grown in medium containing hypoxanthine, aminopterin, and thymidine (HAT medium) (2), only those cells containing HGPRT (i.e., normal parental cells and hybrids) survive. Since normal lymphocytes die after a few days in culture, growth in HAT medium will select for hybrids.

ANTIBODY-SECRETING HYBRIDS

In order to express a differentiated cell function, the two parental cells should be at a similar stage of differentiation. The fusion of unlike cells frequently results in the "extinction" of differentiated function (2,3). Thus, antibody secretion is only maintained if normal antibody-secreting cells are fused with myeloma cells.

The general strategy for production of antibody-secreting hybrids, described more fully elsewhere (1,4) is as follows. Mice are immunized with the desired antigen (or a mixture containing the desired antigen), and, shortly after boosting, the spleen cells are fused with azaguanine-resistant myeloma cells by means of PEG. The cells are then cultured in HAT medium. In the first few days, there is massive cell death, but at 10–14 days after fusion hybrid colonies begin to appear. The culture medium is then tested for antibody to the desired antigen, and positive cultures are cloned by limiting dilution. Positive clones may then be grown in bulk cultures or injected into histocompatible mice where they will grow as tumors. The antibodies may be recovered from culture supernates or from serum or ascites fluid of tumor-bearing mice.

During growth of hybrids there is a tendency for chromosome loss (2). Since the loss of antibody secretion probably allows more rapid growth, cultures may be overgown by nonproducing variants. The best solution to this problem seems to be to clone early and reclone periodically.

PRODUCTION OF HYBRIDS

USE OF NS-1 AS PARENT

The parental cell line used was the NS-1 variant of the P3 (MOPC 21) line (5). Cells of the NS-1 line are resistant to azaguanine, and do not synthesize the MOPC 21 γ_1 heavy chain. Although NS-1 synthesizes the MOPC 21 κ chain, it is not secreted. NS-1-derived hybrid cell lines secreting the normal parental spleen cell immunoglobulin also secrete hybrid molecules containing the MOPC 21 κ chain. Thus, if the synthesis of light chains from each parental cell occurs at similar rates, and if pairing is random (1), about 25% of antibody molecules will possess only the spleen cell light chain, 25% will possess only the MOPC 21 κ chain, and 50% will possess one of each of the light chains. If the MOPC 21 line were used rather than NS-1, only 6.25% of secreted molecules would be expected to be derived entirely from the spleen cell parent.

EFFECT OF THE IMMUNIZATION PROTOCOL

In early experiments, we examined the effect of various forms of immunization on the production of antibody-secreting hybrids. BALB/c mice were immunized with C57BL/10 (Ig^b) anti-B. *pertussis*–pertussis complexes, an immunization that generates anti-allotype antibodies (6). There was no clear-cut effect of the different immunization protocols on the number of culture wells with hybrid growth, but there was a marked improvement in the number of wells with anti-Ig-1b antibody when hybridization was performed 3 days after boosting rather than 6 or 8 days. There was also a much greater number of wells secreting anti-Ig-1b antibody when the mice were primed and boosted once, as opposed to more prolonged immunization. No other anti-allotype positive wells were found.

It is thus our impression that the immunization regimen is best kept short and the hybridization performed 3 days after the last boost. Similarly, good results were obtained in antispleen cell alloantigen immunizations when the mice were primed with 2×10^7 spleen cells per animal, followed by a similar boost 3 weeks later, and hybridization 3 days after the boost.

CULTURE CONDITIONS

Details of the hybridization protocol and cell culture conditions are given elsewhere (4,7). In brief, NS-1 cells from log-phase cultures were fused with immune spleen cells at a 1 : 4 or 1 : 2 ratio, using 50% PEG (BDH Chemicals Ltd., Poole, England) and 3×10^8 cells in 1 ml of serum-free RPMI-1640 medium. Cells were plated out into 96-well microculture plates in RPMI-1640 with 15% FCS, and subjected to progressive HAT selection over a 2 week period. During the second to fourth weeks, depending on the rate of cell growth, supernates were tested for antibody activity (see below). Cells from active wells were transferred to 1 ml cultures, together with 5×10^6 thymocytes as feeders, and then expanded into larger flasks (50–100 ml). Because of the problem of chromosome loss alluded to earlier, we chose to freeze aliquots of cells at this early stage, so that active clones could be rescued at a later stage if necessary.

Cloning was generally performed by limiting dilution in microculture plates, using 10^6 thymocyte "feeder" cells per well, and three different dilutions of cells such that each well contained an average of 10, 2, or 0.5 hybrid cells. When the cloning plates showed evidence of vigorous growth, cells from a group in which 20–50% of wells were positive for growth were tested for antibody, and positive cultures expanded as previously. Cells were always diluted gradually; generally not more than a tenfold increase in volume between serial expansions. Loss of production of specific antibody occurred frequently, but in general it was possible to "rescue" failing lines by recloning and re-expansion of the cultures. It was generally observed that those hybrid cell lines that maintained antibody production in 1 ml and flask cultures had high cloning efficiencies and good recoveries of antibody-producing clones.

After cloning, aliquots of cells were frozen, and mice were injected with $2–5 \times 10^6$ cells per mouse. About 90% of clones produced tumors (hybridomas) within 10–30 days, and of these about 90% produced myeloma-like proteins of the desired antibody activity.

ANTIBODY ASSAY

Reactivity against soluble immunoglobulin allotypes was measured by a solid-phase radioimmunoassay using antigen-coated plates (6). Purified myeloma proteins were adsorbed onto wells of flexible plastic microtiter plates (Cooke Lab. Prod., Alexandria, VA), the excess washed off, and any remaining nonspecific binding sites saturated with BSA. Plates were reacted with 5–20 μl of culture supernate for 1 hr at room temperature, washed, and held with ^{125}I-labeled purified anti-Ig-1b or anti-Ig-4b antibodies (6).

Antibodies to spleen cell alloantigens were detected by reacting 4×10^5 spleen cells with culture supernates in wells of microtiter plates, washing, and incubation with ^{125}I-anti-allotype antibodies or with ^{125}I-staphylococcal protein A (8). Virtually all of the antibodies detected with the anti-allotype reagent were also detected with protein A. In addition, the protein A detected several clones that were not detected with the anti-allotype reagents (especially IgG$_{2b}$ and IgG$_3$). We did not screen for IgM antibodies.

ANTIBODIES TO ALLOANTIGENS OF THE MAJOR HISTOCOMPATIBILITY COMPLEX

The production of strong and specific alloantibodies to products of the major histocompatibility complex (MHC) requires selection of the appropriate mouse strains (both with regard to the H-2 haplotype and background genes controlling overall immune responsiveness), careful selection of mice producing high titer antibody, and a considerable amount of luck (9). In addition, such antisera very frequently contain high titer antibodies to proteins of murine leukemia virus. Viral antigens are frequently present on the surface of neoplastic (10,11) and even normal (10) cells, and may seriously confuse the interpretation of serological data (11). The availability of homogeneous, high titer monospecific antibodies to products of the MHC would greatly facilitate studies of MHC-linked alloantigens on normal and neoplastic cells.

Two hybridizations were performed with spleen cells from mice immunized with allogeneic cells. In one hybridization (H10), donor

TABLE I

Linkage Analysis of Hybrid Cell Antibody Reactivity

Strain	H-2	Ig	BALB anti-CKB (H11) (anti-H-2^k, Ig^b, . . .)						CWB anti-C3H (H10) (anti-H-2^k, Ig^a)			
			11-1[a]	11-2[a]	11-3[a]	11-4[b]	11-5[b]	11-6[b]	10-1[a]	10-2[a]	10-3[c]	10-4[c]
C3H	k	a	+	+	+	+	+	−	+	+	n.d.	n.d.
CWB	b	b	−	−	−	−	−	+	+	−	n.d.	n.d.
CKB	k	b	+	+	+	n.d.	n.d.	n.d.	+	+	+	−
CSW	b	a	−	−	−	n.d.	n.d.	n.d.	+	−	−	+

[a] ^{125}I-protein A;   [b] ^{125}I-anti-Ig-1a + anti-Ig-4a;   [c] ^{125}I-anti-Ig-1b + anti-Ig-4b.

cells were from CWB (H-2^b, Ig^b) mice which were immunized with C3H (H-2^k, Ig^a) spleen cells. CWB and C3H mice differ only in their alleles at the H-2 complex and also at the heavy chain complex; thus this immunization could produce antibody against products of the MHC or allotypes of IgM or IgD receptors (12). The second hybridization (H11) used BALB/c (H-2^d, Ig^a) spleen cells from mice immunized with CKB (H-2^k, Ig^b) spleen cells. This immunization could potentially elicit antibodies against MHC products, IgM, IgD, or numerous C3H "background" gene products.

LINKAGE ANALYSIS

Screening of supernates from initial microcultures was performed with a cell binding radioimmunoassay as described previously. The availability of the tetralogy of congenic mice on the C3H background (Table I) greatly facilitated linkage analysis. As shown in Table I, the reactivities of five of the H11 and two of the H10 supernatant antibodies are against antigens linked to the MHC, while one antibody each from H10 and H11 seems to react with surface immunoglobulin. The 10.1 hybrid supernate reacted with cells from all four congenic strains, including CWB, the spleen cell donor. This hybrid cell line apparently is producing an autoantibody against an undefined cell surface antigen, and was not studied further.

It is interesting to note that the great majority of H11 hybrids were directed against products of the MHC or the heavy chain complex, and no antibody against "background" gene products was observed. This

TABLE II
MHC Mapping of Hybrid Cell Antibody Reactivity

	K	A	B	J	E	C	S	G	D	I-A(2)[a]	I-A(17)[b]	H-2K[c]
										Reactivity pattern		
CKB	k	k	k	k	k	k	k	k	k	+	+	+
B10.A(4R)	k	k	b	b	b	b	b	b	b	+	+	+
A.TL	s	k	k	k	k	k	k	k	d	+	+	−
B10.S	s	s	s	s	s	s	s	s	s	−	+	−
B10.AQR	q	k	k	k	k	d	d	d	d	+	+	+
B10.T(6R)	q	q	q	q	q	q	q	?	d	−	−	+
B10.A(3R)	b	b	b	b	k	d	d	d	d	−	−	−
C3H.OH	d	d	d	d	d	d	d	d	k	−	−	−

[a] 11-2.12, 11-5.2, 11-1.23.   [b] 10-2.16, 10-3.6, 11-3.25.   [c] 11-4.1.

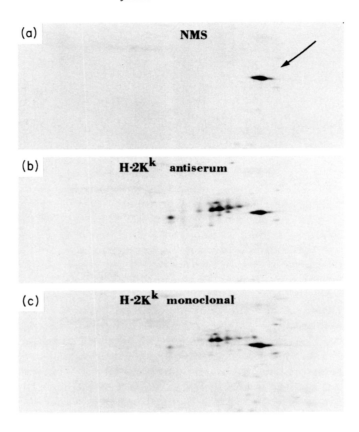

Fig. 1. Autoradiograms of 2-D gels of H-2K^k antigens. Proteins were precipitated from NP-40 extracts of ^{35}S-methionine-labeled CKB spleen cells by (a) normal mouse serum, (b) (A.TL × C3H.OL) anti-C3H, and (c) antibody from clone 11-4.1. The first-dimension separation was by nonequilibrium pH gradient electrophoresis (acidic proteins are on the right and basic proteins on the left). The second-dimension separation was by SDS–PAGE (from top to bottom). Both separations were done under reducing conditions. Only the relevant portions of the autoradiograms are shown. The position of actin is indicated by the arrow.

finding is consistent with previous biochemical analyses of several noncongenic mouse alloantisera (12,13).

A more detailed analysis of the seven MHC-linked clones was carried out using H-2 recombinant mice (Table II). The reactivity of six of the antibodies is consistent with their detecting I-A^k antigens; the remaining antibody apparently reacts with H-2K^k antigens. None of these antibodies detected H-2D, T1a, or other I subregion products.

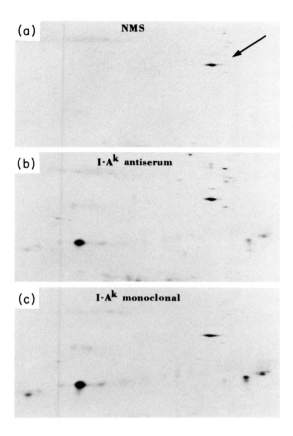

Fig. 2. Autoradiograms of 2-D gels of I-A^k antigens. Proteins precipitated from (a) C3H extract by normal mouse serum, (b) B10.A(4R) extract by A.TH anti-A.TL, and (c) C3H extract by antibody from clone 10-2.16 were electrophoresed as described in the legend to Fig. 1.

It should be noted that clone 11-1.23 was erroneously typed as an anti-H-2K (7), due to an unexplained false negative on A.TL. This clone is, in fact, positive on A.TL, and also positive on B10.AQR, yet negative on B10.T(6R) (Table II). Thus, the reactivity must be assigned to I-A.

BIOCHEMICAL ANALYSIS

To confirm the reactivities of the anti-MHC antibodies, proteins were labeled biosynthetically with ^{35}S-methionine, immunoprecipitated, and analyzed by two-dimensional (2-D) polyacrylamide gel electrophoresis (PAGE) (14,15). The first dimension separates the proteins on the basis of their net charge, by means of a technique or nonequilibrium pH-gradient electrophoresis (16). The second dimension was conventional SDS–PAGE, using the Laemmli discontinuous buffer system (14). Earlier studies have shown that this form of analysis produces patterns that are characteristic of both the region or subregion coding for the precipitated antigen and the haplotype (14,15).

Figures 1 and 2 show the excellent correspondence between the gel patterns obtained with monoclonal and conventional antibody. Antibody from the cloned anti-H-2K hybrid cell line 11-4.1 precipitates

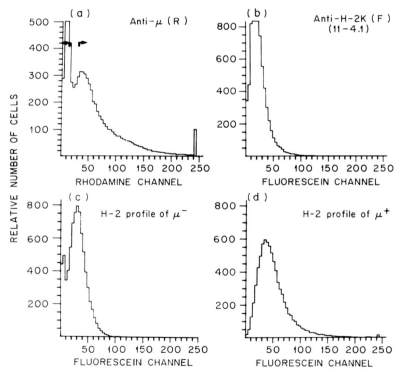

Fig. 3.   Anti-H-2K and anti-μ chain immunofluorescence histograms. C3H spleen cell stained with rhodamine (R*) conjugated rabbit anti-μ and anti-H-2K antibody from clone 11-4.1, followed by fluorescein (F*) conjugated rabbit anti-γ, were analyzed by means of the FACS: (a) R-anti-μ profile, (b) F*anti-H-2K profile, (c) F*anti-H-2K profile of μ^- cells (cells to the left of channel 15 in (a), indicated by the left arrow), and (d) F*anti-H-2K profile of μ^+ cells (cells to the right of channel 30 in (a), indicated by the right arrow).

molecules from ^{35}S-methionine-labeled CKB extracts identical to those precipitated by an alloantiserum (A.TL × C3H.OL)F$_1$ anti-C3H, which is directed against H-2K^k. Similarly, antibody from clone 10-2.16 precipitated the same set of I-A^k molecules from C3H extracts as does A.TH anti-A.TL (anti-I^k) alloantiserum from B10.A(4R).

Previous work (16a) has shown that antisera against the I-A subregion precipitate three distinct families of molecules in the 25,000–33,000 molecular weight range: a basic set, an intermediate set, and an acidic set. The intermediate spot is seen in precipitates of all I-subregions and haplotypes, and shows no evidence of polymorphism. The acidic and basic sets show mobilities characteristic of each I-A haplotype. It is thought that these spots represent three discrete gene products. All three sets are precipitated by antibody from clone

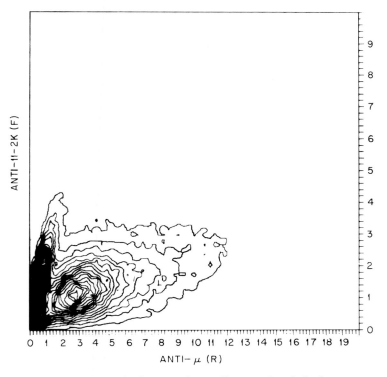

Fig. 4.   Contour map in which C3H spleen cells stained with rhodamine-anti-μ and anti-H-2K antibody from clone 11-4.1, followed by fluorescein-conjugated rabbit anti-γ, were analyzed by means of the FACS and data plotted using a computer program written by W. Moore. The interval between adjacent contours is 25 cells. A total of 10,000 cells were analyzed.

10-2.16. Since it is unlikely (though not impossible) that the three molecules have in common the antigenic determinant recognized by clone 10-2.16, the three chains probably exist as a tri-molecular complex on the cell surface. Anti-I-A molecules produced by clones 10-3.6 and 11-5.2 precipitate the same molecules as 10-2.16, adding support to this concept. These data illustrate the power of monoclonal antibodies in the analysis of the fine structure of complex cell surface molecules.

ANALYSIS BY TWO-COLOR IMMUNOFLUORESCENCE USING THE FLUORESCENCE-ACTIVATED CELL SORTER (FACS)

The cell subpopulations recognized by the hybrid cell antibodies were analyzed by two-color fluorescence using the fluorescence-

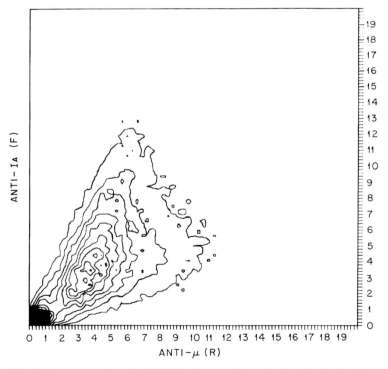

Fig. 5. Contour map in which C3H spleen cells stained with rhodamine-anti-μ and anti-Ia antibody from clone 10-2.16, followed by fluorescein-conjugated rabbit anti-γ, were analyzed by means of the FACS, and the data plotted as in Fig. 4. Virtually all μ^+ cells are I-A$^+$.

activated cell sorter (FACS) as previously described (17). Spleen cells from C3H (H-2^k) mice were stained with rhodamine-anti-μ to stain most B cells, followed by either anti-H-2K^k (11-4.1) or anti-I-A^k (10-2.16), followed by a fluorescein-conjugated rabbit anti-γ. Results are shown in Figs. 3–5. The anti-H-2K hybrid stains most of the spleen cells, although there appears to be a small subpopulation of cells with little or no H-2K or μ. These may represent nonlymphoid cells. Figure 3 also shows that B cells possess slightly more H-2K than do T cells. On the other hand, the anti-I-A^k antibodies stained virtually all of the μ^+ cells, but did not detectably stain μ^- cells (Fig. 5).

PURIFICATION AND CHAIN COMPOSITION OF HYBRID CELL ANTIBODIES

The great majority of hybrid cell lines bound staphylococcal Protein A, as detected in the cell binding assay. Thus, affinity chromatography on protein A–Sepharose (8,18) provided a simple and efficient one-step procedure for isolation of antibody from culture supernates or serum. In accordance with recently published work (18) all mouse IgG subclasses were found to bind at pH 8.0 (although we prefer pH 8.6 which provides more firm binding of IgG$_1$). Selective elution of IgG subclasses was obtained by stepwise elution at pH 6.0 (IgG$_1$), 4.0 (IgG$_{2a}$), and 2.2 (IgG$_{2b}$). Yields from culture supernates were typically 10–20 μg/ml, but were sometimes as high as 50 μg/ml. There was no detectable binding of proteins from the FCS in the culture medium. Figure 6 shows the degree of purity obtainable.

In order to analyze the antibody heavy and light chain composition, hybrid cell antibodies were also analyzed by 2-D PAGE. A typical pattern is shown in Fig. 7. Normal mouse IgG purified from whole serum by affinity chromatography on protein A-Sepharose is heterogeneous in charge. In contrast, IgG$_1$ from mice bearing the MOPC 21 tumor is much simpler. The presence of two to three spots for each chain probably reflects post-translational modifications such as deamidation, and causes movement towards the more acidic end of the gel. A similar analysis of IgG isolated from the clone 10-3.6 is shown in Fig. 7. As expected from the contribution of the NS-1 parent, one of the two light chain spots corresponds to the position of the MOPC 21 κ chain. On the other hand, the single pair of heavy chain spots is distinct from the expected position of the MOPC 21 heavy chain, which is absent.

The isolated proteins were tested for isotype using subclass-specific sera. In every case, light chains were κ in type. The heavy chain types are listed in Table III.

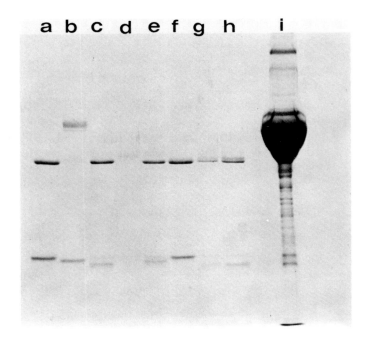

Fig. 6. SDS–PAGE of reduced immunoglobulins. (a) MOPC 21; (b) C.BPC-112; (c) 11-4.1; (d) 11-5.2; (e) 10-4.22; (f) 11-3.24; (g) 11-2.13; (h) 11-2.12; (i) 11-6.3. Samples (a) and (b) were isolated from serum of tumor-bearing mice by ion exchange chromatography and gel filtration. Samples (c)–(h) were isolated from culture supernates by affinity chromatography on protein A–Sepharose. Sample (i) consisted of culture fluid from clone 11-6.3.

TABLE III

Monoclonal Antibodies to H-2K and Ia Antigens

			Cytotoxicity	
Clone	Isotype	Specificity	Titer $(\times 10^3)$	Maximum lysis (%)
11-1.23	γ_{2a}	I-A(2)	10	69
11-2.12	γ_3	I-A(2)	5	68
11-5.2	γ_{2b}	I-A(2)	5,000	71
10-2.16	γ_{2b}	I-A(17)	10,000	70
10-3.6	γ_{2a}	I-A(17)	4	54
11-3.25	γ_{2b}	I-A(17)	75	68
11-4.1	γ_{2a}	H-2K(new)	200	98

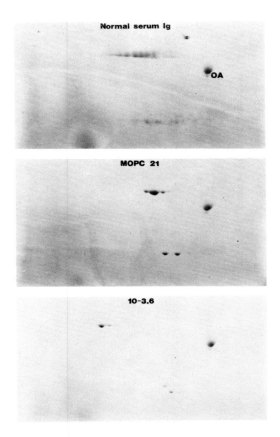

Fig. 7. 2-D PAGE analysis of light and heavy chains from (a) normal BALB/c serum Ig purified on protein A–Sepharose; (b) MOPC 21 myeloma protein; (c) antibody from clone 10-3.6 (anti-I-A^k) purified from culture supernates on protein A–Sepharose. The gels were run as described in the legend to Fig. 1, and the proteins visualized by Coomassie Blue staining. Ovalbumin (OA), 45,000 daltons, was added as a molecular weight marker.

ANTIBODIES TO IMMUNOGLOBULIN ALLOTYPES

IgD ALLOTYPES

In addition to the antibodies reacting with MHC determinants obtained from the H10 and H11 hybridizations, two cultures were found to react with lymphocyte surface antigens linked to the heavy chain complex (see Table I). Since these antibodies potentially could recognize allotypic determinants on either IgM or IgD receptors (12,13), further experiments were carried out to identify the antigen.

BIOCHEMICAL ANALYSIS

Spleen cells from BALB/c (Ig^a) or BAB/14 (Ig^b) mice were surface radio-iodinated with ^{125}I by the lactoperoxidase technique, and the membrane proteins solubilized in the non-ionic detergent NP-40. Antigens were precipitated and analyzed by SDS–PAGE. Results are shown in Fig. 8.

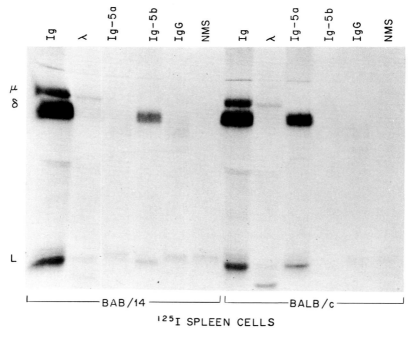

Fig. 8. Autoradiogram of SDS–PAGE analysis of immunoprecipitates of NP-40 solubilized BALB/c (Ig^a) and BAB/14 (Ig^b) spleen cells, labeled with ^{125}I by the lactoperoxidase technique. Reactivities of antibodies used for immunoprecipitation are indicated at the top of the gel. Anti-Ig-5a is from clone 10-4.22 and anti-Ig-5b from clone 11-6.3. Fixed *S. aureus* bacteria were used to bring down the antigen–antibody complexes. Since the 11-6.3 antibody (IgG$_1$) does not bind strongly to *S. aureus* protein A, a small amount of rabbit anti-mouse γ chain was added to facilitate binding of the 11-6.3 complexes to the bacteria.

When antibody from clone 10-4.22 was tested against BALB/c spleen cells, bands corresponding in mobility to δ and light chains were seen. No bands were seen using BAB/14 cells. Conversely, clone 11-6.3 precipitated δ and light chains from BAB/14 cells but not from BALB/c cells. Thus, it was concluded that both the clones producing antibodies against allotype-linked surface structures were recognizing allotypic determinants of δ chain. Clone 10-4.22 recognizes the Ig-5^a allele and 11-6.3 the Ig-5^b allele.

FACS ANALYSIS

Clones 10-4.22 and 11-6.3 were analyzed by two-color fluorescence using the FACS as described earlier. Results are shown in Fig. 9. Several conclusions may be drawn. The great majority of μ^+ cells were

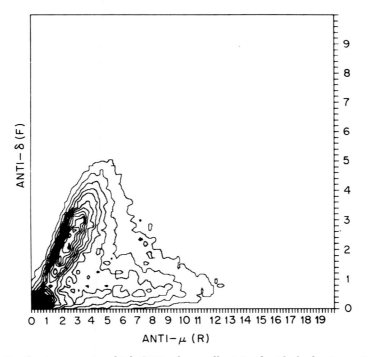

Fig. 9. Contour map in which C3H spleen cells stained with rhodamine-anti-μ and anti-Ig-5a (anti-δ) antibody from clone 10-4.22, followed by fluorescein-conjugated rabbit anti-γ, were analyzed by means of the FACS, and data plotted as in Fig. 4. Three predominant populations are seen: T cells ($\mu^-\delta^-$) lie near the origin; the majority of B cells are $\mu^+\delta^+$, while a minority of B cells are $\mu^+\delta^-$.

TABLE IV
Genetic Analysis of Anti-IgD Antibodies

	BALB/c a	B10 b	DBA/2 c	AKR d	A/J e	CE f
			Ig Haplotype			
NMS	−	−	−	−	−	−
11-6.3[a]	−	+	−	−	−	−
NMS	−	−	−	−	−	−
10-4.22[b]	+	−	+	+	−	+

[a] Second-step was ^{125}I-anti-Ig-4a.
[b] Second-step was ^{125}I-protein A.

also δ^+. No cells were seen which possessed IgD but not IgM. There was, however, a distinct set of cells which possess IgM but not IgD. These cells may represent a mixture of immature and activated B cells (12). Among the $\mu^+\delta^+$ cells, there was positive correlation between the amount of μ and the amount of δ. Finally, the mean intensity of μ staining on the $\mu^+\delta^-$ cells was greater than that of the $\mu^+\delta^+$ cells.

SPECIFICITY ANALYSIS

The monoclonal anti-IgD allotype antibodies simplify the analysis of Ig-5 antigenic specificities, since unlike alloantisera (12) they can be used on any strain possessing an appropriate Ig-5 allele, regardless of background. Two Ig-5 specificities have been described using conventional antisera. Specificity 1 is present on cells of Ig^a and Ig^e haplotype, but not on Ig^b (12). Specificity 2 is present on Ig^b but not on Ig^e (12). Specificity 3 is defined by the H6/31 monoclonal antibody (19), which

TABLE V
IgD Specificities

	1	2	3	4
a	1	−	−	4
b	−	2	3	−
c	n.d.	−	−	4
d	n.d.	−	−	4
e	1	−	3	−
f	n.d.	−	−	4

reacts with Ig[b] and Ig[e] haplotypes, but not Ig[a] (T. Pearson and L. A. Herzenberg, unpublished). Specificity 4 is defined by clone 10-4.22, which reacts with Ig[a] but not Ig[b] or Ig[e] (Tables IV and V). Thus, hybrid cell antibodies provide a powerful means of analysis of the complexity of antigenic determinants on single molecules, and of dissecting the nature of genetic polymorphisms.

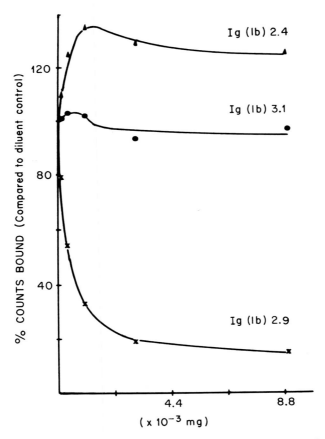

BLOCKING OF ^{125}I–Ig (Ib) 2.9 BINDING TO
Ig–Ib (C.BPC101) MYELOMA PROTEIN

Fig. 10. Anti-Ig-1b blocking curve. Various concentrations of unlabeled Ig-1b 2.4, 3.1, and 2.9 were used (abscissa) to block the subsequent binding of ^{125}I-Ig-1b 2.9. One hundred percent of counts bound represents the number of ^{125}I-Ig(1b)2.9 bound when medium (1% BSA-PBS, pH 7.5) was used in the blocking step of the assay.

TABLE VI
Monoclonal Antibodies to
Immunoglobulin Allotypes

Clone	Isotype	Specificity
Ig(1b)1.7	γ_{2a}, γ_3	Ig-1b
Ig(1b)2.4	γ_3	Ig-1b
Ig(1b)2.9	γ_{2a}	Ig-1b
Ig(1b)3.1	γ_1	Ig-1b
10-4.22	γ_{2a}	Ig-5a
11-6.3	γ_1	Ig-5b

Ig-1 (γ_{2a}) ALLOTYPES

The value of monoclonal antibodies in the analysis of antigenic specificities is also illustrated by five clones producing antibody against the Ig-1b allotype. These five clones [Ig-1b, 1.2, 1.7, 2.4, 2.9, and 3.1] were obtained from BALB/c mice immunized with immunoglobulins from C57BL/10 mice, as described earlier. Specificity analysis was carried out by a binding assay in which the antigen (C.BPC101 IgG_{2a} myeloma protein) was bound to flexible plastic plates. The plates were then incubated with unlabeled antibody (inhibitor), followed by ^{125}I-labeled antibody. Each antibody was capable of blocking itself (i.e., the labeled and unlabeled antibodies competed for the same sites, as expected). However, Ig(1b)2.9 was *not* blocked by Ig(1b)3.1, and the binding of Ig(1b)2.9 was slightly but reproducibly *enhanced* by Ig(1b)2.4 (Fig. 10). These results suggest the presence of at least two antigenic specificities on Ig-1b which are not on Ig-1a. Conventional antisera distinguish only one specificity between these alleles.

The nature of the antibody-induced enhancement of binding is not understood, and is currently under investigation. We favor the idea that antibody induces a conformational change in the antigen which facilitates binding. The chain composition and reactivities of the anti-allotype clones are given in Table VI.

CONCLUSIONS

There are many advantages of monoclonal antisera over conventional antisera (1,4). Especially important are: (a) the need to purify the antigen is eliminated; (b) the specificity, titer, and yield of antibody are extremely high; (c) problems of reproducibility are eliminated.

Increasing clinical applications will be found for monoclonal antibodies in addition to their use in the research laboratory. The use of monoclonal antibody against HLA antigens will greatly add to the precision of tissue typing, and monoclonal antibodies against drugs or hormones will improve and simplify radioimmunoassay procedures.

Macromolecular antigens often possess multiple antigenic determinants. Thus, a single antigen molecule may be capable of binding simultaneously several different antibodies from a conventional antiserum. In contrast, a given monoclonal antibody may be expected to interact with a *single* antigenic determinant. If all of a given species of surface molecule were equally accessible to antisera, this property would allow quantitation of surface molecules (20).

Moreover, the number of monoclonal antibody molecules bound per cell may be much less than that bound by conventional antisera. Directly conjugated fluorescent monoclonal antibodies have given relatively weak staining. Attention will have to be paid to ways of improving fluorescence intensity. The hapten-sandwich technique of Wofsy and colleagues (21,22) should provide the necessary amplification, although it may be anticipated that some monoclonal antibodies may have their combining site damaged by haptenation.

Precipitation would seem impossible where the antigen has only one antigenic site per molecule. Even when there are two sites (e.g., IgG$_\gamma$ chain allotypes), only linear arrays rather than lattices would be formed. However, the anti-Ig-1b monoclonal antibodies form strong precipitation lines in Ouchterlony analysis. This phenomenon is currently being investigated. Possible explanations include (a) precipitation occurring with long chains of antigen–antibody complexes or (b) presence of multiple identical antigenic determinants in each heavy chain, reflecting origin of the domains by gene duplication.

The inability of monoclonal antibodies to bind more than one determinant has implications for functions involving cross-linking, such as capping, complement fixation, and precipitation. If the density of a cell surface antigen is low, or if it is not favorably oriented, or if it exists only as a monomer, complement fixation by monoclonal antibody may be inefficient. However, the anti-H-2 and anti-Ia hybrid antibodies have extremely high cytotoxic titers. Monoclonal antibodies may also be useful in resolving the question of which immunoglobulin subclasses fix complement.

The extreme specificity of monoclonal antibodies should allow much more detailed analysis of cell surface proteins than is possible with conventional antibodies. The precise correspondence between antigen and antibody should allow the dissection of molecular complexes, such as histocompatibility antigens and Ia antigens. The use of allo-immunizations rather than xeno-immunizations, while restricting analysis to those molecules which are polymorphic, facilitates gene mapping, and will probably lead to the definition of many new loci.

Antibodies have been used widely to study the conformation of protein antigens (23). Monoclonal antibodies may extend the value of this approach, as illustrated in the case of the anti-Ig$_{1b}$ allotype antibodies. Finally, the production of homogeneous antibodies to haptens and fluorophores should allow a better understanding of the antibody combining site.

ACKNOWLEDGMENTS

This work was supported by grants from the National Institutes of Health: GM-17367, CA-04681, HD-01287, AI-08917. Dr. J. W. Goding is a C. J. Martin Fellow of the National Health and Medical Research Council of Australia; Dr. P. P. Jones is a Fellow of the National Science Foundation. The authors wish to thank Mr. F. T. Gadus and Mr. T. Tsu for their excellent technical assistance, Dr. D. B. Murphy for performing the cytotoxicity assays, Dr. S. J. Black for the biochemical analysis of the two anti-IgD clones, and Ms. Jean Anderson for skilled assistance in preparation of the manuscript.

REFERENCES

1. Köhler, G., and Milstein, C. (1975) *Nature (London)* **266**, 550–552.
2. Ringertz, N. R., and Savage, R. E. (1976) "Cell Hybrids." Academic Press, New York.
3. Iverson, G. M., Goldsby, R. A., and Herzenberg, L. A. (1978) *In* "Lymphocyte Hybridomas" (F. Melchers, N. L. Warner, and M. Potter, eds.). Springer-Verlag, Berlin **81**: 192–194.
4. Herzenberg, L. A., Herzenberg, L. A., and Milstein, C. (1978) *Handb. Exp. Immunol. 3rd Ed.* 12.1–12.23.
5. Köhler, G., Howe, S. C., and Milstein, C. (1976) *Eur. J. Immunol.* **6**, 292–295.
6. Herzenberg, L. A., and Herzenberg, L. A. (1978) *Handb. Exp. Immunol. 3rd Ed.* 12.1–12.23.
7. Oi, V. T., Jones, P. P., Goding, J. W., Herzenberg, L. A., and Herzenberg, L. A. (1978) *In* "Lymphocyte Hybridomas" (F. Melchers, N. L. Warner, and M. Potter, eds.). Springer-Verlag, Berlin and New York **81**: 115–129.
8. Goding, J. W. (1978) *J. Immunol. Methods* **20**, 241–253.
9. Klein, J. (1975) "Biology of the Mouse Histocompatibility-2 Complex." Springer-Verlag, Berlin and New York.
10. Ledbetter, J., Nowinski, R. C., and Emery, S. (1977) *J. Virol.* **22**, 65–73.
11. Wettstein, P. J., Krammer, P., Nowinski, R. C., David, C. S., Frelinger, J. A., and Shreffler, D. C. (1976) *Immunogenetics* **3**, 507–516.
12. Goding, J. W., Scott, D. W., and Layton, J. E. (1977) *Immunol. Rev.* **37**, 152–186.
13. Goding, J. W. (1978) *Contemp. Top. Immunobiol.* **8**, 203–243.

14. Jones, P. P. (1978) *J. Exp. Med.* **146**, 1261–1279.
15. Jones, P. P., Murphy, D. B., and McDevitt, H. O. (1978) *In* "Ir Genes and Ia Antigens" (H. O. McDevitt, ed.), pp. 203–213. Academic Press, New York.
16. O'Farrell, P. Z., Goodman, H. M., and O'Farrell, P. H. (1977) *Cell* **12**, 1133–1142.
16a. Jones, P. P., Murphy, D. B., and McDevitt, H. O. (1978) *J. Exp. Med.* **148**, 925–939.
17. Loken, M. R., Parks, D. R., and Herzenberg, L. A. (1977) *J. Histochem. Cytochem.* **24**, 899–907.
18. Ey, P. L., Prowse, S. J., and Jenkin, C. R. (1978) *Immunochemistry* **15**, 429–436.
19. Pearson, T., Galfré, G., Ziegler, A., and Milstein, C. (1977) *Eur. J. Immunol.* **7**, 684–690.
20. Williams, A. F., Galfré, G., and Milstein, C. (1977) *Cell* **12**, 663–673.
21. Cammisuli, S., and Wofsy, L. (1976). *J. Immunol.* **117**, 1695–1704.
22. Wofsy, L., Henry, C., and Cammisuli, S. (1978) *Contemp. Top. Mol. Immunol.* **7**, 215–237.
23. Atassi, M. Z. (1977) "Immunochemistry of proteins," Vol. 2. Plenum, New York.

PART VI

IMMUNOGLOBULIN IDIOTYPES

Idiotype-Specific Suppression Mediated by B Cells

ALFRED NISONOFF

Rosenstiel Basic Science Research Center
Brandeis University
Waltham, Massachusetts

INTRODUCTION

Antibodies formed to certain antigens by individual mice of the same strain share idiotypic determinants. This is by no means a universal finding, but it is common enough so that a number of systems of this type have been investigated extensively (1). The system we have been studying involves the production of antibodies to the p-azophenylarsonate group in the A/J strain (2). When an A/J mouse is immunized with KLH-p-azophenylarsonate (KLH-Ar), approximately 20–70% of the anti-Ar antibodies produced share a common idiotype with the anti-Ar antibodies produced in another mouse of the same strain. The remainder of the anti-Ar population consists of a large number of "private" idiotypes, some of which cannot be detected by a sensitive assay in other mice of the same strain (3,4). Thus one may consider the anti-Ar response as consisting of two components: one comprising a cross-reactive idiotype present in a substantial concentration in all mice of that strain, and the other consisting of a variety of private idiotypes, some of which cannot be detected in other mice. In a study of this question (4) a panel of 181 mice was hyperimmunized and tested for the presence of four private idiotypes, each arising in a mouse suppressed with respect to the common idiotype and then immunized with KLH-Ar. Three of the four "private" idiotypic antibodies, isolated by isoelectric focusing, could not be detected at a significant level in any of the 181 mice by a sensitive radioimmunoassay. The fourth idiotype was present in very low concentration, in

335

about 28% of the panel. The 181 mice, all of which produced high levels of anti-Ar antibodies, included animals that were suppressed or nonsuppressed with respect to the common idiotype. An hypothesis to account for the striking difference between the two classes of antibodies (2) is that the cross-reactive idiotype is encoded by germ-line genes whereas the private idiotypes arise through a large number of somatic events (4) (such as mutation, recombination or deletion of DNA, and repair with error), so that the probability of recurrence of the same series of events in another mouse is small.

In the case of anti-Ar antibodies, we have found strong *intrastrain* cross-reactions only in strains that are closely related to A/J (A/He, A/WySn, AL/N). For example, the anti-Ar antibodies produced in one BALB/c mouse do not share idiotype to a substantial extent with the anti-Ar antibodies produced in another BALB/c mouse. The absence of strong intrastrain cross-reactions applies to six other strains that we have studied which are unrelated to the A strains (5).

The fact that every mouse of the A/J strain produces a common idiotype made it possible to attempt suppression of this idiotype by administration of rabbit anti-idiotypic antibodies. This proved to be feasible in adult as well as neonatal mice (6). At about the same time Cosenza and Köhler demonstrated suppression *in vitro* of the production of anti-phosphocholine antibodies of a particular idiotype in BALB/c mice (7). Suppression of idiotypes *in vivo* has also been carried out by Strayer *et al.* (8), by Eichmann (9), and by Bordenave (10), who suppressed secondary idiotypic responses in individual rabbits.

When an adult A/J mouse is treated with rabbit anti-idiotypic antibodies, the state of idiotypic suppression persists in nearly all mice for at least 2 months. At the end of 22 weeks, about 60% of the suppressed mice had recovered from the suppressed state (11). These experiments were carried out by delaying the administration of antigen for various intervals after the injection of anti-idiotypic antibodies. If, however, antigen is administered within 2 weeks after the anti-idiotype, and antigen is then given periodically, the state of suppression persists indefinitely; we have never seen recovery from the suppressed state of a mouse once immunization has been started. We now believe that two mechanisms, involving T or B cells, respectively, account for the permanence of this suppressed condition. It was first shown by Eichmann (12) that idiotypically suppressed mice generate suppressor T cells which can adoptively transfer the suppressed state into a sublethally irradiated syngeneic recipient. We subsequently found that administration of antigen after suppression with anti-idiotype results in the formation of large numbers of suppressor T cells which can be identified by their capacity to form rosettes with autologous RBC coated with the idiotype, i.e., the suppressor cells generated by this mechanism have anti-idiotypic receptors (13,14).

A second role of antigen in inducing a permanently suppressed state will be the major topic of this presentation. This mechanism involves "clonal dominance" by B cells having anti-Ar receptors which lack the common idiotype. Such secondary cells can be generated in large numbers in an idiotypically suppressed A/J mouse that is hyperimmunized against the phenylarsonate group, or by immunizing a mouse of a strain that does not produce the idiotype. Such B cells have now been shown to be capable of adoptively transferring the idiotypically suppressed state to another mouse without the intervention of suppressor T cells. For convenience in this discussion the common idiotype will be referred to as CRI (cross-reactive idiotype).

RESULTS AND DISCUSSION

The experiments described next, carried out in collaboration with B. M. Eig and S-T. Ju (15), were designed to minimize the possibility of any involvement of idiotype-specific suppressor T cells. They made use of a congenic strain of mouse, C.AL-20, that was provided by Dr. Michael Potter. These mice possess genes controlling heavy chain allotypes of the AL/N strain on a BALB/c background. AL/N mice have heavy chain allotypic determinants that are closely related to those of the A/J strain, and produce anti-Ar antibodies with the CRI characteristic of A/J mice. It was also found that the CRI is produced by C.AL-20 mice; this provided some of the earliest evidence for the linkage of idiotype and heavy chain allotype (16,17).

The experimental procotol consisted first in immunizing BALB/c mice with KLH-Ar. Spleen cells, or spleen cells treated with anti-Thy 1.2 and complement, from immunized BALB/c mice were transferred into sublethally irradiated (200 rad) C.AL-20 recipients. The latter were then immunized with KLH-Ar, edestin-Ar, or BGG-Ar until a substantial titer of anti-Ar antibodies was present in their serum. The sera were then assayed for content of anti-Ar antibodies and for CRI. The assay for anti-Ar antibodies was that of Klinman et al. (18) in which the wells of a polyvinyl microtiter plate are first coated with BSA-Ar, then saturated with an unrelated protein. Upon addition of mouse serum containing anti-Ar antibodies, some of these antibodies are bound to the plate. After washing, the wells are exposed to ^{125}I-labeled specifically-purified rabbit anti-mouse IgG. The uptake of radioactivity is a function of the amount of anti-Ar antibodies present in the serum. The system is calibrated by using a serum of known anti-Ar content, as determined by precipitin analysis.

The assay for the cross-reactive idiotype makes use of ^{125}I-labeled anti-Ar antibodies bearing the idiotype and an antiglobulin reagent. The labeled specifically purified anti-Ar antibody is mixed with rabbit anti-idiotypic antiserum, followed by sufficient goat antirabbit Fc to precipitate all of the rabbit antibodies present. CRI in an unlabeled sample is estimated by its capacity to inhibit precipitation of the radioactive ligand. The data to be reported are expressed in terms of weight of anti-Ar antibody in a given serum required to cause 50% inhibition of precipitation of the radioactive ligand.

The data in Table I show the effect of transfer of spleen cells from BALB/c mice immunized with KLH-Ar into C.AL-20 mice that had received 200 rad 4 hr before the adoptive transfer. Subsequently each recipient mouse was immunized with four i.p. inoculations of 0.25 mg of KLH-Ar in CFA over a 24-day period and bled 1 week later. Data are expressed in terms of ng of anti-Ar antibody required for 50% inhibition of binding in the radioimmunoassay.

TABLE I

Inhibition of CRI in C.AL-20 Mice by Transfer of Spleen Cells from BALB/c Mice Immunized with KLH-Ar

Donor of cells transferred	No. of recipient mice	No. of cells transferred $\times 10^{-6}$	Anti-Ar Ab required for 50% inhibition[a] (ng)	
			Median value	Range
None	19	None	280	41–1,200
Nonimmune BALB/c	5	10	96	38–190
	5	50	140	39–1,900
	5	75	500	110–2,000
BALB/c immunized with KLH	4	10	75	49–110
	3	50	150	41–260
	4	75	330	70–4,800
BALB/c immunized with KLH-Ar[b]	5	10	>13,000–>25,000	
	4	50	>24,000–>29,000	
	10	100	>9,000–>15,000	

[a] 10 ng of labeled ligand were used in the radioimmunoassay.

[b] A single pool of donor cells was used. Donors had been immunized by four weekly i.p. inoculations of 0.25 mg of antigen in complete Freund's adjuvant (volume ratio of antigen to adjuvant 1:1). Adoptive transfers were carried out 2 weeks after the last injection.

The results obtained with the fourth group of mice (Table I) indicate that prior immunization of the donors with KLH-Ar caused virtually complete suppression of the idiotype in the immunized recipients.

Ten million transferred cells were sufficient to completely suppress the idiotype. In contrast, 10×10^6 or 50×10^6 cells from nonimmune BALB/c mice or from BALB/c mice immunized with KLH did not prevent the appearance of the idiotype. The transfer of 75×10^6 nonimmune or KLH-immune cells did cause a significant reduction in the fraction of the anti-Ar antibody population which possessed the CRI upon subsequent immunization, although the degree of suppression was not comparable to that resulting from the transfer of KLH-Ar immune cells. This finding can probably be explained on the basis that the BALB/c cells transferred included primary B cells with anti-Ar receptors, which lack the idiotype, and which competed for antigen with B cells in the recipients.

Another set of experiments was carried out in which 20×10^6 KLH-Ar immune BALB/c cells were transferred into C.AL-20 recipients. The experiments were carried out as described above, except that the donor cells were treated with anti-Thy 1.2 and complement prior to the transfer. Each of the five C.AL-20 recipients, upon immunization with KLH-Ar, was completely suppressed with respect to the cross-reactive idiotype (15).

This finding strongly suggests that the suppression of the idiotype was due to B cells and not to T cells. Furthermore, since BALB/c mice do not synthesize antibodies with the cross-reactive idiotype, one would not expect them to generate idiotype-specific suppressor T cells. (In addition, the production of idiotype-specific suppressor T cells requires priming with anti-idiotypic antibody.)

The possibility was considered that BALB/c mice produced carrier-specific suppressor T cells which in some manner interfered preferentially with the production of the idiotype in the C.AL-20 recipients. In an effort to rule this out, additional experiments were performed in which the BALB/c donors were primed with BGG-Ar rather than KLH-Ar and the C.AL-20 recipients were then immunized with KLH-Ar, i.e., with a carrier different than that used for priming the donors.

The results in Table II indicate that suppression of idiotype was observed under these conditions as well. Thus, the carrier used for priming the donors does not appear to be relevant. This again supports the conclusion that suppression is attributable to B cells.

TABLE II

Inhibition of Cross-Reactive Idiotype in C.AL-20 Mice by Adoptive
Transfer of Spleen Cells from BALB/c Mice Immunized with BGG-Ar[a]

Donor of cells transferred	No. of recipient mice	No. of cells transferred $\times 10^{-6}$	Anti-Ar Ab required for 50% inhibition (ng)
None	5	None	30, 30, 40, 40, 60
BALB/c immunized with BGG	3	10	150, 470, 850
	3	50	31, 110, 690
	2	75	600, 2,000
BALB/c immunized with BGG-Ar	5	1	20, 60, 80, 100, 120
	1	10	1,500
	4	10	>5,000–>13,000
	1	50	6,600
	4	50	>7,000–>35,000
	3	75	>4,500–>8,500

[a] Footnotes as in Table I.

Two factors which could account for these results are, first, the numerical superiority of B cells with anti-Ar receptors, transferred from immunized mice, as compared to the very small number of virgin B cells with anti-Ar receptors that would be expected to be present in the C.AL-20 recipients. Perhaps an equally important factor is the greater ease of triggering of memory cells as compared to primary B cells (19–24). These two properties together may account for the virtually complete suppression of idiotype. (It should be noted that the data reflect the percentage of anti-Ar molecules which carry the idiotype.) Once established the ratio of anti-Ar antibodies with and without the CRI might tend to be quite stable. However, the possibility that some type of active suppression is mediated by B cells cannot be ruled out.

To investigate the persistence of the suppressed state, the last group of mice in Table I was allowed to rest for 5 months. They were then injected with 0.25 mg of KLH-Ar i.p. in CFA and bled 1 week later. The idiotype could not be detected in the anti-Ar antibodies of any of nine surviving mice; the amounts tested range from 7,500 to 38,000 ng. As in each of the experiments described, 10 ng of ^{125}I-labeled ligand was used in the radioimmunoassay.

It should be noted that the antibodies with CRI have a somewhat lower average affinity than the remainder of the anti-Ar antibody population (25). This may be a factor in the failure of the idiotype to emerge on prolonged immunization.

Evidence for clonal dominance has also been obtained by transferring B cells from idiotypically suppressed, hyperimmunized A/J mice into nonimmune A/J recipients that had received 200 rad. Such experiments were carried out, first, in collaboration with K. Ward and H. Cantor (26). Splenic lymphocytes from a suppressed, hyperimmunized mouse, which was actively producing high titers of anti-Ar antibodies lacking the cross-reactive idiotype, were treated with anti-Thy 1.2 and complement. The remaining viable cells were assessed as being over 95% Ig-positive by immunofluorescence. In a series of adoptive transfer experiments it was shown that the number of remaining T cells was far below the threshold necessary to adoptively transfer the suppressed state. However, the irradiated A/J recipients of B cells, upon hyperimmunization with KLH-Ar, were found to be completely suppressed by the adoptive transfer of 1×10^6, 3×10^6, or 10×10^6 anti-theta treated cells. Actually the B cells were two to three times as potent as nylon wool-purified T cells in adoptively transferring the suppressed state.

A related set of experiments was carried out in collaboration with Dr. Frances L. Owen (27). Again, A/J mice that had been suppressed with respect to the CRI and then hyperimmunized were used as a source of B cells. In this case, however, B cells were specifically purified over a column of Sephadex G-200 to which BGG-Ar had been conjugated using cyanogen bromide. After washing the beads the lymphocytes were recovered by exposure to $0.1~M$ sodium p-aminophenylarsonate. The cells were then treated with anti-Thy-1.2 plus complement, which did not kill a significant percentage of the cells. It was found that 1×10^5 or 2×10^5 cells caused more than 90% suppression of the idiotype in ten of twelve recipient A/J mice; in nearly all of the ten mice the idiotype was not detectable. As in earlier experiments, the recipients received 200 rad prior to the adoptive transfer and were subsequently hyperimmunized with KLH-Ar.

The data presented establish the phenomenon of clonal dominance as a mechanism of suppression of idiotype by B cells. In addition, an idiotypically suppressed, hyperimmunized mouse contains substantial numbers of idiotype-specific suppressor T cells (12–14). It is apparent that these two mechanisms acting in conjunction must act as a powerful influence in maintaining the idiotypically suppressed state.

ACKNOWLEDGMENT

This work was supported by grants AI-12907 and AI-12895 from the National Institutes of Health.

REFERENCES

1. Weigert, M., and Potter, M. (1977) *Immunogenetics* **5**, 491.
2. Kuettner, M. G., Wang, A., and Nisonoff, A., (1972) *J. Exp. Med.* **135**, 579.
3. Hart, D. A., Pawlak, L. L., and Nisonoff, A., (1973) *Eur. J. Immunol.* **3**, 44.
4. Ju, S.-T., Gray, A., and Nisonoff, A. (1977) *J. Exp. Med.* **145**, 540.
5. Pawlak, L. L. (1972) Ph.D. Thesis, University of Illinois College of Medicine, Urbana.
6. Hart, D. A., Wang, A. C., Pawlak, L., and Nisonoff, A. (1972) *J. Exp. Med.* **135**, 1293.
7. Cosenza, H., and Köhler, H. (1972) *Science* **176**, 1027.
8. Strayer, D. S., Lee, W. M. F., Rowley, D. A., and Köhler, H. (1975) *J. Immunol.* **114**, 728.
9. Eichmann, K. (1974) *Eur. J. Immunol.* **4**, 296.
10. Bordenave, G. R. (1975) *Immunology* **28**, 635.
11. Pawlak, L. L., Hart, D. A., and Nisonoff, A. (1973) *J. Exp. Med.* **137**, 1442.
12. Eichmann, K. (1975) *Eur. J. Immunol.* **5**, 511.
13. Owen, F. L., Ju, S.-T., and Nisonoff, A. (1977) *Proc. Natl. Acad. Sci. U.S.A.* **74**, 2084.
14. Owen, F. L., Ju, S.-T., and Nisonoff, A. (1977) *J. Exp. Med.* **145**, 1559.
15. Eig, B. M., Ju, S.-T., and Nisonoff, A. (1977) *J. Exp. Med.* **146**, 1574.
16. Pawlak, L. L., Hart, D. A., Nisonoff, A., Mushinski, E. B., and Potter, M. (1973) *Specific Recept., Antibodies, Antigens, Cells, Int. Convocation Immunol. [Proc.], 3rd, 1972* p. 259.
17. Pawlak, L., Mushinski, E. B., Nisonoff, A., and Potter, M. (1973) *J. Exp. Med.* **137**, 22.
18. Klinman, N. R., Pickard, A. R., Sigal, N. H., Gearhart, P. J., Metcalf, E. S., and Pierce, S. K. (1976) *Ann. Immunol. (Paris)* **127c**, 489.
19. Fazekas de St. Groth, S., and Webster, R. G. (1966) *J. Exp. Med.* **124**, 331.
20. Eisen, H. N., Little, R. J., Steiner, L. A., Simms, E. S., and Gray, W. (1969) *Isr. J. Med. Sci.* **5**, 338.
21. Deutsch, A., Vinit, M.-A., and Bussard, A. E. (1973) *Eur. J. Immunol.* **3**, 235.
22. Siskind, G. W., and Benacerraf, B. (1969) *Adv. Immunol.* **10**, 1.
23. Klinman, N. R. (1972) *J. Exp. Med.* **136**, 241.
24. Davie, J. M., and Paul, W. E. (1972) *J. Exp. Med.* **135**, 643.
25. Kapsalis, A. A., Tung, A.S. and Nisonoff, A. (1976) *Immunochemistry* **13**, 783.
26. Ward, K., Cantor, H., and Nisonoff, A. (1978) *J. Immunol.* **120**, 2016.
27. Owen, F. L., and Nisonoff, A. (1978) *J. Exp. Med.* (in press).

Regulation of the Immune System by Idiotype–Anti-Idiotype Interaction in the Rabbit and the Mouse

PIERRE-ANDRÉ CAZENAVE AND
CHRISTIAN LE GUERN
Service d'Immunochimie Analytique
Institut Pasteur
Paris, France

INTRODUCTION

The number of idiotypic determinants (idiotopes) being of the same order of magnitude as the number of combining sites (paratopes), it has been proposed that every immunoglobulin is an anti-idiotypic antibody directed against an idiotope present in the same individual. Interactions between idiotopes and anti-idiotypic antibodies within the repertoire of a given individual could lead to a functional network (1–4).

Several experiments have suggested that anti-idiotypic antibodies play a role to regulate the synthesis of antibodies against which they are directed (5,6).

In recent studies from our laboratory (7) and from Urbain's group (8), evidence for such a regulation has been presented. Rabbit I was immunized against an antigen (AgX) to produce anti-AgX Ab1 antibody. Ab1 were then injected in another rabbit (rabbit II) which produced anti-idiotypic antibodies (designated by Ab2) against Ab1. The Ab2 antibodies were injected into other rabbits (rabbit III) which produced anti-idiotypic antibodies (designated by Ab3) against Ab2. Rabbits III were then immunized against AgX to produce anti-AgX

343

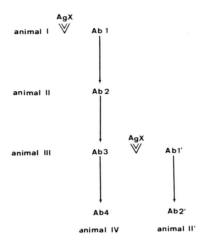

Fig. 1. Summary of the different immunizations.

antibodies designated by Ab1′ (the different immunizations are summarized in Fig. 1). In the ribonuclease system (7) and in the *Micrococcus* system (8), Ab1′ synthesized by rabbits III cross-react with the
anti-idiotypic antibodies Ab2 showing an idiotypic similarity between
Ab1′ and Ab1 despite the possibility for rabbits III immunized against
AgX to be capable of producing a wide range of different anti-AgX
antibodies with a wide range of different idiotypes. The idiotypic similarity between Ab1 and Ab1′ has been confirmed in the *Micrococcus*
system (9) and in the ribonuclease system [Figs. 2 and 3]: Ab1 cross-

Ab1(966)   Ab1′(821)   Ab1′(822)

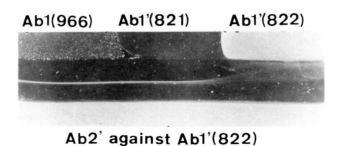

Ab2′ against Ab1′(822)

Fig. 2. Reaction in agar gel (10) in a cell with parallel walls (11) of Ab2′ antibody
(lower layer) with three preparations of anti-ribonuclease antibodies: Ab1(966),
Ab1′(821) and Ab1′(822). Ab2′ antibody has been prepared against Ab1′(822). 966 was
rabbit I, 821 and 822 were rabbits III in the ribonuclease system (7).

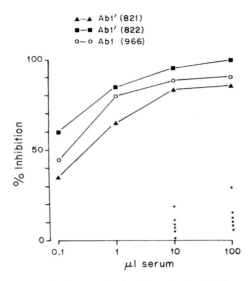

Fig. 3. Inhibition by Ab1(966), Ab1'(821), and Ab1'(822) sera of the binding of ^{125}I-labeled Ab1'(822) to insolubilized Ab2' antibody directed against Ab1'(822). Inhibition values obtained with anti-ribonuclease sera from unrelated rabbits are represented by stars.

reacts with anti-idiotypic antibody (Ab2') prepared against Ab1' in rabbit II' (Fig. 1).

These results suggest: (a) that rabbits, at least with the same allotypes, possess a closely related idiotypic repertoire, and (b) that the immune system is a network of variable domains. By suitable manipulations of the immune system, a private idiotype can become a "public" idiotype.

These observations raise numerous questions. Elements of experimental answers to three of them are presented in this paper:

(1) Can the results obtained in the rabbit be obtained in other species?

(2) What is the influence of allotypic background on this phenomena?

(3) What is the idiotypic relationship between Ab1 and Ab3?

IDIOTYPIC MANIPULATION OF THE MOUSE IMMUNE SYSTEM

In the mouse, we have tried to favor expression of Ab1 by inducing an immune response (Ab3) against the suppressor Ab2.

Several systems are studied in our laboratory; we present results obtained in the DNP system with MOPC 460 myeloma protein as Ab1 (C. Le Guern, B. Mariamé, and P.-A. Cazenave, unpublished).

MOPC 460 protein ($\alpha\kappa$) of BALB/c origin exhibits an anti-DNP (and anti-TNP) activity (12). Ab2 anti-M460 antibodies have been prepared as previously described (13,14) in several inbred strains of mice, including BALB/c and DBA/2 strains. Ab2 antibodies have been isolated on a column of AH-Sepharose (15) with the covalently attached Fab fragment of MOPC 460. M460 idiotype-Ab2 reaction and its inhibition were studied using an indirect precipitation method (16). It has been shown by suitable inhibitions that Ab2 antibodies of BALB/c and DBA/2 origins are directed against ligand-modifiable idiotopes.

1411-F6(51) hybridoma protein from BALB/c origin directed against a M460 ligand-modifiable idiotope (17) has been also used as Ab2.

Anti-idiotypic antibodies against M460 have been prepared in rabbits. Rabbit antisera were absorbed on immunoadsorbents of immunoglobulin fraction of McPC 870 ($\alpha\kappa$) ascite and immunoglobulin fraction of normal BALB/c serum. Rabbit anti-idiotypic antibodies have been also isolated by elution with DNP-glycine from their combination with insolubilized M460 Fab fragment.

After immunization against DNP-ovalbumin (DNP-OVA) conjugate, a part of anti-DNP antibodies synthesized by BALB/c mice are idiotypically similar to M460. Similar results have been obtained in another laboratory (18). The M460 idiotype positive population of BALB/c anti-DNP antibodies is only a minor component of the whole response to DNP group (2–4 μg per ml of immunized BALB/c sera). M460 idiotype is also found in BALB/c mice immunized against TNP-Ficoll.

The different anti-idiotypic sera do not detect M460 idiotype (or a cross-reacting one) in the sera of DBA/2 mice immunized against DNP-OVA.

Idiotypic analysis of anti-DNP antibodies obtained against DNP-OVA in different strains of mice, in several congenic lines, and in progeny (F1, F2, and backcrosses) of BALB/c × DBA/2 crosses show that the gene which governs the expression of M460 idiotype is linked to the genes which govern the expression of *CH* allotypes.

DBA/2 mice are immunized against Ab2 antibody prepared in DBA/2 (each mouse is immunized against the Ab2 antibody isolated from the serum of *one* individual Ab2-producing mouse). Most of them produce Ab3. Then, they are immunized against DNP-OVA to produce anti-DNP Ab1' antibody.

DBA/2 Ab1' sera inhibit the binding of ^{125}I-labeled M460 Fab to rabbit anti-idiotypic serum (Fig. 4). This inhibition is complete. Moreover, the inhibition curve obtained with M460 protein and the inhibition curves obtained with the different Ab1' DBA/2 sera are closely parallel, showing that a population of Ab1' antibody would be idiotypically identical to M460 protein, 2–4 μg/ml of M460 idiotype can be detected in DBA/2 mice III sera.

Ab1' DBA/2 sera adsorbed with DNP-lysine-Sepharose (19) fail to inhibit the binding of labeled M460 Fab to anti-idiotypic antibodies (Fig. 5) showing that M460 idiotype-like material found in Ab1' sera belongs to the anti-DNP antibody population.

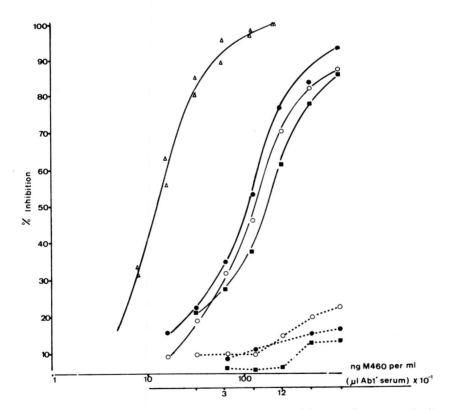

Fig. 4.   Inhibition of the binding of ^{125}I-Fab M460 to rabbit anti-idiotypic antibodies by 7 S M460 protein ($\triangle$——$\triangle$) and by sera from DBA/2 mice III after immunization against DNP-OVA (———). Controls: DBA/2 normal serum (----------) and sera from DBA/2 mice immunized against DNP-OVA.

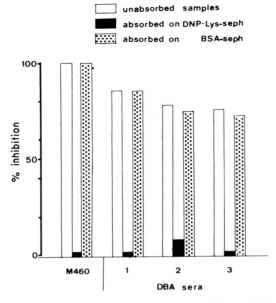

Fig. 5. Inhibition of the binding of ^{125}I-Fab M460 to rabbit anti-idiotypic antibodies by: 7 S M460 protein (10 ng) and individual sera (2 μl) from three DBA/2 mice III immunized against DNP-OVA. The samples used for inhibition were either unabsorbed, or absorbed on DNP-lysine-Sepharose, or absorbed on BSA-Sepharose.

Similar results can be obtained with a different carrier and a T-independent antigen: when DBA/2 mice III are immunized against TNP-Ficoll.

Preliminary data indicate that M460 idiotype can be also induced in mice III belonging to other strains than DBA/2 (C57B1/6, NZB).

These results extend those obtained in the rabbit (7,8). By suitable manipulations, a BALB/c anti-DNP public idiotype undetected in a normal anti-DNP response of DBA/2 mice can become public in this strain.

It is worthy to note that in the rabbit systems studied (*Micrococcus* and ribonuclease), Ab1′ idiotypic specificity is only similar but not identical to the Ab1 one. In the mouse DNP system, we have seen that DBA/2 anti-DNP Ab1′ appears to be identical to Ab1 (M460). In this system, BALB/c and DBA/2 mice seem to be more genetically similar than are two rabbits, chosen at random, in the *Micrococcus* and the ribonuclease systems. It is also possible that the structural gene responsible for the synthesis of M460 idiotype is well preserved in the mouse species. In collaboration with Dr. L. Thaler (Université de

Montpellier, France), we are now working on wild mice belonging to two species and to different subspecies with the aim of analyzing the idiotypic similarity between M460 and the anti-DNP Ab1' that we hope to obtain in these animals.

VH ALLOTYPIC BACKGROUND AND NETWORK

As the structures which correlate with a series allotypic specificities (20) are located on the VH domain of rabbit immunoglobulins (21,22), it is of interest to analyze the influence of a allotypic background in the regulation by Ab3 of Ab1 idiotype expression. Several experiments on this subject are now in progress in our laboratory. Some results are presented here (P.-A. Cazenave, unpublished).

Rabbit I, rabbit II, and rabbit III with the same *a1/a101* genotype have been used (the pecking order is a101 > a1) (23). After immunization against *Micrococcus lysodeikticus* rabbit I produced a restricted heterogeneous anti-micrococcal carbohydrate Ab1 with a⁻ (a minus) phenotype against which Ab2 have been prepared in rabbit II.

Six rabbits III, which have been immunized against Ab2 and have produced Ab3 antibodies, are immunized against *Micrococcus lysodeikticus* and produce antimicrococcal carbohydrate Ab1'. A part of the Ab1' antibodies synthesized by rabbits III cross-react with Ab2. Such a cross-reaction cannot be found with antimicrococcal carbohydrate sera produced in unrelated rabbits or even in rabbits belonging to the same families than the rabbits I, II and III.

In some rabbits III, Ab1' which cross-react with Ab2 are mainly a⁻. In other rabbits III, a⁻ Ab1' molecules are also associated with a1⁺ Ab1' molecules but never with a101⁺ Ab1' molecules. Both a⁻ and a1⁺ Ab1' cross-react with Ab2 showing an idiotypic similarity between a1⁺ Ab1', a⁻ Ab1' and a⁻ Ab1. This observation is in good agreement with a previous one of an idiotypic similarity between a⁻ and a3⁺ antibodies produced by one rabbit against streptococcal carbohydrate (24). In one rabbit III, Ab1' are exclusively a1⁺.

This set of experiments suggests that the gene (or the group of genes) governing the expression of a1 allotype and the gene (or group of genes) governing the expression of idiotypic specificity present on a⁻ molecules are linked.

What is more important is that these experiments suggest an influence of the VH allotypic background on the idiotype anti-idiotype regulation of the immune system. Preliminary data indicate that this influence is significant not only at the level of Ab1' but also at the level of Ab3: in the system described above, Ab3 are a^- or $a1^+$, never $a101^+$. Experiments are now in progress to study, in the same system, the idiotype and the *VH* allotype of Ab1' antibodies induced in rabbits III with *a101/a101, a3/a3,* or *a3/a101* genotype.

COMPARISON BETWEEN IDIOTYPE OF Ab1 AND IDIOTYPE OF Ab3

When two Ab2 (Ab2(A) and Ab2(B)) against the same Ab1 are prepared in two different rabbits A and B, the reaction between labeled Ab2(A) and Ab3 prepared against Ab2(A) is inhibited (at least partially) by Ab2(B) (7). Two explanations can be given for this observation:

(i) Ab1 and Ab3 possess similar idiotypic specificities: anti-idiotypic Ab2(B) antibody directed against Ab1 recognize one or several idiotopes on Ab3 molecules. Ab2(B) acts as antibody in the inhibition of the Ab2(A)–Ab3 reaction.

(ii) Ab2(A) and Ab2(B) possess similar idiotypic specificities: Ab2(B) idiotype cross-reacts with Ab3 directed against Ab2(A) idiotype. In this hypothesis Ab2(B) acts as antigen in the reaction with Ab3.

To favor the hypothesis (i), an analogy has been drawn (9) between the Ab1–Ab2–Ab3 interactions and the results obtained by Sege and Peterson (25). The retinol binding protein (RBP) is able to form a dimer with prealbumin and anti-idiotypic antibodies against anti-RBP antibodies interact with prealbumin. It seems to us that an important restriction to this analogy is the lack of anti-AgX antibody function for Ab3. In the two systems studied in the rabbit and in the mouse DNP system, it is impossible at this time to detect any antibody activity in Ab3 serum against the antigen which has induced the synthesis of Ab1 in animal I.

An argument in favor of the hypothesis (ii) is that, in a network mechanism, Ab3 must suppress Ab2' activity in the animal III to allow the emergence of Ab1' idiotype after immunization of the animal III against AgX and consequently Ab3 must recognize Ab2'. This implies that Ab2' in the animal III and Ab2 synthesized by rabbit II possess some degree of idiotypic similarity. The consequence would be that public idiotypes must be found in antibodies of different rabbits against the same idiotype. Until recently public idiotypes has not been described in the rabbit. However, we have found rabbit anti-allotypic public idiotypes in the three systems studied at this time: anti-a1, anti-b4, and anti-b6 (25a).

To study the idiotypic relationship between Ab1 and Ab3, Ab4 has been prepared against Ab3 in animal IV (Fig. 1). In the rabbit *Micrococcus* system, Ab4 combines with Ab1 showing an idiotypic similarity between Ab1 and Ab3(9). In the rabbit ribonuclease system, Ab4 precipitate Ab3 but not Ab1, it binds labeled Ab3 but not labeled Ab1.

The two results are not contradictory in the two hypotheses considered above. In hypothesis (i), Ab1 and Ab3 exhibit an idiotypic cross-reactivity, for instance Ab1 possesses x and y idiotopes, Ab3 x and z idiotopes. Ab4 in the *Micrococcus* system would be directed against x-like idiotope when, in the ribonuclease system, Ab4 would be directed against z-type idiotope.

If Ab1 and Ab3 have similar idiotypic specificities the idiotypic network can be viewed as being made up of small idiotypic communities (26) and a structure of such a small community in the form of a small circular network (Fig. 6).

In hypothesis (ii), Ab1 and Ab3 possess different idiotypic specificities. If clones which recognize different epitopes bear idiotopes similar to Ab1 idiotopes, they are under the control of Ab2 suppressive activity. The synthesis of Ab3 in animal III results in depression of Ab2 elements (antibody or cells or both). This results in an increase of the synthesis of all Ab1 idiotypelike antibodies independent of their antigen reactivities (1). This set of antibodies with similar idiotypic specificities are designated by Ab1′x (Fig. 7).

Ab3 used to prepare Ab4 are isolated on Ab2 immunoadsorbent. In hypothesis (ii), the putative Ab1′x antibodies bind to Ab2 and are isolated with Ab3. In this hypothesis, Ab4 obtained in the rabbit *Micrococcus* system could be directed against these Ab1′x antibodies and

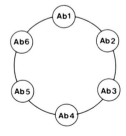

Fig. 6. Closed network: cycle of interacting antibodies and lymphocytes with Ab1, Ab2, Ab3 . . . activities.

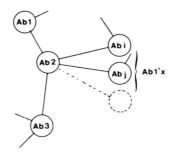

Fig. 7. Opened network: Ab2 antibody (or cell) has a suppressive activity not only on Ab1 antibody (or cell) but also on Abi, Abj . . . antibodies (or cells), Abi, Abj . . . having no detectable antibody activity against AgX antigen.

the Ab4 antibodies obtained in the ribonuclease system against Ab3.

In the mouse M460 system, we are studying the possibility for Ab3 sera to contain Ab1′x antibodies. Ab2 antibodies prepared in mice could recognize Ab1′x and, as antigen, are recognized by Ab3. Rabbit anti-idiotypic antibodies directed against M460 could recognize Ab1′x

TABLE I
Concentration of M460 Idiotype in Different Strains of Mice III

Strain	Ab2 used to induce Ab3 response	Number of mice	Concentration[a] of M460 idiotype (μg/ml)
BALB/c	BALB/c Ab2[b]	5	0.3,0.3,0.3,1.2,1.0
BALB/c	1411-F6(51)Ab2[c]	5	1.0,0.7,0.9,7.0,1.5
DBA/2	DBA/2 Ab2[b]	5	0.9,2.5,1.0,1.6,4.0
DBA/2	1411-F6(51)Ab2	5	0.5,0.4,0.6,0.3,0.3
C57B1/6	1411-F6(51)Ab2	6	0.2,0.2,0.2,0.8,1.2,0.2[d]
BALB/c	nil	5	<0.01
DBA/2	nil	5	<0.01
C57B1/6	nil	5	<0.01

[a] Determined by inhibition of the indirect precipitation of ^{125}I-Fab M460 by rabbit anti-idiotypic antibodies (16), a reference curve is built with 7 S M460 protein as inhibitor.

[b] Ab2 is isolated from the serum of one mouse immunized against M460 protein

[c] Hybridoma molecule from BALB/c origin (17)

[d] The concentrations of M460 idiotype in the sera of C57B1/6 mice III are below the real values because the slope of inhibition curves obtained with these sera is lower than the slope of the inhibition curve obtained with M460 protein.

and do not recognize Ab3 if Ab3 idiotypic specificity is different from M460 idiotypic specificity. Moreover these antibodies are not recognized, as antigen, by Ab3.

In the Ab3 producing DBA/2, BALB/c and C57B1/6 mice III, we have been able to detect M460-like idiotype by means of rabbit anti-idiotypic antibodies (Table I). The concentration of this idiotype is too low to be compatible with the expected concentration of Ab3 antibodies. This result could suggest that Ab1'x would be present in these mice III. Similar results have been obtained in mice III producing Ab3 against 1411-F6(51) hybridoma Ab2.

Work is now in progress in collaboration with Dr. G. Buttin (Université Pierre et Marie Curie, Paris) to try to select hybridoma cells obtained by fusion of mice III spleen cells which could synthesize such Ab1'x antibody.

CONCLUSION

Results summarized in this paper show that by suitable manipulation of the immune system, a rabbit private idiotype can become a public idiotype in this species and that BALB/c strain public idiotype undetected in a normal response of DBA/2 mice can become public in DBA/2 strain.

This suggests that the structural gene governing the synthesis of an idiotype might be present in animals which do not express this idiotype in "normal" conditions. The interpretation of an idiotype as a marker for a V region structural gene must be made with caution and the existence of genes regulating the expression of antibody structural genes must be considered in the discussion of the results on the idiotypes genetics. Other experiments lead to similar conclusions (27).

The results summarized in this paper suggest that the immune system is a network of V domains. But, what is the physiological significance of this phenomena?

Several experiments indicate that cells secreting auto-anti-idiotypic antibodies appear as part of the normal immune response against a given antigen:

In the mouse, auto-Ab2 anti-T15 antibodies have been detected during the response of BALB/c to phosphorylcholine (28,29). Cells with anti-E109 auto-Ab2 activity have also been detected during the response of BALB/c to levan and a roughly inverse correlation between the frequency of anti-E109 PFC and the fraction of anti-levan PFC that secretes E109 idiotype has been found (30).

In the rabbit tobacco mosaïc virus system, cells with auto-Ab2 activity have been found, the kinetics of appearance and disappearance of these cells show an inverse relationship between antibody affinity or concentration and the presence of lymphocytes bearing auto-Ab2 receptors in the peripheral blood (31).

In recent experiments we have shown in the mouse M460 system that T cells with suppressive activity against M460 idiotype are present in normal BALB/c mice (32). These cells have been shown to bear auto-Ab2 receptors and these receptors are recognized by Ab3 antibody.

ACKNOWLEDGMENTS

We are indebted to Drs. J. Oudin, N. Jerne, and J. Urbain for helpful discussions. The expert technical assistance of Miss Danielle Voegtlé is gratefully acknowledged. This work was supported by grants from the Centre National de la Recherche Scientifique (ER 67 and ATP "Bases structurales et fonctionnelles de la réponse immunitaire" n° 3613) and from Université Pierre et Marie Curie.

REFERENCES

1. Jerne, N. K. (1974) *Ann. Immunol. (Paris)* **125c**, 373–389.
2. Jerne, N. K. (1974–1975) *Harvey Lect.* **70**, 93–110.
3. Lindenmann, J. (1973) *Ann. Immunol. (Paris)* **124c**, 171–184.
4. Urbain, J. (1976) *Ann. Immunol. (Paris)* **127c**, 357–374.
5. Rodkey, L. S. (1974) *J. Exp. Med.* **139**, 712–720.
6. Eichmann, K., and Rajewsky, K. (1975) *Eur. J. Immunol.* **5**, 661–666.
7. Cazenave, P.-A. (1977) *Proc. Natl. Acad. Sci. U.S.A.* **74**, 5122–5125.
8. Urbain, J., Wikler, M., Franssen, J. D., and Collignon, C. (1977) *Proc. Natl. Acad. Sci. U.S.A.* **74**, 5126–5130.
9. Urbain, J. (1979) *Proc. Eur. Immunol. Meet., 4th,* (in press).
10. Oudin, J. (1946) *C.R. Hebd. Seances Acad. Sci.* **222**, 115–118.
11. Oudin, J. (1955) *Ann. Immunol. (Paris)* **89**, 531–555.
12. Jaffe, B. M., Eisen, H. N., Simms, E. S., and Potter, M. (1969) *J. Immunol.* **103**, 872–874.
13. Sirisinha, S., and Eisen, H. (1971) *Proc. Natl. Acad. Sci. U.S.A.* **68**, 3130–3135.
14. Sakato, N., and Eisen, H. N. (1975) *J. Exp. Med.* **141**, 1411–1426.
15. Cambiaso, C. L., Goffinet, A., Vaerman, J. P., and Heremans, J. F. (1975) *Immunochemistry* **12**, 273–278.
16. Kuettner, M. G., Wang, A. L., and Nisonoff, A. (1972) *J. Exp. Med.* **135**, 579–595.
17. Buttin, G., Le Guern, C., Phalente, L., Lin, E. C. C., Medrano, L., and Cazenave, P.-A. (1978). *Curr. Top. Microbiol. Immunol.* **81**, (in press).
18. Rosenstein, R. W., Zerdis, J. B., and Richards, F. F. (1977) *Immunogenetics* **5**, 505.
19. Goetzl, E. J., and Metzger, H. (1970) *Biochemistry* **9**, 1267–1278.
20. Oudin, J. (1960) *J. Exp. Med.* **112**, 107–124 and 125–142.

21. Mole, L. E., Geier, M. D., and Koshland, M. E. (1975) *J. Immunol.* **114**, 1442–1448.
22. Porter, R. R. (1974) *Ann. Immunol. (Paris)* **125c**, 85–91.
23. Brézin, C., and Cazenave, P.-A. (1976) *Ann. Immunol. (Paris)* **125c**, 333–346; to be published.
24. Kindt, T. J., Klapper, D. G., and Waterfield, M. D. (1973) *J. Exp. Med.* **137**, 636–648.
25. Sege, K., and Peterson, P. A. (1978) *Nature (London)* **271**, 167–168.
25a. Cazenave, P.-A. and Roland, J. (1978) In preparation.
26. Herniaux, J. (1977) *Immunochemistry* 14, 733–739.
27. Weigert, M., and Potter, M. (1977) *Immunogenetics* 5, 491–524.
28. Köhler, H. (1975) *Transplant. Rev.* 27, 24–56.
29. Cosenza, H. (1976) *Eur. J. Immunol.* 6, 114–116.
30. Bona, C., Lieberman, R., Chien, C. C., Mond, J., House, J., Green, I., and Paul, W. E. (1978) *J. Immunol.* **120**, 1436–1442.
31. Tasiaux, N., Leuwenkroon, R., Bruyns, C., and Urbain, J. (1978) *Eur. J. Immunol* (in press).
32. Bona, C., Le Guern, C., Hooghe, R., Cazenave, P.-A., and Paul, W. G. (1978) To be published.

Ontogeny of Clonal Dominance

HEINZ KÖHLER, DAVID KAPLAN, RUTH KAPLAN,
JOHN FUNG, AND JOSÉ QUINTÁNS

Department of Pathology
La Rabida–University of Chicago Institute
University of Chicago
Chicago, Illinois

INTRODUCTION

Typically antibody responses are made by a large number of different B-cell clones. The heterogeneous or polyclonal character of these responses can easily be demonstrated by a variety of techniques such as isoelectric focusing or hapten binding studies. Only in a few instances do the produced antibodies against a given antigen exhibit restricted heterogeneity. An important factor of inducing restricted responses seems to be the nature of the antigen. Thus, most restricted responses observed in rabbits (1) and mice (2,3) are directed against epitopic structures which are presented in repetitive fashion on the carbohydrate backbone.

A major advance in the search for clonally restricted responses was the use of murine myeloma proteins as references to which induced antibodies could be compared. In such studies one utilizes an anti-idiotypic anti-serum raised against a given myeloma idiotype. If the induced antibodies are identical or similar enough to the reference myeloma protein, the anti-idiotypic antibody will show various degrees of cross-reactivity. The first well-documented example (4) for idiotypic cross-reaction between a myeloma protein and an induced antibody was given in studies of the response of BALB/c mice to the small hapten phosphorylcholine (PC). BALB/c mice, when immunized with PC-containing antigen, produce anti-PC antibodies which are more than 95% of a given BALB/c myeloma idiotype. This idiotype is

357

the most common in a family of PC-binding BALB/c myeloma proteins and is referred to as T15 (5).

Another well-studied example for cross-reacting idiotypes is the response of BALB/c mice to dextran (6). Here, however, the anti-dextran response is not monoclonal since three different idiotypes have been described using anti-idiotypic antisera against three dextran binding myeloma proteins (7).

The expression of only one idiotype in the response to PC is not due to the lack of other PC-binding idiotypes in the repertoire of the BALB/c mouse. Studies of the precursors for anti-PC antibodies in neonatal BALB/c have shown the presence of several non-T15 anti-PC-producing B cells which are normally not expressed in the adult BALB/c mouse (8). However these non-T15 clones become activated after the T15 idiotype had been suppressed during the neonatal period (9,10). Evidently, a selection process occurs in developing BALB/c mouse which leads to the known dominance of the T15 idiotype in the adult BALB/c.

In the following, the factors and the mechanisms which are operating in the ontogeny of a dominant clone will be analyzed. In this context it might be illuminating to recall two findings on the clonal development of the T15 idiotype which underscore the importance of the early postnatal period for the T15 idiotype ontogeny. The T15 clone can be chronically suppressed with small amounts of anti-T15 anti-idiotype antibodies (11). And second, the T15 idiotype clone responds late on ontogeny (8). Both findings seem to indicate that the development of the T15 dominance requires a unique step in the development which marks the transition from clonal heterogeneity to clonal dominance. Obviously, this developmental step does not occur in most other responses which are of heterogeneous character.

LOSS OF CLONAL DOMINANCE AFTER ADOPTIVE TRANSFER

The response capabilities of maturing B cells can be probed in three general ways: measuring the response of neonatal animals *in vivo, in vitro,* or after transfer of neonatal or fetal cells into lethally radiated hosts. By using these methods it became evident that responses to a variety of different antigens can be obtained in mice after adoptive transfer of immature liver or spleen cells (12–14). With the exception of the anti-PC response, the reconstituted responses are produced by several different clones. No deviations from the "normal" maturation

could be detected using the criteria of response magnitude or maturation in these transfer experiments. Thus, adoptive transfer of immature
cells is an accepted approach to study the maturation process. A nota-
ble exception to these findings is the reconstituted response to PC
which seems not to follow the blueprint of maturation taking place *in
vivo* (15).

We have tested the capacity of mature and immature cells to restore
the response to PC and to TNP in a simple adoptive transfer. Lethally
irradiated BALB/c mice were reconstituted with four different cell
populations: (1) adult BALB/c spleen cells, (2) adult BALB/c bone
marrow cells, (3) neonatal BALB/c spleen cells, and (4) neonatal
BALB/c liver cells. As seen in Fig. 1 the adult spleen cell population
reconstituted equally well the response to PC and TNP. However,
none of the other cell populations could reconstitute the response to
PC while the response to TNP was restored. This failure of cells from
generative B-cell organs to reconstitute the anti-PC response was totally unexpected and is not due to changes of the response kinetics or
the lack of mature thymocytes (15,16). The failure to reconstitute
anti-PC response can be explained in two ways. Either the precursor

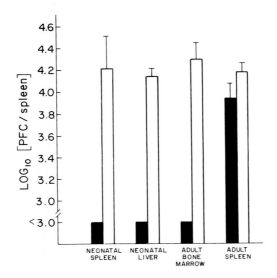

Fig. 1.   Normal adult BALB/c mice were lethally irradiated and reconstituted with
1×10^7 neonatal spleen or liver cells from animals less than 48 hr old, or with 1×10^7 adult
bone marrow or spleen cells. Fifteen days after transfer the recipients were immunized
with R36A and TNP-Ficoll. The PFC responses ($\log_{10}$ of geometric mean and standard
error) to PC (solid bars) and to TNP (open bars) were measured 5 days later.

or progenitor cells for an anti-PC response are not present in neonatal lymphatic tissues and in adult bone marrow, or the maturation of present but nonresponding cells cannot take place in the reconstituted host.

Several attempts were made to facilitate the response of transferred immature cells in the recipients. In Table I the failure of different manipulations of the host to reconstitute the anti-PC are shown. It has been suggested that suppressor cells in the neonatal cell population would cause the unresponsiveness (17). Since, in another T-independent response (18), suppressor cells are sensitive to anti-lymphocyte serum (ATS), the recipients were given ATS before reconstitution with neonatal cells. However, this treatment or giving cyclophosphamide which also is known to affect T suppressor cells did not improve the anti-PC response nor did it affect the anti-TNP response. In another experiment neonatal liver cells were mixed with adult spleen cells and transferred to irradiated recipients. No evidence for suppressor cells present in the neonatal cell population was seen since the response of adult spleen cells was not impaired. Furthermore, increasing the level of circulating T15 idiotype by passive administration of T15 ascites or BALB/c anti-PC serum had no effect either. Finally, repeated challenge of the reconstituted host with R36A antigen also failed to induce an anti-PC response.

TABLE I
Effects of Treating the Recipient

Treatment of recipients of 10^7 neonatal BALB/c cells	PFC/spleen[d]	
	Anti-TNP	Anti-PC
None	3.98 ± 0.05	<3.0
Anti-lymphocyte serum (0.2 ml)[a]	3.69 ± 0.09	<3.0
Cyclophosphamide (100 mg/kg)[a]	4.29 ± 0.11	<3.0
HOPC-8 (0.1 ml ascites)[b]	4.53 ± 0.03	<3.0
BALB/c anti-PC (0.2 ml serum)[b]	4.27 ± 0.09	<3.0
Immunizing with R36A[c]	4.68 ± 0.08	<3.0

[a] Three days before lethal radiation the host BALB/c mice were given the indicated amounts of ATS, cyclophosphamide, HOPC-8 ascites, or BALB/c anti-PC serum.

[b] At the day of reconstitution the recipients were injected with HOPC-8 or BALB/c anti-PC serum.

[c] After reconstitution the recipients were immunized on day 10 and 15 with R36A.

[d] Before the third week after reconstitution the recipients, immunized with TNP-Ficoll and R36A, were assayed 4 days later.

TABLE II

Clonotypic Analysis of Lethally Irradiated BALB/c Mice Reconstituted with Syngeneic Cells[a]

Cells transferred	Number of recipient mice	Time of assay (weeks after transfer)	Log_{10} (Direct PFC)			Percentage non-H8 id PFCs
			Anti-TNP	Anti-PC	Non-H8 id anti-PC[b]	
1×10^7 neonatal liver	6	10	4.83 ± 0.16 (64,608)	3.99 ± 0.17 (9,772)	3.86 ± 0.21 (7,244)	74
1×10^7 adult spleen	5	3	4.18 ± 0.09 (15,276)	3.94 ± 0.14 (8,630)	2.51 ± 0.17 (324)	4
1×10^7 adult spleen	5	10	4.35 ± 0.18 (22,387)	3.74 ± 0.05 (5,470)	2.30 ± 0.20 (200)	4

[a] Lethally irradiated BALB/c mice were reconstituted with neonatal liver cells less than 48 hr old or with adult spleen cells. Mice were immunized with R36A and TNP-Ficoll either 3 weeks or 10 weeks after transfer. Direct PFC's were counted 5 days after challenge. The log of the geometric mean and standard error are given with the geometric mean in parenthesis.

[b] Clonotypic analysis was carried out by incorporating a 1:500 dilution of anti-H8 id into the plaquing mixture. Anti-PC PFC's not inhibited by anti-H8 id were 100% inhibited by 10^{-5} M PC.

All responses to PC and TNP in reconstituted recipients, as discussed so far, were measured not later than 3 weeks after transfer. Conceivably, if one allows more time after transfer the anti-PC response might recover. If BALB/c mice reconstituted with neonatal liver cells were assayed for anti-PC responsiveness 10 weeks after transfer they had recovered with a modest anti-PC response (see Table II). But in contrast to the response of animals reconstituted with adult spleen cells the clonotype analysis showed that reconstitution in the neonatal cells did not yield a T15-dominant response (16).

RESCUE OF CLONAL DOMINANCE

Up to this point of our discussion the question is still open as to whether the loss of clonal dominance using fetal or neonatal cells is due to the absence of the T15 clone or its inability to mature in the host. As a first step in resolving this question we analyzed the effects of the age of donor cells on the reconstituted response. Liver and spleen cells from fetuses and neonates of different ages were transferred and the response to PC and TNP was measured in the third week after transfer (Fig. 2). While the reconstituted response to TNP with donor cells of day 13 fetuses was substantial and remained high throughout the different tested donor ages, the response to PC of liver cells appeared only when the inocula came from 3-day-old neonates or when 6-day-old spleen cells were used as donor cells. It seems that the responding donor cell appears first in the neonatal liver and 2–3 days later in the neonatal spleen.

This finding of a late effectiveness of neonatal cells in the transfer of the anti-PC response is compatible with Klinman's (8) data on the late appearance of the T15 clone which were obtained in the splenic foci assay. When we waited even more than 3 months after reconstitution and challenged the reconstituted animals with PC we could not obtain a T15 dominant response (15,16). Thus, it appears that the T15 clone is present in the transferred inoculum but is somehow inhibited to develop into dominance. Therefore, we can ask more specifically: why is the clonal dominance lost and what are the factors which prevent the development of the T15 dominance in the reconstituted host? Since several attempts to treat the recipient in different ways failed (see Table I) we were essentially left to try one remaining manipulation of the host. The rationale for using neonatally suppressed BALB/c mice (11) as recipients was to have the T15 idiotype expression in the adult host matched with the neonatal donor environment. The neonatally

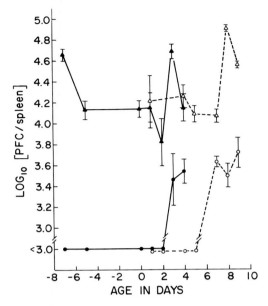

Fig. 2. Lethally irradiated adult BALB/c were reconstituted with syngeneic fetal and neonatal cells of different ages. The recipients were immunized with R36A and TNP-Ficoll 15 days after reconstitution, and the PFC responses were measured 5 days later. The solid lines represent responses of animals reconstituted with liver cells; the dashed lines represent responses reconstituted with spleen cells; the triangles are anti-TNP PFC's, the circles are anti-PC PFC's.

suppressed adult does not express the T15 idiotype and thus simulates the lack of T15 expression in the neonate. The state of suppression is not stable but changes with increasing age of the mouse. During the first few months after neonatal suppression, the T15 clone is completely unresponsive (9–11) while a low non-T15 response can be obtained. In the following phase of recovery from suppression the neonatally suppressed BALB/c regains slowly the T15 idiotype (10). Therefore, we have used neonatally suppressed BALB/c mice of different ages as recipients for the transfer of immature cells. As seen from the data in Fig. 3, there is an age dependence in the capacity of neonatally suppressed recipients to permit development of clonal dominance in adoptive transfer. Though the number of tested neonatally suppressed hosts is not sufficiently large to make definite conclusions it appears that early after neonatal suppression the recipients are not permissive for T15 dominance. It is tempting to speculate that the observed cyclic permissiveness for T15 dominance in neonatally sup-

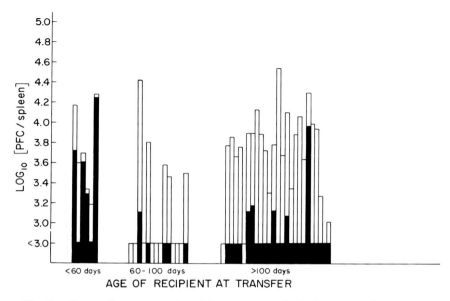

Fig. 3. Neonatally suppressed BALB/c mice were lethally irradiated and reconstituted with syngeneic neonatal cells from animals less than 48 hr old. The recipients were immunized with R36A at different times after reconstitution. The solid portion of the bars represent the amounts of anti-PC PFC's of individual animals which are not of H8 idiotype, the open portions are anti-PC PFC's of H8 idiotype.

pressed recipients correlates with the three phases in the recovery from neonatal suppression.

Assuming that the permissiveness of neonatally suppressed recipients for the T15 dominance is in part determined by a low or suppressed idiotype responsiveness of the host, we used another host having non-T15 dominant idiotype characteristics. The BALB/c congenic CAL-20 mouse carries the A-strain allotype and lacks the T15 dominance. When neonatal liver cells were transferred into CAL-20, several reconstituted animals responded with T15 clonal dominance (Fig. 4). Though the number of experimental animals is small, the mixture of permissive and nonpermissive CAL-20 host is reminiscent of the pattern of permissiveness observed in neonatally suppressed BALB/c hosts of different ages. Although we do not know the reasons which determine the permissiveness for T15 dominance we can at least state that the normal BALB/c host is always nonpermissive while CAL-20 and neonatally suppressed BALB/c mice are permissive though they do not express this faculty at all times. In any case, the important finding obtained from the use of neonatally suppressed BALB/c and

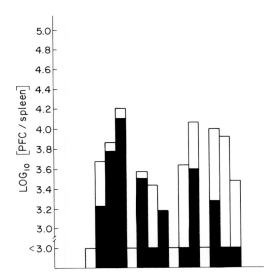

Fig. 4. CAL-20 mice were lethally irradiated and reconstituted with 1×10^7 neonatal BALB/c liver cells. The recipients were immunized with R36A at day 15 after transfer and assayed for anti-PC PFC's 5 days later. The open portion of the bars indicates the amounts of PFC's of individual animals that are of H8 idiotype, the solid portion PFC's of non-H8 idiotype.

CAL-20 mice is that the immature BALB/c contains the T15 progenitor and the non-T15 progenitor clones which can mature in these hosts to respond to a challenge with PC antigens. The reasoning why the progenitors in the neonate are already part of a committed T15 clone will be given in the following discussion.

DISCUSSION

The response to PC in BALB/c mice seems unusual in several aspects; the response to PC is almost entirely of one idiotype, the T15 (2). Anti-T15 idiotypic antibodies given to the neonatal BALB/c suppress the expression of the T15 idiotype chronically (11), and the T15 idiotype dominance is lost upon adoptive transfer (15). We will now attempt to tie these unique findings together and will present a model which describes the differentiation and maturation events responsible for the clonal dominance in the anti-PC response of BALB/c mice.

The critical phase for the development of the T15 dominance evidently is the time between the late fetal and the early postnatal period.

It is at this time of maturation when the T15 dominance appears and when it can be chronically suppressed. The key question is whether the T15 clone appears late, i.e., 5 days after birth (8) or whether the T15 is already present earlier but requires additional differentiation steps before we can observe its response.

We have used neonatally suppressed BALB/c and CAL-20 congenic mice as recipients for fetal and early postnatal cells and have obtained the T15 clonal dominance in the reconstituted response to PC. If the same immature cells are transferred to normal BALB/c the T15 dominance does not develop (15). Inasmuch as the T15 permissive host was manipulated in an idiotype-specific manner the transferred immature cells must be able to sense the idiotype negative environment of the neonatally suppressed BALB/c or of the CAL-20. Therefore, these neonatal cells must have receptors which are idiotype-specific and thus the cells themselves are idiotypically committed. We have referred to this cell type as the progenitor (15). The progenitor is different from the more mature pre-B cell by its inability to be triggered with antigen but is similar to the pre-B cell by virtue of its commitment for a given idiotype. By this criteria the committed progenitor is already the first manifestation of the T15 clone. This reasoning allows us to formulate the following scheme describing the ontogeny of idiotypes: the first step is the commitment of a multipotent stem cell to become an idiotype-specific progenitor. The progenitor, by means of its idiotype-sensitive receptor, can be selected by idiotype-specific factors present in the environment. During this process, progenitor clones are regulated, i.e., suppressed or promoted; the selected progenitor clone undergoes proliferation and maturation and then appears later as predominant precursor clones in the idiotype profile of the response. In the case of the T15 clone the selection process is extremely pronounced, giving rise to the clonal dominance of the T15 idiotype in the response to PC.

We are aware and concerned with the possibility that the fetal or neonatal cell inoculum contains mature precursors in limiting amounts. For example, when we transfer 6×10^7 neonatal liver cells into normal BALB/c, we observed a low anti-PC response, but with 2×10^7 or less cells we obtained only background anti-PC responses of less than 1000 PFC/spleen. Since we have at this point no data on vigorously controlled experiments using a single pool of neonatal cells transferred into large numbers of normal or neonatally suppressed hosts, we cannot formally exclude the presence of small numbers of mature precursors in the inocula. Thus, as far as this hypothetical responding precursor is concerned, our transfer experiments would have to be done under limiting dilution conditions. But on the other hand, this is not the situation for the T15 progenitor which seems to be the predominant cell type in the perinatal BALB/c.

Assuming that the described maturation steps of the T15 idiotype ontogeny occur with some modifications during the maturation of every immune response, one will appreciate the uniqueness of the mechanism which the immune response uses for its development. The essence of this unique developmental pathway is that in the final phase of maturation immune reactions are operating. The selection and promotion of certain idiotype-committed clones seem to involve reactions which are familiar from experiments with anti-idiotype antibodies and cells, i.e., suppression and enhancement of idiotypes. The prerequisite for these idiotype–anti-idiotype interactions is of course a basic library of idiotypes which have already matured and are functionally available. Here again the PC system might give us a first glance at these developmental events. When we measure with sensitive assays the serum levels of idiotype and anti-idiotypes in neonatal BALB/c mice we recognize a peculiar pattern (Fig. 5). Immediately after birth no T15 idiotype is detectable, but anti-idiotypic antibodies are present. With the onset of the T15 idiotype by day 4 or 5 the anti-idiotype disappears. It is tempting to speculate that the early auto-anti-idiotypic antibody (4,19) helps to select and to promote the T15 idiotype to reach clonal dominance. Aside from these speculations

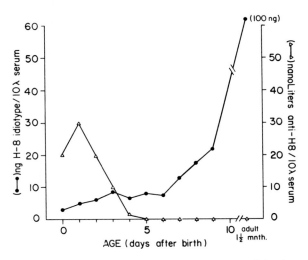

Fig. 5. Neonatal BALB/c mice of different ages were assayed for the presence of the H8 idiotype and anti-H8 antibody using solid phase radioimmunoassays.

on the late phase of the idiotype ontogeny we are on safe ground by knowing that in this period the neonate is exquisitely sensitive to idiotype-specific manipulations such as neonatal idiotype suppression (11) or adoptive transfer (15).

SUMMARY

The response to phosphorylcholine (PC) in BALB/c mice is remarkably restricted to the expression of the T15 idiotype. The development of the T15 clone in ontogeny was studied in an adoptive transfer system. While the transfer of neonatal BALB/c cells into normal lethally radiated syngeneic recipients leads to a loss of the T15 clonal dominance, the use of neonatally suppressed BALB/c or CAL-20 mice as recipients permits the appearance of the T15 dominance in the response to PC. It is proposed that the maturation of idiotype committed progenitor cells to responding precursors is under idiotype-specific regulation.

ACKNOWLEDGMENTS

This work was supported by grants AI-11080 to H. K. and AI-14530 to J. Q.; J. Q. is recipient of a Research Career Development Award AI-00268 and a Basil O'Connor grant from the March of Dimes. D. K. is a Lederer Fellow; R. K. is supported by training grant 1-T32 HD-07009 and J. F. by training grant T32-GM0 7281.

REFERENCES

1. Krause, R. M. (1970) *Adv. Immunol.* **12**, 1.
2. Cosenza, H., and Köhler, H. (1972) *Science* **176**, 1027.
3. Weigert, M. G., Cesari, I. M., Yonkovich, S. J., and Cohn, M. (1970) *Nature (London)* **228**, 1045.
4. Köhler, H. (1975) *Transplant. Rev.* **27**, 24.
5. Potter, M., and Lieberman, R. (1970) *J. Exp. Med.* **132**, 737.
6. Carson, D., and Weigert, M. (1973) *Proc. Natl. Acad. Sci. U.S.A.* **70**, 235.
7. Hansburg, D., Briles, D. E., and Davie, J. M. (1977) *J. Immunol.* **119**, 1406.
8. Sigal, N. H., Pickard, A. R., Metcalf, E. S., Gerhart, P. J., and Klinman, N. (1977) *J. Exp. Med.* **146**, 933.
9. Augustin, A., and Cosenza, H. (1976) *Eur. J. Immunol.* **6**, 497.
10. Accolla, R. S., Gearhart, P. J., Sigal, N. H., Cancro, M. P., and Klinman, N. R. (1977) *Eur. J. Immunol.* **7**, 876.
11. Strayer, D. S., Lee, W., Rowley, D. A., and Köhler, H. (1975) *J. Immunol.* **114**, 722.
12. Rosenberg, Y. L., and Cunningham, A. J. (1976) *J. Immunol.* **117**, 1618.

13. Nossal, G. J. V., and Pike, B. L. (1973) *Immunology* **25**, 33.
14. Goidl, E., and Siskind, G. W. (1974) *J. Exp. Med.* **140**, 1285.
15. Kaplan, D. R., Quintáns, J., and Köhler, H. (1978) *Proc. Natl. Acad. Sci. U.S.A.* **75**, 1967.
16. Köhler, H., Kaplan, D., and Quintáns, J. (1978) *Fed. Proc., Fed. Am. Soc. Exp. Biol.* **37**, 1679.
17. Mosier, D. E., and Johnson, B. M. (1975) *J. Exp. Med.* **141**, 216.
18. Baker, P. J., Stashak, D. W., Ambsbaugh, D. F., and Prescott, B. (1974) *J. Immunol.* **112**, 404.
19. Strayer, D. S., and Köhler, H. (1976) *Cell. Immunol.* **25**, 294.

Anti-(T,G)-A--L Idiotypes: Initial Studies of Genetic Control and Cellular Expression

SETH H. PINCUS, ALFRED SINGER,
RICHARD J. HODES, AND HOWARD B. DICKLER
Immunology Branch, National Cancer Institute
National Institutes of Health, Bethesda, Maryland

INTRODUCTION

Idiotypic determinants are immunologically defined markers that distinguish antibodies of different specificities, presumably on the basis of variable region structural differences (1). As such, they represent clonally expressed markers. Recent evidence has indicated that idiotypic determinants identical or cross-reactive with those on antibody are also present on T lymphocytes (2–4). Since T lymphocytes may play a role in *H-2* linked genetic control of the immune response [reviewed in Benacerraf and Katz (5)], it would be of interest to examine the expression of idiotypes on T cells where the response to antigen is under *H-2*-linked immune response (*Ir*) gene control.

The antigenic properties of the synthetic polypeptide poly-L-(Tyr, Glu)-poly-DL-(Ala)--poly-L-(Lys), designated (T,G)-A--L*, have been extensively studied. Reactivity to (T,G)-A--L is under the control of immune response (*Ir*) genes that map to the *Ir*-1 locus of the *H-2* complex (6). This antigen has been used in studies attempting to characterize the roles of different cell populations in both primary (7,8)

---

* Abbreviations used in this paper: Ir, immune response; KLH, keyhole limpet hemocyanin; (T,G)-A--L, poly-L-(Tyr, Glu)-poly-DL-(Ala)--poly-L-(Lys); TNP, trinitrophenyl.

and secondary (7,9) responses. In addition, a (T,G)-A--L specific T cell helper factor has been described (10). An antiserum directed against anti-(T,G)-A--L idiotypic determinants might therefore be helpful in further clarifying the cellular interactions involved in the immune response to this antigen.

In this paper the production and specificity of antisera reacting with the idiotypes of anti-(T,G)-A--L antibodies from C57BL/10 and C3H.SW mice are described. Also, it is demonstrated that a gene or genes closely linked to the heavy chain allotype locus determine the expression of anti-(T,G)-A--L idiotypes. Lastly, evidence is presented that T cell function can be inhibited by anti-idiotypic antiserum.

PRODUCTION AND SPECIFICITY OF ANTISERA DIRECTED AGAINST ANTI-(T,G)-A--L IDIOTYPES

Immune ascites were prepared against (T,G)-A--L in C57BL/10 and C3H.SW mice by the method of Tung *et al.* (11). Affinity-purified B10 and C3H.SW anti-(T,G)-A--L antibody was prepared by adsorption on to (T,G)-A--L Sepharose and elution with 0.1 M NH$_4$OH. Lewis rats were immunized four times, every other week, with 500 μg of the affinity-purified antibody emulsified in complete Freund's Adjuvant. The rats were then bled at weekly intervals, and the serial bleeds from each rat were pooled. The sera thus prepared reacted only with immunoglobulin by immunoelectrophoretic analysis. These antisera were then exhaustively adsorbed on insolubilized normal globulin from the same strain of mice from which the affinity-purified antibody derived.

A highly sensitive radioimmunoassay was developed to measure the binding of labeled (T,G)-A--L by anti-(T,G)-A--L antibody. Inhibition of this binding was used to detect anti-idiotypic activity. The putative anti-idiotype or normal rat serum was incubated with anti-(T,G)-A--L antibody in microtest tubes. After 10 min radiolabeled (T,G)-A--L was added to the tube and incubated 45 min, following which goat anti-mouse γ-globulin was added. After 2–3 days at 4°C, the total radioactivity in the tube and the radioactivity in the immunoprecipitate were determined. Each determination was done in triplicate and the results expressed as percentage of the total antigen precipitated within the pellet.

The adsorbed Lewis antisera were tested for reactivity with anti-(T,G)-A--L antibodies by measuring the inhibition of (T,G)-A--L binding by such antibodies. Figure 1 shows the effect of Lewis anti-[B10

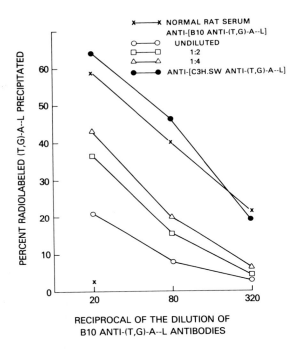

Fig. 1. Inhibition of B10 anti-(T,G)-A--L antigen binding by Lewis anti-[B10 anti-(T,G)-A--L] antibodies. B10 anti-(T,G)-A--L ascites was assayed for binding of radiolabeled (T,G)-A--L at three dilutions in the presence of normal rat serum, Lewis anti-[B10 anti-(T,G)-A--L], and Lewis anti-[C3H.SW anti-(T,G)-A--L]. The binding of antigen by nonimmune sera is designated by X.

anti-(T,G)-A--L] on B10 anti-(T,G)-A--L ascites. In the presence of normal rat serum, at a 1:20 dilution of B10 anti-(T,G)-A--L, 58.5% of the antigen was bound. However, when undiluted Lewis anti-[B10 anti-(T,G)-A--L] was present, only 21% of the label was precipitated. This inhibition was diminished with increasing dilutions of the rat serum, 36.5% of the antigen was bound at a 1:2 dilution and 43% at a 1:4 dilution. Since the curves obtained in the presence of normal rat serum and the various dilutions of rat anti-[mouse anti-(T,G)-A--L] were roughly parallel through the range of B10 anti-(T,G)-A--L dilutions, it was possible to determine the percentage of antibodies inhibited. Thus, equivalent amounts of (T,G)-A--L were bound by the B10 anti-(T,G)-A--L in the presence of undiluted rat anti-[B10 anti-(T,G)-A--L] and in the presence of normal rat serum at dilutions of 1:20 and 1:320, respectively, which is equal to 94% inhibition. Similarly, a

1:2 dilution of the anti-idiotype gave 85% inhibition and a 1:4 dilution 75% inhibition.

The same titrations were performed for C3H.SW anti-(T,G)-A--L and Lewis anti-[C3H.SW anti-(T,G)-A--L] (data not shown). Again, significant inhibition of antigen binding by anti-idiotypic antiserum was seen at all anti-(T,G)-A--L dilutions. In contrast to the B10 titrations, it was found that all dilutions of anti-idiotype up to 1:16 gave equivalent inhibition, approximately 80%. Thus, in the C3H.SW system, the reagent was of higher titer, but was reactive with a somewhat lower proportion of the anti-(T,G)-A--L antibody population.

The specificity of the rat anti-[mouse anti-(T,G)-A--L] for idiotypic determinants on anti-(T,G)-A--L was demonstrated by the following criteria: (1) Demonstration of strain specificity in ascites pools and individual animals, i.e., Lewis anti-[C3H.SW anti-(T,G)-A--L] did not inhibit the binding of B10 antibody to (T,G)-A--L, and vice versa, as demonstrated in Fig. 1 and Table I; (2) Lewis anti-[B10 anti-(T,G)-A--L] failed to inhibit the binding of nuclease by anti-nuclease antibody of the IgCH^b allotype; (3) the anti-idiotypic activity of Lewis anti-[C3H.SW anti-(T,G)-A--L] was removed by adsorption on insolubilized C3H.SW anti-(T,G)-A--L antibody, but not on B10 anti-(T,G)-A--L.

Since the anti-idiotypic antisera were raised and initially tested against the same pools of antibody, it was necessary to test the antisera against anti-(T,G)-A--L antibody from mice who were not members of the initial pools. Animals were scored positive for the expression of an idiotype if the binding of (T,G)-A--L in the presence of anti-idiotype was significantly depressed (as determined by a single tailed Student's t test) when compared to the binding in the presence of normal rat serum. The results of forty-nine B10 and B6, and thirty-six C3H.SW mice so tested are summarized in Table I. Although the majority of mice in each strain share the idiotype(s) defined by the antisera, the

TABLE I
Penetrance of Idiotype Expression in
Individual Mice

Strain	No. expressing B10 idiotype	No. expressing C3H.SW idiotype
B10 and B6	47/49	0/10
C3H.SW	0/11	26/36

penetrance of the C3H.SW idiotype is much lower than that of the B10. As such, the Lewis anti-[B10 anti-(T,G)-A--L] has proven to be the more useful reagent in the genetic and cellular studies that follow. A more detailed description of the techniques and specificity of the reagents is published elsewhere (12).

GENETIC CONTROL OF THE EXPRESSION OF B10 ANTI-(T,G)-A--L IDIOTYPE(S)

It is now generally accepted that a group of genes closely linked to the heavy chain allotype locus is responsible for idiotype determination (13). In order to assess this possibility in the (T,G)-A--L system, the expression of the B10 idiotype was studied in allotype congenic strains of mice in which the B6 allotype locus (and neighboring genes) was bred onto animals of different backgrounds. The CB.20 was derived from BALB/c and the CWB was the result of transferring the IgCH^b locus onto a C3H.SW background. The results are summarized in Table II. Although neither C3H.SW nor BALB/c expresses the B10 idiotype, nine of nine CB.20 and nine out of ten CWB expressed this marker. These data strongly suggest that there is a gene or genes closely linked to the b allotype locus that determines the expression of B10 derived idiotypes. Formal proof requires the analysis of a backcross, for example (BALB/c × B10)F$_1$ × BALB/c, or of recombinant inbred mouse lines (BXH/Ty and CXB/By are particularly suitable). The present data also do not rule out the possibility that other genes not linked to the heavy chain allotype locus also play a role in determination of idiotype. Of particular interest will be the role of *H-2*

TABLE II
Effect of Allotype Linked Genes on the
Expression of B10 Idiotype(s)

Strain	IgCH locus	Percentage expressing idiotype
B10 and B6	b	47/49
C3H.SW	a	0/11
BALB/c	a	0/10
CB.20	b	9/9
CWB	b	9/10

linked genes. Although a number of studies involving antigens under demonstrable *Ir* gene control suggest that *H-2* linked genes play no role in determining idiotype expression (14–17), the question has not been completely resolved, since in all of these studies *Ir* gene control was bypassed in order to raise antibody.

CELLULAR EXPRESSION OF ANTI-(T,G)-A--L IDIOTYPE(S)

The assay chosen to study the effect of the anti-idiotypic sera on cellular function was a primary *in vitro* hapten-carrier response. Unprimed spleen cells were incubated in culture with trinitrophenyl (TNP) derivatives of soluble protein antigens, in this case (T,G)-A--L and keyhole limpet hemocyanin (KLH). After 4 days the number of IgM anti-TNP plaque forming cells (PFC) was determined by a modification of the Jerne technique (18). The generation of such PFC is dependent on both T cells and non-B, non-T adherent radiation-resistant accessory cells in the culture, and follows the genetic patterns established for response to the carrier protein (19). In order to test for the effect of the anti-idiotypic serum on this response, the serum was added to the cells for the duration of the 4-day culture period, the cells were then harvested in the usual manner and assayed for plaques on TNP-sheep red blood cells. To avoid nonspecific effects, the sera were decomplemented, adsorbed on insolubilized normal globulins, insolubilized (T,G)-A--L, and normal spleen cells, and an ammonium sulfate cut prepared, followed by extensive dialysis against phosphate buffered saline.

The effect of the anti-B10 anti-idiotypic antiserum on the response of B10 mice to TNP-(T,G)-A--L and TNP-KLH is demonstrated in Table III. It is apparent that this reagent had a marked inhibitory effect on the response to TNP-(T,G)-A--L at dilutions as low as 0.1%, but had no effect on the response to TNP-KLH at any dilution. Specificity was also observed when this antiserum was tested on different strains (Table IV). The response of C3H.SW or A.BY mice to TNP-(T,G)-A--L was unaffected by the anti-idiotypic serum, with a marked inhibition of the B10 response again noted.

Once the remarkable specificity of this reagent in only inhibiting the response of B10 mice to TNP-(T,G)-A--L had been established, the cellular locus of this effect was evaluated. It seemed likely that T-cell function was being inhibited, since T cells generally determine carrier specificity in a hapten-carrier response (20). In order to determine if

TABLE III

Antigen Specificity of Inhibition of Primary *in Vitro*
Response of B10 Mice by Anti-B10 Anti-Idiotype

Anti-Id (%)	Direct PFC/10^7 cultured cells[a]		
	TNP-(T,G)-A--L	TNP-KLH	No antigen
—	998(1.17)	6241(1.16)	120(1.83)
3	135(1.53)	5574(1.31)	
1	159(1.44)	8687(1.02)	
0.3	152(1.25)	8253(1.15)	
0.1	371(1.26)	5764(1.18)	
0.01	828(1.25)	5302(1.34)	

[a] Geometric means (standard error) of triplicate determinations.

this was correct, graded numbers of nylon wool-purified spleen T cells from B10 and A.BY mice were cultured with B lymphocytes and accessory cells from B10 mice obtained by treatment of spleen cells with rabbit anti-mouse brain antiserum and complement. It had previously been established that B10 B cells and A.BY T cells were capable of collaborating to produce a response (data not shown), that A.BY mice produced anti-(T,G)-A--L antibodies that did not react with the anti-B10 anti-idiotypic serum (data not shown), and that the response of A.BY spleen cells to TNP-(T,G)-A--L was not inhibited by the anti-[B10 anti-(T,G)-A--L] (Table IV). The results of this experiment are shown in Fig. 2. It can be seen that the reagent only had an effect when B10 T cells were cultured with B10 B cells and TNP-(T,G)-A--L. The anti-idiotype had no effect on the response of A.BY T cells and B10 B cells to TNP-(T,G)-A--L or on the response of either of the T cells and B10 B cells to TNP-KLH. Although this experiment seemed to indicate that the effect of the anti-idiotype is on the (T,G)-A--L specific B10 T cells, a possible objection can be raised. It may be argued that the effect is on B10 B cells and that the reason no inhibition of the response of A.BY T cells and B10 B cells is seen is due to non*H-2* allogeneic stimulation of the B10 B cells. Although this appears to be unlikely, since the response in the absence of antigen was not increased, experiments are in progress to formally exclude this possibility.

Additional evidence that B10 T cells bear idiotype(s) defined by this antiserum has been obtained in preliminary experiments where anti-idiotype and complement were used on the T-cell population prior to

TABLE IV
Strain Specificity of Inhibition of Primary *in Vitro* Response to
TNP-(T,G)-A--L by Anti-B10 Anti-Idiotype

Exp.	Anti-Id (%)	Direct PFC/10^7 cultured cells[a]	
		Strain	
A		B10	C3H.SW
	—	1293(1.19)	1394(1.26)
	2.4	240(2.55)	1759(1.26)
	1.0	91(1.52)	1493(1.09)
	0.5	62(1.30)	2108(1.15)
	0.1	542(1.38)	1045(1.18)
	no antigen:	0	104(2.30)
B		B10	A.BY
	—	509(1.09)	406(1.04)
	0.5	98(1.47)	426(1.20)
	no antigen:	0	94(2.69)

[a] Geometric means (standard errors) of triplicate determinations.

the 4-day culture. When treated T cells were added to untreated B cells the response to TNP-(T,G)-A--L, but not to TNP-KLH, was inhibited (data not shown).

There are several possible mechanisms by which the anti-idiotype acting on T cells could induce inhibition of this hapten-carrier response. The two most obvious are the inhibition of idiotype-bearing (T,G)-A--L specific helper T cells or the activation of specific suppressor cells. On the basis of the preliminary cytotoxic experiments noted above, we favor the former possibility, although the latter cannot yet be excluded.

Both the completeness of the inhibition and the potency of the reagent as demonstrated in Tables II and III were impressive. Since the number of T cells that would be expected to bear anti-(T,G)-A--L idiotype(s) is quite low, it should come as no surprise that very small quantities of anti-idiotype contain enough antibody to react with these cells. The 4 day period that the cells and reagent were cultured together provided ample time for the interaction to occur. If it is true that the expression of idiotypes on T cells is of more restricted heterogeneity than is so for antibody, as Krawinkel *et al.* (21) have observed,

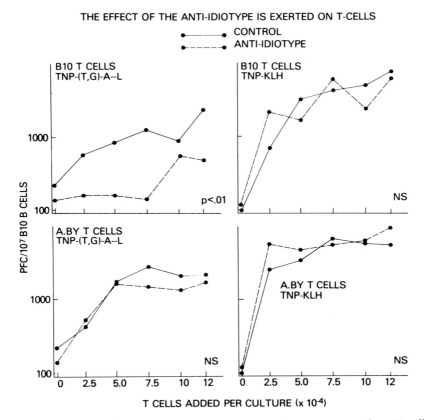

Fig. 2. The inhibitory effect of the anti-B10 anti-idiotype is exerted on T cells. Graded numbers of B10 and A.BY T cells were mixed with 4×10^5 B10 B and accessory cells, and tested for their response to TNP-(T,G)-A--L and TNP-KLH in the presence (----) or absence (——) of Lewis anti-[B10 anti-(T,G)-A--L] antiserum. Statistical significance was determined by a paired Student's t test. Each point represents the geometric mean of triplicate determinations.

then the virtually complete inhibition of the T-cell response is also not unexpected.

Once we have conclusively established that the anti-[B10 anti-(T,G)-A--L] anti-idiotype reacts with T cells, and further, which class of T cells is involved, we hope to explore the genetic basis for the expression of T-cell idiotypes, and the relationship between such idiotypes and *H-2* linked *Ir* gene regulation of the immune response.

ACKNOWLEDGMENTS

We would like to thank Dr. David Pisetsky for invaluable advice. Drs. Roy Riblet and Mel Bosma kindly provided mice for our studies. Our thanks also go to Walter Lyles and Francis Jones for animal care, Karen Hathcock and John Williams for technical support, and Marilyn Schoenfelder for secretarial assistance.

REFERENCES

1. Capra, J. D., and Kehoe, J. M. (1975) *Adv. Immunol.* **20**, 1.
2. Binz, H., and Wigzell, H. (1975) *J. Exp. Med.* **142**, 197.
3. Rajewsky, K., and Eichmann, K. (1977) *Contemp. Top. Immunol.* **7**, 69.
4. Krammer, P. H. (1978) *J. Exp. Med.* **147**, 25.
5. Benacerraf, B., and Katz, D. H. (1975) *Adv. Cancer Res.* **21**, 121.
6. McDevitt, H. O., Deck, B. D., Schreffler, D. C., Klein, J., Stimpfling, J. H., and Snell, G. D. (1972) *J. Exp. Med.* **135**, 1259.
7. Mitchell, G. F., Grumet, F. C., and McDevitt, H. O. (1972) *J. Exp. Med.* **135**, 126.
8. Singer, A., Cowing, C., Hathcock, K. S., Dickler, H. B., and Hodes, R. J. (1978) *J. Exp. Med.* **147**, 1611.
9. Schwartz, R. H., and Paul, W. E. (1976) *J. Exp. Med.* **143**, 529.
10. Taussig, M. J., Mozes, E., and Isac, R. (1974) *J. Exp. Med.* **140**, 301.
11. Tung, A. S., Ju, S. T., Sato, S., and Nisonoff, A. (1976) *J. Immunol.* **116**, 676.
12. Pincus, S. H., Sachs, D. H., and Dickler, H. B. (1978) *J. Immunol.* **121**, 1422.
13. Weigert, M., and Riblet, R. (1978) *Semin. Immunopathol.* (in press).
14. Mozes, E. (1978) *4th Ir Gene Workshop, 1978* p. 475.
15. Fathman, G. C., Pisetsky, D. S., and Sachs, D. H. (1977) *J. Exp. Med.* **145**, 569.
16. Ju, S. T., Kipps, T. J., Thezé, J., Benacerraf, B., and Dorf, M. E. (1978) *J. Immunol.* **121**, 1034.
17. Kipps, T. J., Benacerraf, B., and Dorf, M. E. (1977) *Eur. J. Immunol.* **7**, 865.
18. Hodes, R. J., and Singer, A. (1977) *Eur. J. Immunol.* **7**, 892.
19. Singer, A., Dickler, H. B., and Hodes, R. J. (1977) *J. Exp. Med.* **146**, 1096.
20. Raff, M. C. (1970) *Nature (London)* **226**, 1257.
21. Krawinkel, U., Cramer, M., Melchers, I., Imanishi-Kari, T., and Rajewsky, K. (1975) *J. Exp. Med.* **147**, 1341.

PART VII

ONTOGENY OF
IMMUNOGLOBULIN-SYNTHESIZING
CELLS

B Lymphocyte Development and Activation: Analysis with a Mutant Mouse Strain

WILLIAM E. PAUL, BONDADA SUBBARAO,
JAMES J. MOND, DONNA G. SIECKMANN,
IAN ZITRON, AFTAB AHMED,†
DONALD E. MOSIER, AND IRWIN SCHER† ‡

Laboratory of Immunology
National Institute of Allergy and Infectious Diseases
National Institutes of Health
Bethesda, Maryland
and
†*Department of Clinical and Experimental Immunology and*
‡*Department of Pathology*
Naval Medical Research Institute
Bethesda, Maryland

INTRODUCTION

Although the clonal diversity of B lymphocytes has been recognized for some time, the functional diversity of these cells is only now being appreciated. Progress in this area has been relatively slow because of a limitation in suitable techniques to obtain relatively pure preparations of various B lymphocyte subpopulations. One of the most useful of the available models to dissect B lymphocyte subpopulations has been provided by the CBA/N mouse. This strain has an X-linked mutant gene, *xid* (1), which appears to result in the absence of a mature or late appearing subpopulation of B lymphocytes. The defect of these mice has allowed a preliminary characterization of the functions of the B lymphocytes possessed by CBA/N mice and, by inference, of those B lymphocytes which CBA/N mice lack. Recently, antisera directed at differentiation antigens expressed by B cells lacking in the CBA/N have been prepared. These sera allow a separation of B cell subpopulations of normal strains and thus provide the possibility of decisive assignment of functions to individual cell populations in normal mice. Finally, the ability to specifically deal with individual B lymphocyte subpopulations makes possible a more rational approach to the problem of determining mechanisms of B lymphocyte activation. This communication summarizes progress from our laboratories using the CBA/N model and reports recent work on the role of membrane structures in the activation of one B lymphocyte subpopulation.

THE FUNCTIONAL DEFECT OF CBA/N MICE

CBA/N mice are an NIH subline derived from the CBA/H strain in 1966. These animals were the routinely supplied NIH CBA mouse and were regarded as essentially normal until Baker and his colleagues reported that they were totally unresponsive to type III pneumococcal polysaccharide and that this unresponsiveness was inherited as an X-linked trait (2). More detailed exploration of CBA/N immune responsiveness has demonstrated that these mice make no antibody response whatever to a group of thymus-independent antigens which includes haptenated-Ficoll, levan, dextran, and polyinosinic · polycytidilic acid, as well as type III pneumococcal polysaccharide. On the other hand, they make near normal responses to another set of thymus-independent antigens, which includes trinitrophenyl (TNP)-*Brucella abortus*, TNP-lipopolysaccharide, and TNP-*Nocardia* water-soluble mitogen. On the basis of the relative responsiveness of CBA/N mice, we now have subdivided thymus-independent (TI) antigens into two sets: the TI-1 antigens, to which CBA/N mice are responsive, and the TI-2 antigens, to which they are unresponsive (3). In general, the TI-1 antigens have very large molecular dimensions (i.e., they are particles, or aggregates) and have substantial polyclonal activating capacity. The TI-2 antigens, on the other hand, are of intermediate size (1×10^5 to 2×10^6 daltons) and have little or no activity as mitogens or polyclonal activators. However, one cannot classify TI-1 and TI-2 antigens solely on the basis of polyclonal activation potential, since levan, which is a TI-2 antigen, is an excellent polyclonal activator while TNP-*Brucella abortus*, the prototype TI-1 antigen, is a very weak polyclonal activator.

CBA/N mice can make thymus-dependent antibody responses, but these are not entirely normal in amount and it has been reported that the diversity of their response may be less extensive than normal (4,5).

The inability of mice with the CBA/N immune defect to respond to

TI-2 antigens has been shown to be a property of the lymphoid cells of these mice and not of their developmental microenvironment. The strongest evidence for this comes from studies of development of stem cells from normal and abnormal donors in irradiated abnormal and normal recipients (6). The actual experiments involved the use of off-spring of a cross between CBA/N mothers and DBA/2 fathers. The male progeny are hemizygous for the *xid* gene and express the immunologic defects of the CBA/N while the female offspring are heterozygous (+/*xid*) and are phenotypically normal. F_1 female bone marrow transplanted to a lethally irradiated F_1 male develops normally; the reconstituted recipient is fully responsive to TNP-Ficoll (Table I). On the other hand, irradiated F_1 female recipients of F_1 male bone marrow express the CBA/N immune defect.

The actual defective cell appears to be a B lymphocyte as transfer of Ig-bearing lymphocytes from an F_1 female to a nonirradiated F_1 male allows the recipient to respond immediately to immunization with TNP-Ficoll. As noted below, the reconstituting cells are members of a mature or late developing subset of B lymphocytes which bear the differentiation antigen Lyb 5. Transfer of Ig$^-$ lymphocytes, of thymocytes, or of irradiated spleen cells does not reconstitute responsiveness (6). Similarly, F_1 male spleen cells fail to make *in vitro* primary responses to TNP-Ficoll. B lymphocytes, but not T lymphocytes or macrophages, from F_1 female donors allow responses to occur in cultures of F_1 male spleen cells (7).

Finally, in these reconstitution experiments, it can be shown that it

TABLE I

The CBA/N Immune Defect Is a Property of Their Lymphoid Cells[a]

Donor of bone marrow	Irradiated recipient	Response to DNP-Ficoll
(CBA/N × DBA/2)F$_1$ male xid/ − (defective)	(CBA/N × DBA/2)F$_1$ male xid/ − (defective)	−
(CBA/N × DBA/2)F$_1$ female +/xid (normal)	(CBA/N × DBA/2)F$_1$ female +/xid (normal)	+
(CBA/N × DBA/2)F$_1$ male xid/ − (defective)	(CBA/N × DBA/2)F$_1$ female +/xid (normal)	−
(CBA/N × DBA/2)F$_1$ female +/xid (normal)	(CBA/N × DBA/2)F$_1$ male xid/ − (defective)	+

[a] Recipients were lethally irradiated (1000 R) and received 10^7 bone marrow cells. After a period of 8 weeks to allow repopulation of their lymphoid systems, they were immunized with 100 μg of DNP-Ficoll and the number of spleen cells capable of forming plaques on TNP-sheep erythrocytes enumerated 5 days later.

is the immunologically normal F_1 female cells which actually synthesize the anti-TNP antibody, indicating that the defect of the male is in the precursor of the antibody secreting cell and not in some auxilliary cell.

ANALYSIS OF CBA/N B LYMPHOCYTES

The B lymphocytes of CBA/N mice and of (CBA/N × DBA/2F$_1$ male mice have been studied by a variety of techniques and several interesting features have been noted. First, CBA/N spleens tend to contain fewer nucleated cells than do normal spleens and the fraction of Ig-bearing lymphocytes in these spleen cell populations is approximately 60% of normal. Consequently, their total number of splenic B lymphocytes is often only 30–40% of that of normal mice (8).

The B lymphocytes they possess express certain "abnormalities." The word abnormality is shown in quotation marks because it seems likely to us that CBA/N cells may actually be relatively normal representatives of one set of B cells found in normal strains and, thus, many of the unusual features observed may represent the absence of another population and not a bizarre or aberrant development of the lymphocytes the CBA/N's do possess. We hasten to add that it would be premature to regard CBA/N cells as entirely normal representatives of a putative B cell subset.

Among the abnormalities expressed by CBA/N B lymphocytes are an inability to stimulate *Mls* determined mixed lymphocyte responses, an unusual population distribution in the amount of membrane (m) Ig expressed on lymphocytes, and a ratio of mIgM to mIgD which is very abnormal for adult mice.

The inability of CBA/N cells to stimulate an *Mls* determined mixed lymphocyte response has been studied in depth by Ahmed and Scher (9); it has been shown not to be due to an absence from the CBA/N of the genetic information required to stimulate such mixed lymphocyte responses but rather from a failure of CBA/N cells to express the membrane molecules which stimulate such responses. This illustrates a basic principal of the CBA/N defect; the defective gene, *xid,* is not the structural gene for the Mls antigen nor for many other proteins which appear abnormal in CBA/N mice. Rather, *xid* controls the development of cells which express Mls antigens. Scher *et al.* (10) have shown that in normal mice the B cell which stimulates an *Mls* determined mixed lymphocyte response is a late developing cell with a characteristic amount of mIg which allows its separation from other B lymphocytes of the normal. This illustrates a second principal of the

CBA/N immune defect; the function lacking in CBA/N mice is usually a property of a defined subset of normal B lymphocytes and not of B lymphocytes in general.

CBA/N B lymphocytes have been analyzed in detail for the expression of mIg. When stained with fluoresceinated (Fl) F(ab')$_2$ fragments of anti-Ig and analyzed using the Fluorescence Activated Cell Sorter, their splenic B lymphocytes appear markedly deficient in a population of cells which expresses a low to intermediate amount of mIg and which is dominant in normal adult B lymphocyte populations (11,12). Analysis with Fl anti-μ reveals a greater amount, per cell, of this isotype. The pattern of anti-μ amount in adult CBA/N mice is very similar to that in normal (and CBA/N) neonatal spleen cells. Thus, one abnormal feature of the CBA/N is the failure to show the normal developmental diminution in the density or amount of mIgM which occurs in normal mice.

Closely related to this is an abnormal ratio in mIgM : mIgD on CBA/N B lymphocyte membranes (13). Analysis of the relative amount of radioactivity in μ and δ H chains isolated from cells labeled by the lactoperoxidase-catalyzed iodination procedure reveals that the ratio in CBA/N cells is approximately three times that of normal cells. This also is comparable to findings obtained with cells of relatively young mice. However, since the amount of mIgM on CBA/N B cells is somewhat greater than normal, we do not know whether the abnormal μ : δ ratio actually represents a diminution of mIgD and to what extent CBA/N B cells mimic neonatal cells in expression of mIgD.

FAILURE OF CBA/N B LYMPHOCYTES TO EXPRESS Lyb3 AND Lyb5 ANTIGENS

The concept that CBA/N mice might lack a subpopulation of B lymphocytes suggested that these animals might aid in the preparation of antibodies directed against differentiation antigens unique to the putative deficient subpopulation. Two approaches to preparing such sera have been taken. Huber et al. (14) immunized F$_1$ male mice from a cross of (CBA/N × BALB/c) with BALB/c spleen cells. This F$_1$ anti-parent serum should be able to identify only antigens possessed by the parent and absent from the F$_1$. Other than idiotypes on certain antigen-specific receptors, the principal antigens of this type would be antigens the F$_1$ male did not express because of its defective immunologic status. Sera from such immunized F$_1$ male mice contained γ_1 antibodies which bound to a subset of B lymphocytes. The antigen(s) identified by these sera was found in all strains of mice but tended to be expressed relatively late in postnatal maturation. The antiserum augmented the immune response of mice to low doses of sheep erythrocytes and partially replaced T lymphocyte function in responses of thymus-deprived mice to sheep erythrocytes. Recent chemical studies indicate that the antigen, designated Lyb3, is a membrane protein of approximately 68,000 daltons in size (15).

Our group immunized C57BL/6 mice with lymphoid cells from DBA/2 donors and then extensively absorbed the serum with DBA/2 thymocytes and with spleen cells from (CBA/N × DBA/2)F_1 male donors (16). This absorbed serum no longer was capable of causing complement (C)-mediated lysis of spleen cells from F_1 male mice but could lyse 30–40% of a spleen cells from F_1 female or from DBA/2 mice. Separation of such cells into mIg$^+$ and mIg$^-$ populations by cell sorting revealed that 50–60% of the mIg$^+$ cells were susceptible to lysis but that only 7% of mIg$^-$ cells could be lysed (Table II). When mIg$^+$ cells were separated into complement receptor-bearing (CR$^+$) and complement receptor-lacking (CR$^-$) populations, all the cells which could be lysed were found in the CR$^+$ population. Furthermore, if normal F_1 female spleen cells were exposed to the absorbed serum, designated anti-Lyb5, and C, the $\mu : \delta$ mIg H chain ratios of the remaining cells resembled that of cells from CBA/N mice. This suggests that anti-Lyb5 identifies a membrane alloantigen expressed on a normal cell type deficient in the CBA/N and that removing Lyb5 bearing cells from normal mice leaves them with a cell population which resembles that found in the CBA/N.

Since CR$^+$ lymphocytes and lymphocytes with a "normal" $\mu : \delta$ H

TABLE II

Anti-Lyb5 Identifies a Membrane Alloantigen on a Subset of B Lymphocytes of Mature Mice

Cell type	Cells Lysed by anti-Lyb5.1 (%)
(CBA/N × DBA/2)F_1 male spleen cells	<5
(CBA/N × DBA/2)F_1 female spleen cells	25–30
DBA/2 spleen cells	25–30
F_1 female mIg$^+$ spleen cells	60
F_1 female mIg$^-$ spleen cells	7
F_1 female mIg$^+$CR$^+$ spleen cells	76
F_1 female mIg$^+$CR$^-$ spleen cells	5
DBA/2 (2-week-old) mIg$^+$ spleen cells	20
DBA/2 (adult) mIg$^+$ spleen cells	67

chain ratio tend to appear relatively late in development (17,18), it would be expected that the frequency of Lyb5-bearing cells as a fraction of mIg$^+$ lymphocytes should rise with age. Approximately 20% of mIg$^+$ lymphocytes express Lyb5 at 2 weeks of age whereas in adult mice 50–60% of the Ig$^+$ cells express Lyb5.

Before proceeding with a further characterization of the functions of Lyb5$^+$ and Lyb5$^-$ cell populations, we felt it would be important to characterize the Lyb5 antigen and the anti-Lyb5 serum. We first wished to determine if anti-Lyb5 was directed at a single antigen or if the lytic activity of this serum was due to its possession of antibodies directed at several membrane determinants. To examine this, we prepared an F$_1$ hybrid between C57BL/6 and DBA/2 mice and then bred the F$_1$ mice to C57BL/6. We observed that approximately half (37/76) of the backcross progeny contained lymphocytes which could be lysed by anti-Lyb5 and C while the cells of the remaining animals were not lysed by this reagent (19). This indicated that Lyb5 antigen was controlled by a single genetic region. We have subsequently identified an alternative form of Lyb5, possessed by C57BL/6 mice, allowing us to designate the form of Lyb5 possessed by mice of the "DBA/2 type" as Lyb5.1 and that possessed by mice of "C57BL/6 type" as Lyb5.2.

Treatment of spleen cells from (CBA/N × DBA/2)F$_1$ female donors with anti-Lyb5.1 and C prior to transfer into F$_1$ male recipients abolishes the capacity of the cells to allow recipients to respond to TNP-Ficoll (Table III). Similarly, normal cells treated with anti-Lyb5.1 and

TABLE III
Treatment of F$_1$ Female Cells with Anti-Lyb5.1 and C Ablates their Capacity to Transfer Responsiveness to TNP-Ficoll to F$_1$ Males[a]

Transferred cells		Response
Treatment	Number	Anti-TNP PFC/spleen
Anti-Lyb5.1	2.5 × 10^6	144
and C	5 × 10^6	210
	10 × 10^6	192
Control serum	2.5 × 10^6	757
and C	5 × 10^6	3197
	10 × 10^6	8866
No transferred cells		262

[a] F$_1$ female cells were treated with anti-Lyb5.1 and C or a control serum and C and then transferred to nonirradiated F$_1$ male recipients. The control serum was an anti-Lyb5.1 serum from which all activity was removed by absorbtion with F$_1$ female spleen cells.

C are unresponsive, *in vitro,* to TNP-Ficoll. Thus, it appears likely that the inference is correct that Lyb5[+] cells, which are lacking in CBA/N mice, mediate those B lymphocyte functions which CBA/N cells do not express. A more detailed exploration of the capacity of anti-Lyb5 and C to ablate functions of normal B lymphocytes is now in progress. However, the availability of anti-Lyb5 and anti-Lyb3 provides valuable tools with which to probe B lymphocyte heterogeneity and function.

ANALYSIS OF B LYMPHOCYTE ACTIVATION REQUIREMENTS

In the course of analyzing the activities of anti-Lyb5.1 serum, we made the surprising finding that this serum could cause a 60–80% inhibition of the primary *in vitro* anti-TNP-Ficoll antibody response of spleen cells from most Lyb5.1 possessing strains. The serum had no blocking activity on cells from strains typed as Lyb5.2 (20) (Table IV). Furthermore, if the anti-Lyb5.1 serum was absorbed with spleen cells from normal female progeny of a (CBA/N × DBA/2) cross, both its capacity to lyse Lyb5.1 bearing B lymphocytes and to block TNP-Ficoll responses was lost.

The blocking activity has several other interesting features. The

TABLE IV
Anti-Lyb5 Antisera Inhibits *in Vitro* Response to TNP-Ficoll[a]

	Inhibition of anti-TNP PFC response (% ± S.E.)	
Donor of spleen cells	TNP-Ficoll	TNP-BA
Lyb5.1 strains[b] (DBA/1; DBA/2; CE/J; C3H/HeJ; and (CBA/N × DBA/2)F$_1$ female)	63 ± 3	−1 ± 7
Lyb5.2 strains (C57BL/6; CBA/J; BALB/c; AKR/J; SJL/J; B10.D2)	8 ± 4	−16 ± 8

[a] Spleen cells (1×10^6) were cultured in microtiter wells in the presence of 1% anti-Lyb5.1 or control serum and TNP-Ficoll (10^{-3} μg/ml) or TNP-*Brucella abortus* (TNP-BA) (1 : 200 dilution of stock).

[b] Responses to TNP-Ficoll of cells from one strain, AL/N, which typed as Lyb5.1, were not blocked by antiserum.

serum blocks responses to TNP-Ficoll but not to TNP-*Brucella abortus* (Table IV); furthermore, the serum has been shown to block responses to several TI-2 antigens but not to TI-1 antigens (21). This suggests that a membrane alloantigen recognized by anti-Lyb5.1 serum is critical to responses to TI-2 antigens, while it is not essential for responses to TI-1 antigens. This is, of course, quite consistent with the finding that CBA/N mice can respond to TI-1 but not TI-2 antigens.

Responses of spleen cells from F_1 hybrids between C57BL/6 and DBA/2 are also blocked by anti-Lyb5.1. Since these mice are heterozygous and should thus express both allelic forms of the alloantigen in question, this result suggests that anti-Lyb5.1 serum blocks not by preventing the binding of some other moiety to a membrane structure but by delivering an inhibitory or suppressive signal.

We also studied the inheritance of the membrane antigen important in the blocking of anti-TNP-Ficoll antibody responses by anti-Lyb5.1. The same (C57BL/6 × DBA/2)F_1 × C57BL/6 backcross mice used previously for analysis of inheritance of the Lyb5.1 antigen by cytolysis with antibody and C were studied. We found that approximately 50% of the backcross mice possessed spleen cells, the responses of which were blocked by antibody. However, the capacity of spleen cells to be lysed by anti-Lyb5.1 and C and to be blocked in responsiveness to TNP-Ficoll were inherited independently (Table V). No significant linkage was noted. Thus, the blocking activity of anti-Lyb5.1 serum must be due to the presence of antibody to another

TABLE V
Blocking Activity of Anti-Lyb5.1 Antiserum Is Due to an Antibody against a Distinct Alloantigen

Cross	(C57BL/6 × DBA/2)F_1 × C57BL/6	
	$Lyb5^b/Lyb5^a$	$Lyb5^b/Lyb5^b$
	$Blocking^-/Blocking^+$	$Blocking^-/Blocking^-$
	Lyb5.1 status as determined by cytolysis with antiserum + C	
	Lyb5.1$^+$	Lyb5.1$^-$
Blocking type Blocking$^+$	23	17
Blocking$^-$	14	22

$$\chi^2 = 2.84$$
$$p > 0.05$$

alloantigen which we tentatively designate Lyb7. A linkage analysis involving approximately sixty individual backcross mice indicates that the *Lyb7* gene is linked to the genes determining Ig H chain constant regions (IgC_H genes); it appears to map approximately 10–15 centimorgans from the gene controlling the allelic forms of IgG_{2a}. Preliminary analysis of "Lyb7 type" and *Ig5* [IgD] alleles also reveals recombination events between the genes for these molecules indicating that the capacity of anti-Lyb7 to block TNP-Ficoll responses cannot be due to contamination with anti-δ. Although the association of *Lyb7* and the *IgC_H* region may be fortuitous, the placement of a gene for a molecule involved in regulation of B lymphocyte activation near the genetic region specifying immunoglobulin H chain structure is exceptionally provocative and might represent genetic linkage because of some type of coregulated function.

The analysis of the CBA/N system has led us to two further findings which are of considerable interest in regard to B lymphocyte activation. The first of these concerns the activation of B lymphocytes by exposure to anti-Ig antibodies. Although it has been known for some time that certain anti-Ig antibodies could cause *in vitro* proliferation of rabbit lymphoid cells, it was generally held that such activation did not occur when B lymphocytes of other species were cultured with anti-Ig. Several recent reports have challenged this concept. Results from our laboratory indicate that specifically purified goat anti-mouse μ is a powerful stimulant of B lymphocyte proliferation (22). The responsive cells are Ig^+, Thy 1^-; T lymphocytes are not required for the proliferative response and macrophages can be extensively depleted without diminishing the resultant response (23). Proliferation is also caused by anti-κ antibodies but it is substantially less vigorous. These proliferative responses are first obtained using spleen cells of 3–4-week-old mice, and adult responsiveness is attained by 8 weeks of age. Strikingly, cells from mice with the CBA/N immune defect make no proliferative response whatever to anti-μ or anti-κ (Table VI). Additional experiments indicate that treatment of normal adult spleen cell populations with anti-Lyb5.1 and C destroys the cells which respond to anti-μ. Thus, anti-μ interaction with mIgM of $Lyb5^+$ B lymphocytes constitutes a signal for the extensive proliferation of these cells. By itself, interaction of anti-μ with mIg^+ B lymphocytes causes no synthesis of Ig, indicating that the signal generated in this manner does not cause complete B lymphocyte differentiation into antibody-secreting cells. Based on published studies of Kishimoto and Ishizaka (24) and on preliminary work in our laboratory, T lymphocyte help should cause the $Lyb5^+$ cells, proliferating in response to anti-μ, to

TABLE VI
Lymphocytes from Mice with the CBA/N Immune Defect
Fail to Proliferate in Response to Anti-μ[a]

Cell Donor	Proliferative response (Uptake of ^{3}H-TdR; Δ CPM)	
	Anti-μ (100 μg/ml)	LPS (50 μg/ml)
(CBA/N × DBA/2)F$_1$ male *xid/* − (defective)	1,000	78,000
(CBA/N × DBA/2)F$_1$ female +/*xid* (normal)	155,000	130,000

[a] Spleen cells from F$_1$ male and female mice were cultured with anti-μ or lipopolysaccharide (LPS); incorporation of tritiated thymidine (^{3}H-TdR) was determined on the third day of culture.

complete their differentiation. These results strongly suggest that the IgM receptor of the Lyb5$^+$ cell can receive positive stimulatory signals and is not simply a "tolerance-inducing" receptor. However, we should note that this does not rule out such a role for the mIgM of Lyb5$^-$ cells. Indeed, since these cells dominate in neonatal mice, it is conceivable that interaction of thymus-dependent antigens or of TI-2 antigens with μ^+ δ^- Lyb5$^-$ cells may lead to tolerance induction. However, it appears that such cells can respond to TI-1 antigens (3).

A final point to be considered is the role of mIgD in activation of Lyb5$^+$ cells. In order to examine this point, we evaluated the response of spleen cells from normal mice to TNP-Ficoll in the presence or absence of an alloanti-δ reagent and compared this to the effect of this reagent on responses to TNP-BA. Since the response to TNP-Ficoll is entirely dependent on Lyb5$^+$ B lymphocytes, any difference in susceptibility to anti-δ would suggest distinctive roles for IgD in Lyb5$^+$ and Lyb5$^-$ B cells.

An alloanti-δ reagent was prepared using an approach analagous to that reported by Goding *et al.* (25). C57BL/Ka mice were immunized with spleen cells from BALB/c donors. After extensive immunization, sera were obtained which had considerable activity against the IgD of BALB/c mice (Ig 5.1) and which could be studied in the absence of antibody directed at other BALB/c membrane antigens by using it with spleen cells of B.C8 mice. The latter are allotype congenic mice possessing background genes from C57BL/Ka and *IgC*$_H$ and *IgV*$_H$ genes from BALB/c. When tested on this strain, the sera behaves as if it

TABLE VII
Anti-δ Inhibits Anti-TNP Responses to TNP-Ficoll[a]

| Donor of cells | Antibody | Anti-TNP antibody response (PFC/10⁶ cells) | |
		TNP-Ficoll $(10^{-2}\ \mu g/ml)$	TNP-BA (5×10^{-5})
B.C8	Normal ascites	324	192
	Anti-δ	79	175
C57BL/Ka	Normal ascites	195	n.d.
	Anti-δ	273	n.d.

[a] Spleen cells (10^6) were cultured in microtiter wells with TNP-Ficoll ($10^{-2}\ \mu g/ml$) or a 5×10^{-5} dilution of working stock of TNP-BA in the presence of anti-δ ascitic fluid or a control ascites. The number of direct anti-TNP PFC was measured on day 4 for TNP-Ficoll and day 3 for TNP-BA. Data adapted from reference (26).

were a monospecific anti-δ antibody. Culture of B.C8 spleen cells with a final concentration of 1 or 2% of the anti-δ reagent markedly inhibits responses to TNP-Ficoll but has essentially no effect on the response to TNP-*Brucella abortus* (26; Table VII). The alloanti-δ serum has no effect on responses of C57BL/Ka spleen cells to TNP-Ficoll or TNP-*Brucella abortus,* indicating that its effects are specific.

This result strongly suggests that mIgD plays a critical role in the activation of Lyb5⁺ cells by TNP-Ficoll. It might be argued that the alloanti-δ could be contaminated with small amounts of anti-Lyb5 antibody and that the latter antibodies actually blocked the response. We do not believe that this can explain our results since a monoclonal anti-Ig 5.2 antibody, produced by a hybridoma, caused a striking inhibition of the response of C57BL/6 spleen cells to TNP-Ficoll but did not effect their response to TNP-*Brucella abortus.* We are grateful to Leonore Herzenberg and her colleagues for making this reagent available to us.

CONCLUSION

The analysis of B lymphocyte activation has been a tantalizing prospect for both immunologists and cell biologists because these cells have the unique characteristics of possessing a well-characterized receptor and displaying a clear inducible response to a specific stimulant. Despite the apparent simplicity of B lymphocyte systems, progress in understanding the activation process has been relatively slow. The current studies suggest that an important key to clarifying this issue is a fuller appreciation of B lymphocyte heterogeneity and of the structural characteristics of various classes of antigens which can directly activate B lymphocytes. As in so many other biological systems, animals with specific genetic defects provide powerful systems in which to test various ideas about heterogeneity and activation of B lymphocytes. The experiments described here involving the CBA/N system, have allowed the identification of two principal B lymphocyte subsets and the characterization of the activation requirements for one of them. It is clear that further progress in this area will depend on more complete exploitation of the existing systems and on the use of new genetic systems involving defects at other steps in lymphocyte development and activation.

Our current analysis leads to the conclusion that Lyb5$^+$ cells can be activated to proliferate solely by the binding of anti-μ to cell membrane IgM; that this, by itself, does not initiate Ig synthesis but that, with appropriate T lymphocyte help, Ig synthesis does occur. Moreover, both IgD and Lyb5, as membrane molecules, play important but still poorly understood roles in the regulation of B lymphocyte activation. Current efforts in our laboratories are focused on delineating the nature of the controls exerted by these receptors and at a more complete understanding of the functions of the two principal B lymphocyte classes.

ACKNOWLEDGMENTS

Donna G. Sieckmann was the recipient of a postdoctoral fellowship from the Arthritis Foundation. The work described here was supported in part by the Naval Medical Research and Development Command, Work Unit Nos. M0095-PN. 001-1030. The opinions or assertions contained herein are the private ones of the authors and are not to be construed as official or reflecting the views of the U.S. Navy Department or the naval service at large. The experiments reported herein were conducted according to the principles set forth in the "Guide for the Care and Use of Laboratory Animals," Institute of Laboratory Animal Resources, National Research Council, DHEW publication No. (NIH)74-23.

REFERENCES

1. Berning, A., Eicher, E., Paul, W. E., and Scher, I. (1978) *Fed. Proc., Fed. Am. Soc. Exp. Biol.* **37**, 1396.
2. Amsbaugh, D. F., Hansen, C. T., Prescott, B., Stashak, P. W., Barthold, D. R., and Baker, P. J. (1972) *J. Exp. Med.* **136**, 931–949.

3. Mosier, D. E., Zitron, I. M., Mond, J. J., Ahmed, A., Scher, I., and Paul, W. E. (1977) *Immunol. Rev.* **37**, 89–104.
4. Gershon, R. K., and Kondo, K. (1976) *J. Immunol.* **117**, 701–702.
5. Scher, I., Berning, A. K., and Asofsky, R. (1979) *J. Immunol*, in press.
6. Scher, I., Steinberg, A. D., Berning, A. K., and Paul, W. E. (1975) *J. Exp. Med.* **142**, 637–650.
7. Cohen, P. L., Scher, I., and Mosier, D. E. (1976) *J. Immunol.* **116**, 301–304.
8. Scher, I., Ahmed, A., Steinberg, A. D., and Paul, W. E. (1975) *J. Exp. Med.* **141**, 788–803.
9. Ahmed, A., and Scher, I. (1976) *J. Immunol.* **117**, 1922–1926.
10. Scher, I., Ahmed, A., and Sharrow, S. O. (1977) *J. Immunol.* **119**, 1938–1942.
11. Scher, I., Sharrow, S. O., Wistar, R., Jr., Asofsky, R., and Paul, W. E. (1976) *J. Exp. Med.* **144**, 494–506.
12. Scher, I., Sharrow, S. O., and Paul, W. E. (1976) *J. Exp. Med.* **144**, 507–518.
13. Finkelman, F. D., Smith, A. H., Scher, I., and Paul, W. E. (1975) *J. Exp. Med.* **142**, 1316–1321.
14. Huber, B., Gershon, R. K., and Cantor, H. (1977) *J. Exp. Med.* **145**, 10–20.
15. Cone, R. E., Huber, B., Cantor, H., and Gershon, R. K. (1978) *J. Immunol.* **120**, 1733–1740.
16. Ahmed, A., Scher, I., Sharrow, S. O., Smith, A. H., Paul, W. E., Sachs, D. H., and Sell, K. W. (1977) *J. Exp. Med.* **145**, 101–110.
17. Gelfand, M. C., Elfenbein, G. J., Frank, M. M., and Paul, W. E. (1974) *J. Exp. Med.* **139**, 1125–1141.
18. Vitetta, E. S., Melcher, U., McWilliams, M., Phillips-Quagliata, J., Lamm, M., and Uhr, J. W. (1975) *J. Exp. Med.* **141**, 206–215.
19. Subbarao, B., Ahmed, A., Paul, W. E., Scher, I., Lieberman, R., and Mosier, D. E. (1979) Submitted for publication.
20. Subbarao, B., Mosier, D. E., Ahmed, A., Scher, I., and Paul, W. E. (1978) *Fed. Proc., Fed. Am. Soc. Exp. Biol.* **37**, 1754.
21. Subbarao, B., Mosier, D. E., Ahmed, A., Mond, J. J., Scher, I., and Paul, W. E. (1979) *J. Exp. Med.* **149**, 495–506.
22. Sieckmann, D. G., Asofsky, R., Mosier, D. E., Zitron, I. M., and Paul, W. E. (1978) *J. Exp. Med.* **147**, 814–829.
23. Sieckmann, D. G., Scher, I., Asofsky, R., Mosier, D. E., and Paul, W. E. (1978) *J. Exp. Med.* **148**, 1628–1643.
24. Kishimoto, T., and Ishizaka, K. (1975) *J. Immunol.* **114**, 585–591.
25. Goding, J. W., Warr, G. W., and Warner, N. L. (1976) *Proc. Natl. Acad. Sci. U.S.A.* **73**, 1305–1309.
26. Zitron, I. M., Mosier, D. E., and Paul, W. E. (1977) *J. Exp. Med.* **146**, 1707–1718.

Influence of Thymus Cells on the Ontogeny of B-Lymphocyte Function

GREGORY W. SISKIND

Division of Allergy and Immunology
Department of Medicine
Cornell University Medical College
New York, New York

INTRODUCTION

In this report we will describe a cell transfer system which we have developed for use in studies of the ontogeny of B-lymphocyte function. With this system we have shown that the B-cell population from immature mice produces a response of low affinity and restricted heterogeneity of affinity. In the LAF_1 mouse, the B-cell population matures to be able to produce an adultlike, heterogeneous, high affinity antibody response relatively abruptly between 7 and 10 days of age. Evidence has been obtained that this is an induced differentiation event and that its occurrence requires the presence of "mature" thymus cells or some factor produced by them. The differentiation of the B-cell population to be able to produce a normal, high affinity, heterogeneous response appears to be regulated by the maturation of the thymus cell population to be capable of inducing this differentiation event. Thus, a role for the thymus in B-cell differentiation is proposed.

METHODS AND RATIONALE

EXPERIMENTAL DESIGN AND CELL TRANSFER TECHNIQUES

A cell transfer system has been developed to study the ontogeny of B-cell function (1). Lethally irradiated (800 R), 6–8-week-old, LAF_1

397

male mice (Jackson Laboratories, Bar Harbor, Maine) were used as cell transfer recipients. Each recipient receives 1×10^8 thymus cells, from a pool of thymuses, from 3–4-week-old syngeneic donors. Recipients also receive a source of syngeneic B cells from an individual donor of known age. The source of B cells is the liver when fetal or neonatal (within 18 hr of birth) donors are studied, and spleen or bone marrow with older mice. With fetal and neonatal donors a single liver, suspended in physiologic salt solution, is injected intravenously into an individual recipient. Approximately 5×10^7 spleen cells from a single donor are injected into an individual recipient. This represents roughly one-third of an adult spleen or a whole spleen from a donor under 2 weeks of age. Cells are injected into recipients approximately 3 hr after irradiation. In some experiments the recipients are thymectomized approximately 1 month before cell transfers.

IMMUNIZATION

Mice are immunized 1 day after cell transfer by the intraperitoneal injection of 2,4-dinitrophenylated bovine gamma globulin (DNP-BGG) emulsified in Freund's complete adjuvants. A dose of 500 mg is usually given in a total volume of emulsion of 0.2 ml.

ASSAY OF ANTI-DNP PLAQUE FORMING CELLS (PFC) AND PFC AFFINITY DISTRIBUTION

The anti-DNP plaque forming cell (PFC) response is assayed (2,3) by a slide modification (4) of the Jerne technique (5) using trinitrophenylated sheep red blood cells (6). Indirect PFC are developed by the addition of appropriately diluted rabbit anti-mouse immunoglobulin antiserum. The distribution of PFC with respect to the affinity of the anti-DNP antibody which they are secreting is determined from the inhibition of plaque formation by various concentrations of free hapten (DNP-ϵ-amino-N-caproic acid) (2,5,7).

RATIONALE OF EXPERIMENTAL DESIGN

The cell transfer system is designed to permit the evaluation of the function of B cells, from donors of various ages, in an adult *in vivo* environment, in the presence of adult helper T cells and other accessory cells. Differences in the responses of such animals can presumably be attributed to differences in the functional capacity of the B-cell populations with which they were reconstituted. It has been shown (8) that mice reconstituted, in this manner, with adult spleen cells as the source of B cells, produce a normal response to DNP-BGG with respect to affinity and heterogeneity of affinity. That is, the response is qualitatively indistinguishable from that of similarly immunized intact animals. The PFC responses of the reconstituted animals are, however, somewhat lower in magnitude and somewhat slower to develop than the responses of normal animals. These differences do not interfere with the interpretation of the studies reported here which are primarily concerned with heterogeneity of affinity. It is worth noting that heterogeneity of affinity represents a probe of the degree of polyclonality of the antibody response, since individual clones secrete a homogeneous antibody product.

RESULTS AND DISCUSSION

IMMUNE RESPONSE BY THE IMMATURE B-CELL POPULATION

It was found that mice reconstituted with fetal or neonatal liver, as a source of B cells, produce a response of low affinity and restricted heterogeneity of affinity as compared with mice reconstituted with B cells from adult donors (1). That is, the anti-DNP response of mice reconstituted with immature B cells is lacking in high affinity PFC. It was shown that between 7 and 10 days of age, the splenic B-cell population of LAF_1 mice acquires the capacity to reconstitute irradiated animals so that they are able to produce a heterogeneous, high affinity, PFC response to DNP-BGG (Fig. 1). The B-cell population of the bone marrow matures in this regard about 3 days later than that of the spleen. This may merely reflect the migration of mature peripheral B cells to the bone marrow. It was further found (Table I) that the B-cell population of day 16 fetal donors produces only direct PFC, while mice reconstituted with B cells from day 17 fetal donors produce both direct and indirect PFC. Thus, two differentiation events were identified in the functional ontogeny of the B-cell population. Between day 16 and 17 of fetal life the B-cell population acquires the capacity to produce indirect PFC and between day 7 and 10 after birth, the splenic B-cell population acquires the capacity to produce an adultlike, heterogeneous, high affinity PFC response.

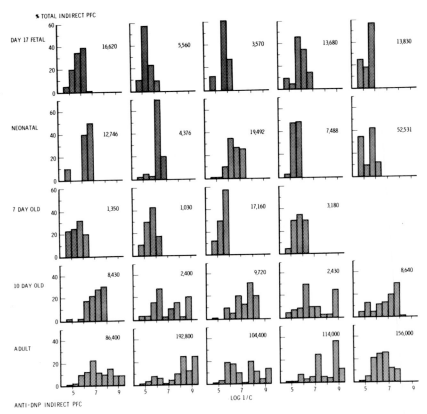

Fig. 1. Ontogeny of the capacity of the B-cell population to reconstitute lethally irradiated syngeneic mice to give a normal, heterogeneous, high affinity, anti-DNP PFC response to DNP-BGG. Each histogram illustrates the distribution of affinities of indirect PFC in the spleen of an individual LAF_1 mouse. The percentage of the total population of PFC which is present in each subpopulation is indicated in the ordinate. The log of the inverse of the free hapten concentration used in the plaque inhibition assay is indicated in the abscissa. Affinity increases to the right. Lethally irradiated mice received 1×10^8 adult thymus cells plus a source of B cells from various aged donors (indicated to the left of each row). The number of indirect PFC/spleen is indicated in the right upper corner of each histogram. Each recipient received B cells from an individual donor. Recipients were immunized with 500 μg DNP-BGG in CFA, intraperitoneally, 1 day after cell transfer and were assayed 3 weeks thereafter.

TABLE I

TABLE I
Maturation of the Capacity of the B-Cell Population of LAF$_1$ Mice to Produce Indirect PFC in Response to DNP-BGG^a

Age of fetal liver donor	Number of animals	Direct anti-DNP PFC/spleen	Indirect anti-DNP PFC/spleen
14 days	15	1113	575
16 days	4	1035	525
18 days	7	1091	4895

^{a} Irradiated mice were reconstituted with 1×10^8 adult thymus cells and liver from fetal donors of the age indicated. Animals were immunized 1 day after cell transfer and were assayed at 3 weeks after immunization.

EFFECT OF POLYCLONAL B-CELL ACTIVATORS ON THE IMMUNE RESPONSE OF THE IMMATURE B-CELL POPULATION

The question which was next considered is whether the immature B-cell population lacks the information required to synthesize high affinity antibody or rather possesses this information, but fails to express it. Two approaches to answering this question were adopted. First, if the B-cell population had the information required to synthesize high affinity antibodies, it might be "turned on" to do so by a polyclonal B-cell activator such as endotoxin (LPS) or dextran sulfate. Second, if the high affinity B-cell population can respond to antigen, but cannot secrete antibody, it might be possible to demonstrate a high affinity memory cell population by boosting.

It was found (3) that mice reconstituted with neonatal liver as the source of B cells will produce a normal, adultlike, high affinity PFC response to DNP-BGG if 10 μg of LPS are injected at the same time as the antigen. This finding suggests that the immature B-cell population has all the information required to produce high affinity antibody, but fails to express this information upon exposure to antigen. Mice reconstituted with B cells from 16 day fetal donors will also produce a high affinity, heterogeneous response if LPS is injected together with antigen. However, animals reconstituted with B cells from day 14 fetal donors produce a low affinity response of restricted heterogeneity, even if LPS is administered. In contrast, 100 μg dextran sulfate, administered together with antigen, did convert the response of mice reconstituted with liver from day 14 fetal donors to a heterogeneous, high affinity, adultlike character. Thus, a third differentiation event (Table II) was identified in the ontogeny of B-cell function. Between day 14 and 16 of fetal life, the B-cell population acquires the capacity

TABLE II
Differentiation Events in the Functional Maturation of the
B-Lymphocyte Population[a]

Age	Differentiation Event
Day 14–16 of gestation	B-cell population acquires the capacity to react with LPS to give a heterogeneous high affinity PFC response to concomitantly administered antigen
Day 16–17 of gestation	B-cell population acquires the capacity to produce indirect PFC
Day 7–10 after birth	B-cell population acquires the capacity to produce a heterogeneous, high-affinity PFC response

[a] Based on studies in LAF_1 mice using DNP-BGG as antigen. Lethally irradiated mice were reconstituted with adult thymus plus a source of B cells from donors of various ages. Animals were immunized 1 day after cell transfer and were assayed for anti-DNP PFC and PFC affinity distribution 3 weeks after immunization.

to respond to LPS so as to produce a heterogeneous high affinity response to concomitantly administered antigen. In addition, the results suggest that the day 14 fetal B-cell population contains all of the information required to produce a high affinity heterogeneous response comparable to that produced by the adult B-cell population.

SECONDARY RESPONSE BY MICE RECONSTITUTED WITH IMMATURE B-CELL POPULATIONS

It was found (3,9) that animals reconstituted with B cells from day 14 fetal donors were capable of giving a typical high affinity secondary response if boosted with DNP-BGG 3 weeks after the primary injection of antigen. High affinity cells were present in high incidence 5 days after boosting. The secondary response was indistinguishable from a secondary response by mice reconstituted with adult spleen as the source of B lymphocytes. It should be noted that 5 days after primary immunization, the anti-DNP PFC response is still of low affinity in both normal intact animals and in irradiated animals reconstituted with adult spleen and thymus cells (8). Thus, the presence of high affinity PFC 5 days after boosting mice reconstituted with day 14 fetal liver indicates that a high affinity "memory" cell population was expanded during the primary response. These results are consistent with the data on the effects of dextran sulfate described above. Both observations support the hypothesis that the day 14 fetal B-cell population contains, within the limits of discrimination of the PFC inhibition assay, all of the information required to produce high affinity antibodies. In addition, the data on the secondary response imply that not only does the B-cell population of the day 14 fetal donors possess all the information required to synthesize high affinity antibodies, but cells capable of producing high affinity antibodies can be selectively stimulated to proliferate. This implies that the full catalog of B-cell specificities is present in the day 14 fetal mouse. In addition, the data suggest that in the day 14 fetus, antigen binding receptors (cell-associated antibodies) are already present on the surface of B cells and that B cells are capable of responding to antigen with proliferation to establish a B memory cell population. It would appear reasonable to hypothesize that the differentiation event which takes place between 7 and 10 days of age in LAF$_1$ mice involves the acquisition of the capacity of activated B cells to become antibody-secreting cells (i.e., PFC).

MATURATION OF THE CAPACITY OF THE B-CELL POPULATION TO PRODUCE A HETEROGENEOUS ANTIBODY RESPONSE IN DIFFERENT STRAINS OF MICE

Studies, comparable to those described in detail above on LAF$_1$ mice, were carried out on five additional strains of mice of various H-2 types (10). The results are briefly summarized in Table III. The general pattern of maturation of the B-cell population, from being able to produce an anti-DNP PFC response of low affinity and restricted heterogeneity to being capable of producing a heterogeneous high affinity response, was seen in every strain studied. The age at which this differentiation event occurred in different strains varied widely (from day 18 of fetal life to 4 weeks after birth). Similarly, the age of acquisition of the capacity to produce indirect PFC was different in different strains. There was no apparent association between H-2 type and the age when the differentiation of the capability of producing a high affinity, heterogeneous response took place.

MATURATION OF THE CAPACITY OF THE B-CELL POPULATION TO GIVE A HETEROGENEOUS, RELATIVELY HIGH AFFINITY PFC RESPONSE TO DIFFERENT ANTIGENS

The ontogeny of the capacity to give a heterogeneous antibody response was studied using five T-dependent antigens and three

TABLE III
Differentiation of the Functional Capacity of the B-Cell Population
in Different Strains of Mice to Respond to DNP-BGG[a]

Strain	Acquisition of the capacity to produce a heterogeneous, high affinity, anti-DNP PFC response	Acquisition of the capacity to produce indirect anti-DNP PFC
A/HeJ (H-2^A)	Day 15–18 of gestation	Day 15–18 of gestation
AKR (H-2^K)	Day 15–18 of gestation	Day 15–18 of gestation
C57L/J (H-2^B)	Day 15–18 of gestation	Day 15–18 of gestation
DBA/1J (H-2^q)	Birth–10 days after birth	Day 15–18 of gestation
LAF$_1$ (H-2^{A,B})	7–10 days after birth	Day 16–17 of gestation
C57B1/6 (H-2^B)	21–28 days after birth	Birth–7 days after birth

[a] Lethally irradiated mice were reconstituted with 1×10^8 adult thymus cells plus a source of B cells from donors of various ages. They were immunized 1 day after cell transfer and their response was assayed 3 weeks after immunization.

T-independent antigens (11). In every case, a shift from the capacity to produce only low affinity antibodies to the capacity to produce a highly heterogeneous, high affinity population of antibody molecules was observed. Even with the T-independent antigens, which tend to stimulate less high affinity antibody synthesis, a shift from a highly restricted to a more heterogeneous response could be detected. Thus, this differentiation sequence in the function of the B-cell population appears to be a general property seen with many, or perhaps all, antigens. As indicated in Table IV, with four of the five T-dependent antigens studied, differentiation to be capable of producing a high affinity, heterogeneous response took place between 7 and 10 days of age in the splenic B-cell population. Maturation of the response to the T-dependent antigen BGG took place just slightly later: between 10 and 14 days of age. In each case, the B-cell population of the bone marrow acquired the ability to give a heterogeneous, high affinity response several days later than that of the spleen. The significance of this finding is not clear, but it might merely reflect the recirculation of mature peripheral B cells from the spleen to the bone marrow. In

TABLE IV

Acquisition of the Capacity of the B-Cell Population of the Spleen and
Bone Marrow of LAF$_1$ Mice to Produce a Heterogeneous, Relatively
High Affinity PFC Response to Different Antigens[a]

Antigen[b]	Age of acquisition of the capacity to give a heterogeneous, relatively high affinity PFC response	
	Splenic B-cell population (age in days)	Bone marrow B-cell population (age in days)
DNP-BGG (T-dependent)	7–10	10–14
Fluorescein-BGG (T-dependent)	7–10	10–14
DNP-KLH (T-dependent)	7–10	10–14
Dansyl-KLH (T-dependent)	7–10	10–14
BGG (T-dependent)	10–14	14–18
TNP-BA (T-independent)	21–28	21–28
DNP-Ficoll (T-independent)	21–28	21–28
TNP-PA (T-independent)	21–28	21–28

[a] Lethally irradiated mice were reconstituted with 1×10^8 adult thymus cells plus a source of B cells from donors of various ages. The mice were immunized with the indicated antigen 1 day after cell transfer and assayed 2–3 weeks later.

[b] BA, *Brucella abortus*; BGG, bovine gamma globulin; DNP, 2,4-dinitrophenyl group; KLH, keyhole limpet hemocyanin; PA, polyacrylamide beads; TNP, 2,4,6-trinitrophenyl group.

marked contrast to the results with the five T-dependent antigens, the capacity of the B-cell population to produce a heterogeneous, relatively high affinity, adultlike response to three T-independent antigens matured considerably later: between 21 and 28 days of age.

These results indicate that the differentiation event being studied is a general property of the maturation of the functional capabilities of the B-cell population in that similar results were obtained with eight antigens. In addition, the marked difference in the time of maturation of the response to T-dependent and T-independent antigens suggests that different subsets of B cells may respond to these different classes of antigens and that these different B subsets mature at different times. Clearly, the data do not prove this hypothesis and it is possible that the same population of B cells responds to the different classes of antigen, but that they mature to be capable of producing high affinity antibody-secreting cells to different classes of antigens at different times. This latter possibility seems intuitively more complex and, therefore, less likely.

EVIDENCE THAT THE ACQUISITION, BY THE B-CELL POPULATION, OF THE CAPACITY TO PRODUCE A HETEROGENEOUS HIGH AFFINITY PFC RESPONSE IS AN INDUCED DIFFERENTIATION EVENT

Liver cells from neonatal or day 15 fetal LAF_1 mice were transferred into lethally irradiated syngeneic recipients together with 10^8 adult thymus cells. The animals were immunized with DNP-BGG at various times thereafter. Thus, the duration of residence in an adult recipient, together with adult thymus cells, which is required for the immature B-cell population to acquire the capacity to produce a heterogeneous, high affinity response, was determined. The B-cell populations from both day 15 fetal donors and neonatal donors acquire the capacity to respond in a heterogeneous, high affinity, adultlike manner within 3 days of residence in the cell transfer recipient (12).

The results suggest that the differentiation of the B-cell population to be capable of producing a heterogeneous, high affinity PFC response is an induced event. That is, it is not regulated by a cell clock within the B lymphocytes, but is induced by some factor in their environment. In addition, the results suggest that the B-cell population present in the day 15 fetal mouse is already capable of responding to the inducer and of thereupon differentiating to be capable of producing a high affinity, heterogeneous response. This implies that the immaturity of the day 15 fetal B-cell population is due to a lack of inducer activity in the fetal animal.

THYMIC CELL DEPENDENCE OF THE MATURATION OF THE B-CELL POPULATION TO PRODUCE A HETEROGENEOUS, HIGH AFFINITY, PFC RESPONSE

Parking experiments, such as that described immediately above, were carried out to determine if the presence of adult thymus cells influenced the rate of differentiation of the B-cell population to become capable of producing a heterogeneous, high affinity PFC response. Lethally irradiated thymectomized mice were reconstituted with day 15 fetal B cells alone or together with 1×10^8 adult thymus cells. Recipients were immunized with DNP-BGG at various times thereafter. All animals received 1×10^8 adult thymus cells, intravenously, one day prior to immunization so as to provide helper T-cell activity. It was found (13) that, in the absence of adult thymus cells, fetal B cells could be parked for up to 3 weeks and still remain immature in that they produced a response of restricted heterogeneity and low affinity. Studies for longer than 3 weeks were not carried out.

The results indicate that some cell in the adult thymus, or a factor produced by it, is required for (induces) or facilitates the differentiation of the B-cell population to be capable of responding to form high affinity antibody-secreting cells. Preliminary results, obtained in collaboration with Dr. David Sherr, suggest that adult thymus cells retained within a millipore chamber, implanted intraperitonally, are capable of inducing the differentiation of the B-cell population to produce high affinity antibody-secreting cells. The results imply that this differentiation event is induced by a diffusable factor produced by thymus cells.

MATURATION OF THE CAPACITY OF THE THYMUS TO INDUCE THE DIFFERENTIATION OF THE B-CELL POPULATION TO BE CAPABLE OF PRODUCING HETEROGENEOUS, HIGH AFFINITY PFC

If, as the data presented above suggest, thymus cells (or a factor produced by them) induce the differentiation of the B-cell population, and the day 15 fetal B-cell population is already capable of responding to this factor, then one would hypothesize that it is the maturation of the thymus which regulates the maturation of the B-cell population to be capable of producing a heterogeneous, high affinity PFC response. This hypothesis was tested by reconstituting lethally irradiated, thymectomized mice with day 15 fetal liver and 2×10^7 thymus cells from various aged donors. The recipients were held for 6 days, were all given 10^8 adult thymus cells to provide helper T-cell activity, and were immunized with DNP-BGG one day later. It was found (14) that animals reconstituted with T cells from 7-day-old or younger donors produced responses of low affinity and restricted heterogeneity. In contrast, mice receiving thymus cells, at the time of the initial cell transfer, from donors which were 10 days old or older, produced high affinity, heterogeneous PFC responses.

Thus, the results are consistent with the hypothesis that the thymus serves to regulate this step in the differentiation of the B-cell population. After the thymus matures to be capable of inducing the differentiation of the B-cell population to be capable of producing a heterogeneous, high affinity PFC response, then a mature B-cell population is observed.

CONCLUSIONS

1. A cell transfer system was developed for use in studying the ontogeny of the functional capabilities of the B-cell population.

2. Three differentiation points were identified in the ontogeny of B-lymphocyte function (listed in Table I).

3. The data are consistent with the view that all of the information required to synthesize the complete array of anti-DNP antibodies is already present in the B-cell population of the day 14 fetal LAF_1 mouse (within the limits of resolution of the inhibition of PFC assay of antibody affinity).

4. In contrast with the B-cell population of adult mice, the immature B-cell population produces a PFC response, to a variety of antigens, which is of low affinity, restricted heterogeneity of affinity, and lacks high affinity antibody secreting cells.

5. Maturation of the capacity to produce a high affinity heterogeneous PFC response is an induced differentiation event which occurs between 7 and 10 days of age in the LAF_1 mouse. The day 15 fetal B-cell population is already capable of responding to the inducer and of differentiating to be capable of producing a heterogeneous, high affinity PFC response.

6. It is suggested that the differentiation event which leads to the ability to produce high affinity PFC represents the acquisition of the capacity of B cells to become high rate antibody-secreting cells. Immature B cells can be selectively stimulated by antigen to become memory cells.

7. The age at which the B-cell population acquires the capacity to give a heterogeneous, high affinity response varies in different strains.

8. With five T-dependent antigens, the splenic B-cell population acquires the capacity to produce a heterogeneous response between 1 and 2 weeks of age. With three T-independent antigens, this capacity is not acquired until 3–4 weeks of age. This suggests that different B-cell subpopulations might respond to T-dependent and T-independent antigens and that these subpopulations mature at different times.

9. Evidence was presented to support the hypothesis that thymus cells, or a factor produced by them, are required for (induce) or facilitate the differentiation of the B-cell population to be capable of producing a high affinity, heterogeneous PFC response. This differentiation of the B-cell population appears to be regulated by the maturation of the thymus cell population. Thus, the thymus cell population acquires the capacity to induce (or facilitate) the maturation of the B-cell population to produce a heterogeneous, high affinity, PFC response between 7 and 10 days of age. A role for the thymus in regulating the differentiation of the B-cell population is, therefore, proposed.

ACKNOWLEDGMENTS

Supported in part by a research grant from the National Institutes of Health, U.S.P.H.S., Number AI-11694.

REFERENCES

1. Goidl, E. A., and Siskind, G. W. (1974) *J. Exp. Med.* **140**, 1285.
2. Szewczuk, M. R., Halliday, M., Soybel, T. W., Turner, D., Siskind, G. W., and Weksler, M. E. (1977) *J. Exp. Med.* **145**, 968.
3. Goidl, E. A., Klass, J., and Siskind, G. W. (1976) *J. Exp. Med.* **143**, 1503.
4. Dresser, D. W., and Greaves, M. F. (1973) *In* "Handbook of Experimental Immunology" (D. M. Weir, ed.), 2nd ed., Vol. □, p. 271. Blackwell, Oxford.
5. Jerne, N. K., Nordin, A. A., and Henry C. (1963) *In* "Cell-Bound Antibody" (B. Amos and H. Koprowski, eds.), p. 109. Wistar Inst. Press, Philadelphia, Pennsylvania.
6. Rittenberg, M. B., and Pratt, K. L. (1969) *Proc. Soc. Exp. Biol. Med.* **132**, 575.
7. Andersson, B. (1970) *J. Exp. Med.* **132**, 77.
8. Goidl, E. A., Barondes, J. I., and Siskind, G. W. (1975) *Immunology.* **29**, 629.
9. Szewczuk, M. R., Sherr, D. H., Cornacchia, A., Kim, Y. T., and Siskind, G. W. (1978) *J. Immunol.* (in press).
10. Sherr, D. H., Szewczuk, M. R., Kim, Y. T., Sogn, D., and Siskind, G. W. (1979) In preparation.
11. Sherr, D. H., Szewcyuk, M. R., Cusano, A., Rappaport, W., and Siskind, G. W. (1979) *Immunology* (in press).
12. Sherr, D., Szewczuk, M. R., and Siskind, G. W. (1977) *J. Immunol.* **119**, 1674.
13. Sherr, D. H., Szewczuk, M. R., and Siskind, G. W. (1978) *J. Exp. Med.* **147**, 196.
14. Szewczuk, M. R., Sherr, D. H., and Siskind, G. W. (1978) *Eur. J. Immunol.* **8**, 370.

Pre-B Cells: Normal Morphologic and Biologic Characteristics and Abnormal Development in Certain Immunodeficiencies and Malignancies

MAX D. COOPER AND ALEXANDER R. LAWTON

The Cellular Immunobiology Unit of the Tumor Institute
University of Alabama in Birmingham
Birmingham, Alabama

INTRODUCTION

With the recognition in 1965 that immunocompetent cells develop along two distinct pathways of lymphoid differentiation and that B cells do not share the thymic derivation of T cells, we and others began experimental attempts to locate the microenvironment(s) in which B-cell formation begins in mammals. The main stimulus for this search was the idea that many of the genetic decisions that B cells must take in order to achieve clonal diversity were likely to be made in their generation site. In support of this notion, the bursa was shown to control generation of immunoglobulin isotype diversity for chicken B cells.

It is now evident that in mammals differentiation along B-cell lines is initiated in fetal liver; later in development, bone marrow assumes the function of generating clones of B cells. The mammalian cells in which antibody synthesis begins differ in important ways from their more mature B-cell progeny. Pre-B cells, as they are called, contain

411

cytoplasmic IgM but, unlike their avian bursal-cell counterparts, appear to lack functional surface antibody receptors. A growing body of evidence suggests that clonal diversity is initiated among Pre-B cells. It therefore seems all the more important to define the genetic and metabolic events occurring in Pre-B cells in relation to new information about the nature of changes in immunoglobulin genes that take place between undifferentiated cells and mature plasma cells (see chapter by Tonegawa). Moreover, it is evident that many of the defects involved in antibody deficiency diseases and in "B" malignancies are manifested at the Pre-B cell level.

HISTORICAL PERSPECTIVE OF THE IDENTIFICATION OF PRE-B CELLS

Our attention was first focused on gut-associated lymphoepithelial tissues (GALT) as possible mammalian bursa-equivalent sites because of morphologic similarities with the avian bursa and the belief that local mesenchymal cell–epithelial cell interactions were important for induction of primary lymphoid differentiation. Although reduction of antibody responses in rabbits after removal of GALT seemed to support this thesis, subsequent studies showed this to be an erroneous conclusion. Largely because in studies of collaborative responses of T and B cells to antigens, bone marrow proved to be a good source for B cells relatively uncontaminated by T cells, bone marrow was assumed to be the site of B-cell origin.

Extensive studies of lymphoid cell kinetics in adult rodents, begun in 1964 by Osmond, Everett and others (1–3), revealed that bone marrow produces and exports large numbers of small lymphocytes; the T or B-cell nature of these was then unknown. Lafleur et al. who first used the term precursor B cells, observed in 1972 that rapidly-sedimenting, surface Ig$^+$ lymphoid cells from marrow and spleen required a few days of residence in irradiated recipients before they became able to cooperate with mature T cells in an antibody response (4–6). In 1974, Osmond and Nossal observed that about half of the small lymphocytes in mouse marrow had highly variable but detectable amounts of surface(s) Ig (7). By combining DNA labeling by ^{3}H-thymidine in vivo and antiglobulin-^{131}I binding in vitro, they showed that large sIg$^-$ lymphocytes gave rise to small sIg$^-$ lymphocytes that acquired sIg after 1–2 days (8). Similar studies conducted by Ryser and Vassalli at the same time indicated rapid generation of small sIg$^-$ lymphocytes in mouse marrow that were capable of subsequent expression of sIg and of selective migration to the spleen on infusion into irradiated recipients (9).

Melchers and colleagues (10) observed that large lymphoid cells in marrow and spleen produced 7–8 S IgM that could be detected on their surface by lactoperoxidase-catalyzed radioactive labeling; these cells release 7–8 S IgM very rapidly ($t_{1/2}$ between 1 and 3 hr) in comparison to small lymphocytes ($t_{1/2}$ between 20 and 28 hr). Armed with the knowledge that sIg$^+$ cells could be detected in mouse fetal liver around the sixteenth day of gestation (11), these investigators began ontogenetic studies of cells capable of synthesizing IgM. Large cells capable of 7–8 S IgM synthesis were detected in fetal liver from day 12 to shortly after birth, and small lymphocytes capable of synthesis of 7–8 S IgM were found beginning between 15 and 16 days of gestation.

Owen *et al.* used organ culture experiments to determine which tissues were capable of generating sIg$^+$ B cells (12,13). Fetal liver, spleen, and marrow were shown to have this capacity, while thymus, pancreas, yolk sac, and intestines did not. During the course of these experiments Raff *et al.* discovered that Pre-B cells could be directly identified by immunofluorescent staining of cytoplasmic IgM using purified anti-μ chain or anti-κ chain antibodies (14). Cells containing IgM and lacking detectable surface Ig were observed in mouse fetal liver from the twelfth day of gestation, appeared later and transiently in spleen and became localized in bone marrow after the onset of hemopoiesis in that site. Phillips and Melchers then showed in cell transfer studies that precursor B cells appeared in fetal liver by day 13, whereas none were present in yolk sac (15). Organ cultures of liver from 11-day mouse embryos (i.e., before the appearance of Pre-B cells) were shown to be capable of generating sIgM$^+$ B cells (13). These results firmly established that mammalian fetal liver, like the avian bursa, has the capability of promoting cell differentiation along B-cell lines. Later in development, bone marrow apparently takes over this function. Equally important, the immunofluorescent studies provided a sensitive and direct way of identifying individual Pre-B cells, thus allowing study of their morphology, function, and subcellular constituents in many species.

ONTOGENY, MORPHOLOGY, AND ORGAN DISTRIBUTION OF PRE-B CELLS

Pre-B cells are easily distinguished by immunofluorescence from more mature IgM$^+$-B lymphocytes, -plasmablasts, and -plasma cells.

Unlike Pre-B cells, IgM$^+$ B lymphocytes bear surface IgM that is easily capped, but have no detectable cytoplasmic IgM. IgM$^+$ plasmablasts bear surface IgM that is not easily capped, and stain much more brightly for cytoplasmic IgM than do Pre-B cells. IgM$^+$ plasma cells often bear easily detectable sIgM, stain brilliantly for cytoplasmic IgM, and usually exhibit a distinct morphology.

Pre-B cells are first found in fetal liver at 12, 23, and ~60 days of gestation, respectively, in mice, rabbits, and humans (14,16,17). In all three species, these are large lymphoid cells with a convoluted nuclear contour. A few days after large Pre-B cells appear, small cIgM$^+$.sIg$^-$ lymphocytes can be seen in fetal liver. The latter are morphologically similar to small lymphocytes throughout the body, having a smooth round nucleus and relatively little cytoplasm. Small sIgM$^+$.cIg$^-$ B lymphocytes are first detectable in mouse fetal liver about 5 days after the appearance of large Pre-B cells. In liver of rabbit and human embryos, the lag time between appearance of large Pre-B cells and small B lymphocytes is roughly similar. As hemopoiesis ceases in fetal liver, Pre-B cells disappear, too. Following the onset of bone marrow hemopoiesis, both large and small Pre-B cells appear and persist in the marrow throughout life. Because Pre-B cells are so heterogeneous in size and represent a minor subpopulation of cells in both fetal liver and bone marrow (e.g., ~0.6 and ~6%, respectively, of total nucleated cells and of lymphoid cells in human marrow) (18), it has not yet been possible to purify normal Pre-B cells for examination of their fine structure. Malignant Pre-B cells from a few children with acute lymphoblastic leukemia have been examined by electron microscopy (19). They had vesicular nuclei and irregular nuclear membranes. The cytoplasm contained individual and aggregated ribosomes, a few strands of rough endoplasmic reticulum, numerous mitochondria, and a prominent Golgi apparatus.

Large Pre-B cells have only been found in fetal liver and bone marrow of mice, rabbits, and humans, but small Pre-B cells have occasionally been observed in peripheral tissues. Small Pre-B cells can be seen for a few days in the spleen of perinatal mice, where their presence probably accounts for the ability of fetal spleen cultures to generate sIgM$^+$ B lymphocytes. In young human fetuses, small Pre-B cells have been observed in low frequencies in spleen and lymph nodes. Blood from newborns occasionally may contain significant numbers of small Pre-B cells, and their presence in circulation has been noted in patients after bone marrow transplantation for aplastic anemia. We have also observed small Pre-B cells in human lymph nodes after local antigenic stimulation. Brahim and Osmond have demonstrated migration of newly formed small lymphocytes from mouse bone marrow to lymph nodes during primary immune responses (20). Thus, it appears that antigen stimulation may induce the release of small Pre-B cells from the marrow but the nature of the signal for this emigration has not yet been elucidated.

GROWTH CHARACTERISTICS OF PRE-B CELLS

We have already mentioned labeling studies in which the results indicate that large rapidly dividing sIg⁻ lymphoid cells in adult mouse bone marrow give rise to nondividing, small sIg⁻ lymphocytes that begin to express sIgM within 20 or more hours. In more recent experiments employing direct immunofluorescent identification of Pre-B cells, it was shown that large Pre-B cells are a rapidly dividing population of cells while small Pre-B cells seldom divide (21,22). For example, after a 45 min *in vitro* pulse with ³H-thymidine, ~90% of the large Pre-B cells in human fetal liver and in bone marrow show nuclear incorporation of the radiolabel. Although very few small Pre-B cells incorporate thymidine within 45 min, many acquire the nuclear DNA label after 48 hr in culture. These small Pre-B cells contain less radioactive thymidine, in keeping with their derivation by division of large Pre-B cells.

Osmond has estimated that mouse bone marrow produces ~10⁸ small lymphocytes per day. Even if, as is likely, all of these are not of B-cell lineage and some perish before migration, this implies an impressive production of B cells for export from bone marrow.

EVIDENCE FOR PRECURSOR–PROGENY RELATIONSHIP OF PRE-B CELLS AND B LYMPHOCYTES

There is much indirect evidence in support of the idea of a differentiation sequence of lymphoid stem cell induction to become large Pre-B cells which divide to give rise to small Pre-B cells that serve as the direct precursors of sIgM⁺ B lymphocytes. There is at present no means for direct identification of the stem cell precursor of Pre-B cells, but there is abundant evidence from cell transfer studies for their existence. Results of organ culture studies leave little doubt that fetal liver serves as the initial induction microenvironments for stem cell conversion to Pre-B cells. Bone marrow then becomes the site in which Pre-B cells are generated from Ig⁻ precursors. There is still no direct evidence, however, that bone marrow can initiate the initial commitment of stem cells to differentiate along B-cell lines. Thus we believe it is still possible that committed Ig⁻ progenitors may merely relocate from the fetal liver to bone marrow where conversion to large Pre-B cells can occur.

The kinetic studies combining ³H-thymidine labeling and immunofluorescent identification of Pre-B cells provide strong evidence for the parent–daughter relationship of large Pre-B cells to small Pre-B cells. Along with the ontogenetic sequence of appearance in mice, rabbits, and man (14,16,17), results of the above studies also imply direct conversion of small Pre-B cells into B lymphocytes. Moreover, elimination of Pre-B cells and B lymphocytes in mature mice by a single large dose of cyclophosphamide is followed by the sequential appearance of large Pre-B cells, small Pre-B cells, and then sIgM⁺ B lymphocytes (23).

The most convincing evidence that Pre-B cells give rise to B lymphocytes comes from studies of mice treated from birth with large doses of goat antibodies to mouse μ-chains. Although this treatment effectively aborts development of sIg⁺ B cells of all classes, it does not affect the frequencies of large and small Pre-B cells in bone marrow (23). Cultures of bone marrow, but not spleen cells, from anti-μ suppressed mice give rise within 24 hr to functional sIgM⁺ B lymphocytes, and these increase in number over the next 3 days in culture. Finally, a large proportion of the Pre-B cells in bone marrow samples from patients with IgA myelomas contain the same idiotypic determinants as those expressed by the IgA produced by homologous myeloma plasma cells. The idiotype-positive Pre-B cells in this instance contain μ-chain, but not α-chain determinants (24). Thus it should be possible,

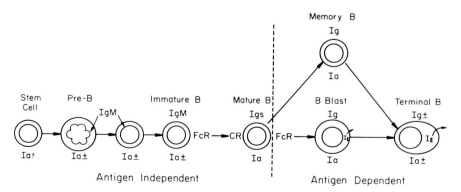

Fig. 1.   Developmental milestones in the life history of B cells.

although perhaps difficult, to formally prove the sequence of B-cell differentiation outlined in Fig. 1 by sequential study of a cloned Pre-B cell.

Indirect methods of identifying sIg⁺ cells have been employed in *in vitro* studies to show that sIg⁻ cells from mouse fetal liver can be induced by lipopolysaccharide to differentiate into sIg⁺ cells (25). However, this result could not be confirmed when direct immunofluorescent methods were used to examine *in vitro* induction of Pre-B cells to B lymphocytes. The inducing agents employed in these studies included dibutyl cyclic AMP, dibutyl cyclic GMP, and cholera toxin over wide dose ranges (26).

SURFACE AND CYTOPLASMIC CONSTITUENTS OF PRE-B CELLS

The existence of surface IgM on Pre-B cells is still a controversial issue. The evidence for this is (i) Melcher's demonstration of rapidly-shed sIgM on a population of large lymphoid cells from bone marrow and *spleen* of normal and nude mice (10), (ii) Lafleur and co-workers' findings that the large precursor-B cells in adult marrow and *spleen* had sIg by immunofluorescence and could be eliminated by antiIg treatment before cell transfer (4–5), and (iii) Rosenberg and Parrish's detection by a sensitive rosetting assay of large sIg⁺ cells in mouse fetal liver beginning on the thirteenth day of gestation (27). In keeping with the observation that the large bone marrow and spleen lymphocytes quickly shed their surface IgM, Rosenberg and Parrish observed that the erythrocytes coated with antimouse Ig were few in number, often present only on one pole of the cell and only transiently adherent to the large lymphoid cells (Y. J. Rosenberg, personal communication). On the other hand, we and others have not been able to detect any surface Ig on large or small Pre-B cells using sensitive radiolabeling and immunofluorescence techniques (8,9,14,16,17). One possible explanation for this failure is that sIgM is shed too quickly from Pre-B cells for detection by these methods. However, sIg on Pre-B cells is still undetectable by immunofluorescence even after the cells are pre-fixed to prevent sIg shedding under conditions that do not modify immunofluorescence staining of B lymphocytes.

A combination of factors could explain the apparent discrepancies in the findings with regard to the presence or absence of sIgM on "Pre-B cells." (1) We could be looking at different cells. This is likely to be a partial explanation since Melchers, Lafleur, Phillips and their colleagues find large (rapidly sedimenting) type I or PB cells with rapid turnover of sIgM in both adult marrow and spleen, whereas we can identify large Pre-B cells only in the bone marrow of adult mice. Moreover, the very high frequency of sIg^+ cells ($>15\%$) found in fetal liver by Rosenberg and Parrish also raises the possibility that they could have been detecting some nonPre-B cells. (2) Another relevant consideration is raised by results of ontogenetic studies of IgM distribution in bursal cells (28). Although the latter differ from mammalian Pre-B cells in that they have functional sIgM receptors detectable by immunofluorescence, they also contain cIgM. The first bursal lymphocytes to appear contain IgM scattered throughout the cytoplasm and lack a detectable Golgi apparatus. Later, with Golgi body development, cytoplasmic IgM becomes concentrated to the perinuclear cisterna and Golgi regions. Bursal cells showing this pattern are followed by development of cells in which IgM is located in vesicles dispersed throughout the cytoplasm. These IgM-laden vesicles merge with the plasma membrane to release their contents by a process that is inhibited by cytochalasin B, a disrupter of the contractable microfilament system. These same developmental patterns of cytoplasmic IgM localization have been seen in mammalian Pre-B cells but are much more difficult to confirm by biochemical studies, as has been possible in chickens (R. M. E. Parkhouse *et al.*, unpublished) owing to the ease of obtaining relatively pure suspensions of bursal lymphocytes at each developmental stage. It is entirely possible that lactoperoxidase might catalyze the labeling of IgM molecules in Pre-B cell vesicles just as they are being released by exocytosis.

Clearly a pressing need is for more precise information regarding the molecular nature of Pre-B IgM and its metabolism and transport. It is evident from already available information, however, that Pre-B cells do not bear *functional* surface IgM receptors. Pre-B cells are neither morphologically nor functionally affected by *in vivo* or *in vitro* exposure to antibodies against IgM determinants; it is only their immature $sIgM^+$ progeny that are eliminated or whose further development is otherwise aborted by this treatment (14,23,29). The absence of functional antibody receptors on Pre-B cells has obvious profound implications with regard to the mechanisms for generation of diversity and for tolerance induction.

Receptors other than immunoglobulins that can be easily found on sIg^+ B lymphocytes are also not expressed in Pre-B cells of mice or humans. In both mice and humans, Pre-B cells lack detectable receptors for activated C3 components and for the Fc portion of IgG (14,22,26). Results of ongoing studies of receptors for Epstein–Barr

virus suggest that these are also missing on human Pre-B cells. Although Ia determinants are not detectable on Pre-B cells or immature
B lymphocytes in mice, this is not the case for "B-cell antigens" in
humans. Human Pre-B cells express the Ia-like determinants detected
by heterologous antibodies to p23-30 antigens (L. B. Vogler, A. Fuks *et
al.*, unpublished). Moreover, human Pre-B cells bear a recently discovered B-cell antigen that has a molecular weight of ~65,000, is distinct from the DR surface component, and is not detected on cells of
the monocyte-macrophage series (30).

ABSENCE OF FUNCTIONAL RESPONSES OF PRE-B CELLS

Since Pre-B cells lack functional immunoglobulin receptors and receptors for C3 and Fc of IgG on their surface, it is not surprising that
the available evidence suggests that they cannot be influenced either
positively or negatively by antibodies to immunoglobulin determinants or by antigens. In addition, extensive studies in mice indicate that
Pre-B cells are unresponsive to the B-cell mitogen, lipopolysaccharide
(29,31). The absence of functional receptors on Pre-B cells, through
which development of immature clones producing potentially useful
antibodies could be prematurely aborted, and the rapid rate of proliferation exhibited by large Pre-B cells make this stage in differentiation
along the B axis an ideal one for the initial expression of clonal
diversity.

EVIDENCE FOR CLONAL DIVERSITY OF PRE-B CELLS

So far μ-chains are the only heavy chain-isotypic determinants that
have been detected in normal Pre-B cells. Biosynthetic studies have
shown that 7–8 S IgM molecules are synthesized by cells in embryonic
fetal liver containing Pre-B cells but lacking in more mature cells of
B-cell lineage. These observations and those indicating that
immunoglobulin-isotype diversity is expressed during B-lymphocyte
maturation suggest that Pre-B cells normally do not develop isotype
diversity. There is evidence that individual Pre-B cells make the deci-
sion as to whether they will express kappa- or lamda-chain genes. A
significant proportion of Pre-B cells in mice and rabbits can be
stained cytoplasmically with fluorochrome-labeled antibodies
specific for kappa-chain determinants (14,16). In preliminary studies
employing differential immunofluorescence, human Pre-B cells that

stained for kappa-chain determinants did not contain detectable lambda-chains, and vice versa (H. Kubagawa *et al.*, unpublished). More substantial evidence has been obtained for allelic exclusion of the kappa-chain allotypes, b^4 and b^5 in Pre-B cells of heterozygous rabbits (16). Individual Pre-B cells in b^4b^5 heterozygous rabbits express detectable amounts of only one of the alternative alleles. The allelic exclusion occurs in both large and small Pre-B cells before and after the development of sIg+ B lymphocytes. In b^4b^5 heterozygous rabbits given alloantibodies specific for the paternal κ-chain allotype, complete suppression of B lymphocytes expressing the paternal allotype could be achieved without affecting expression of that allotype in Pre-B cells.

Two sets of observations by Kubagawa *et al.* suggest that Pre-B cells are clonally diverse with regard to expression of V-region determinants. Pre-B cells staining with idiotype-specific antibodies have been detected in low frequency in human bone marrow samples (32). A high frequency of Pre-B cells staining doubly for μ-chain and myeloma idiotypic-determinants was observed in marrow samples from two patients with IgA myelomas (33). In each of these individuals the idiotype was individually specific for both Pre-B and myeloma plasma cells.

Thus it appears that most of the genetic decisions with regard to immunoglobulin genes are made and/or expressed during this stage of differentiation. This means that in order to understand the molecular basis for generation of clonal diversification, the focus of study must be on Pre-B cells. The mere fact that clonal diversity is generated among cells lacking functional antibody receptors apparently eliminates the possibilities that antigens or V-region epitopes (i) can influence a selective mutational process for the initial generation of V-gene diversity or (ii) can abort the development of clones of Pre-B cells. It is readily apparent that these two conclusions have significant biologic implications.

PRE-B CELLS IN IMMUNODEFICIENCIES

So far integrity of the development of Pre-B cells has only been assessed in human immunodeficiency diseases. Useful information has been obtained in four types of antibody deficiencies (18,33,34). Adults with thymoma and associated hypogammaglobulinemia have too few marrow Pre-B cells to detect. This suggests that stem cells have ceased to give rise to this line of cells, an interpretation consistent with vari-

able cessation of stem cell differentiation along other lym-
phohemopoietic avenues of differentiation in such patients. The basis
for such an acquired stem cell defect of variable severity is unknown.
In contrast, boys with the X-linked form of agammaglobulinemia
(XLA) usually have normal numbers of marrow Pre-B cells despite
their severe deficit of B lymphocytes and other more mature B-cell
progeny. Pre-B cells look normal in such patients, but they divide less
frequently than normal. The abnormality preventing further differentiation of Pre-B cells is still unknown. In one of twelve boys with
congenital agammaglobulinemia, we could find no Pre-B cells. The
same has been true in a few patients with late onset of panhypogam-
maglobulinemia associated with a paucity of circulating B lymphocytes. In fact, there is a high degree of correlation between the frequencies of Pre-B cells in bone marrow and the number of circulating
B lymphocytes when values derived from patients with XLA are excluded (Fig. 2). In our view this is further support for the precursor–
progeny relationship of Pre-B cells and B cells.

It will be of obvious interest to examine Pre-B cells in patients with
other immunodeficiencies, especially those in which clonal and intra-
clonal diversity (heavy chain isotypes) are limited.

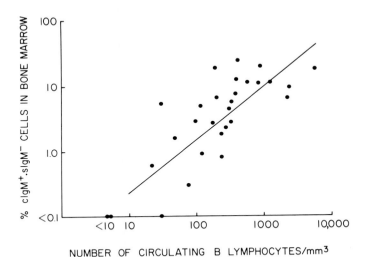

NUMBER OF CIRCULATING B LYMPHOCYTES/mm³

Fig. 2. Relationship between the proportion of human Pre-B cells in bone marrow
and the number of circulating B lymphocytes. These determinations were made in
normal adults and patients of various ages with hematological or immunodeficiency
diseases, excluding X-linked agammaglobulinemia (18). (Reproduced with permission
from The Williams & Wilkins Co.)

MALIGNANCIES INVOLVING PRE-B CELLS

So far Pre-B cells have been shown to be involved in two distinct types of malignancies affecting clones of this lineage. The malignant cells in approximately 20% of patients with acute childhood lymphoblastic leukemia (ALL) exhibit the characteristic phenotype of Pre-B cells (19; L. B. Vogler *et al.*, unpublished). All of the leukemic cells in three of six such patients contained cytoplasmic IgM and bore the "B-cell antigens," p23-30 and BDA, but lacked detectable surface immunoglobulin, C3 and Fc receptors, binding sites for sheep erythrocytes, and T-cell antigens. Most leukemic cells in a fourth individual with ALL had this phenotype but coexisted with a subpopulation of lymphoblasts with trace amounts of sIgM. Malignant ALL cells in the remaining two patients had Fc receptors; in one of these, C3 receptors and trace amounts of sIgM were detectable on leukemic subpopulations. The leukemic cells in all of these patients had typical ALL morphology and lacked E–B nuclear antigen distinguishing them from Burkitt's lymphomalike leukemia. Their paucity of rough endoplasmic reticulum and lack of monoclonal immunoglobulin secretion distinguished them from more mature B-lymphocyte malignancies. The establishment of cell lines of leukemic cells with the Pre-B phenotype should allow detailed study of the IgM molecules produced by Pre-B cells, and of the biosynthesis and fate of these IgM molecules which do not become attached to the cell membrane.

One very interesting feature noted in a few of the malignant Pre-B cells was the coexistence of IgG with IgM and of IgA with IgM. Even though malignant Pre-B cells containing multiple heavy chain isotypes were present in very low frequencies, this suggests that isotype diversification may be possible at a Pre-B cell level. Suffice it to say, Pre-B cell leukemias and corresponding cell lines could be as useful to the study of Pre-B cells as myeloma cells have been in the characterization of plasma cells and their products.

Plasma cell myelomas appear to represent another informative study model of a B-cell malignancy involving Pre-B cells. Highly specific antibodies to idiotypes (Id) expressed by IgA myelomas have been prepared and used to determine the extent of the clonal involvement in two such patients (24). A coexisting excess of IgM-containing, Id⁺ Pre-B cells, and IgA-containing, homologous Id⁺ plasma cells was demonstrated in marrow samples from these patients. We draw three major conclusions from these results: (i) the oncogenic event in multiple myeloma occurs at least as early as the Pre-B cell stage in differentiation; (ii) clonal diversification as expressed by V-region epitope diversity is evident at this stage in the life history of B cells; and (iii) these data provide compelling evidence for the lineal relationship of Pre-B cells and mature B cells.

CONCLUSION

The identification and direct examination of Pre-B cells have furnished new insight into the processes of clonal development and elimination. Because these rapidly dividing, clonally-diverse cells lack functional receptors for antigens and for other known B-cell inducers, most of the mechanisms proposed for driving clonal diversification are made unlikely. Still there must be microenvironmental influences which promote differentiation and proliferation of Pre-B cells, but these have yet to be defined. Klinman has reviewed his reasons for favoring a predetermined permutation pattern of the generation of clonotypes (see chapter by Pierce et al.), and Siskind has countered this argument with data suggesting that the B-cell repertoire is of adult proportions as early as it can be examined in the mouse (see chapter by Siskind). We have reviewed elsewhere the basis for believing that each B stem cell gives rise to multiple B-cell clones, and have proposed a rudimentary model for this (35). We favor the possibility that transcription of the different families of germ line V genes begins at fixed points and proceeds along the cistron in an orderly stepwise fashion, perhaps always using the oldest DNA strand for the change (36). This notion does not preclude the possibility of a hypermutator element that modifies germ line V genes in a more or less patterned way, nor does it preclude the possibility of mutational generation of further clonal diversity among sIg^+ B cells as a result of antigen or idiotypic selection processes. Nevertheless, it does seem clear that these are not the mechanisms involved in the initial expression of clonal diversification. It would therefore seem evident that the problem will need to be resolved by examination of DNA sequences, relocations, mutations, and transcription during and just before the Pre-B cell stages in differentiation. For this, the models provided by immunodeficiencies and malignancies involving B stem cells and Pre-B cells could be invaluable.

ACKNOWLEDGMENTS

We are grateful to our colleagues for sharing their ideas and data and to Summer King and Ann Brookshire for preparing the manuscript. Studies cited from our laboratory were supported by U.S. Public Health Service grants CA 16673 and CA 13148 awarded by the National Cancer Institute, AI 11502 awarded by the National Institute of Allergy and Infectious Diseases, and 5M01-RR32 awarded by the National Institutes of Health. Alexander R. Lawton is recipient of a Research Career Development Award, AI 70780.

REFERENCES

1. Osmond, D. G., and Everett, N. B. (1964) *Blood* **23**, 1–17.
2. Rosse, C. (1971) *Blood* **38**, 372–377.
3. Röpke, C., and Everett, N. B. (1973) *Cell Tissue Kinet.* **6**, 499–507.
4. Lafleur, L., Miller, R. G., and Phillips, R. A. (1972) *J. Exp. Med.* **135**, 1363–1374.
5. Lafleur, L., Underdown, B. J., Miller, R. G., and Phillips, R. A. (1972) *Ser. Haematol.* **5**, 50–63.
6. Lafleur, L., Miller, R. G., and Phillips, R. A. (1973) *J. Exp. Med.* **137**, 954–966.
7. Osmond, D. G., and Nossal, G. J. V. (1974) *Cell. Immunol.* **13**, 117–131.
8. Osmond, D. G., and Nossal, G. J. V. (1974) *Cell. Immunol.* **13**, 132–145.
9. Ryser, J. E., and Vassalli, P. (1974) *J. Immunol.* **113**, 719–728.
10. Melchers, F. H., von Boehmer, H., and Phillips, R. A. (1975) *Transplant. Rev.* **25**, 26–58.
11. Nossal, G. J. V., and Pike, B. L. (1973) *Immunology* **25**, 33–45.
12. Owen, J. J. T., Cooper, M. D., and Raff, M. C. (1974) *Nature (London)* **249**, 361–363.
13. Owen, J. J. T., Jordan, R. K., Robinson, J. H., Singh, U., and Willcox, H. N. A. (1977) *Cold Spring Harbor Symp. Quant. Biol.* **41**, 129–137.
14. Raff, M. C., Megson, M., Owen, J. J. T., and Cooper, M. D. (1976) *Nature (London)* **259**, 224–226.
15. Phillips, R. A., and Melchers, F. (1976) *J. Immunol.* **117**, 1099–1103.
16. Hayward, A. R., Simons, M., Lawton, A. R., Mage, R. G., and Cooper, M. D. (1977) *In* "Developmental Immunobiology" (J. B. Solomon, ed.), pp. 181–188. Elsevier, Amsterdam.
17. Gathings, W. E., Lawton, A. R., and Cooper, M. D. (1977) *Eur. J. Immunol.* **7**, 804–810.
18. Pearl, E. R., Vogler, L. B., Okos, A. J., Crist, W. M., Lawton, A. R., and Cooper, M. D. (1978) *J. Immunol.* **120**, 1169–1175.
19. Vogler, L. B., Crist, W. M., Bockman, D. E., Pearl, E. R., Lawton, A. R., and Cooper, M. D. (1978) *N. Engl. J. Med.* **298**, 872–878.
20. Brahin, F., and Osmond, D. G. (1976) *Clin. Exp. Immunol.* **24**, 515–526.
21. Owen, J. J. T., Wright, D. E., Habu, S., Raff, M. C., and Cooper, M. D. (1977) *J. Immunol.* **118**, 2067–2072.
22. Okos, A. J., and Gathings, W. E. (1977) *Fed. Proc., Fed. Am. Soc. Exp. Biol.* **36**, 1294A.
23. Burrows, P. D., Kearney, J. F., Lawton, A. R., and Cooper, M. D. (1978) *J. Immunol.* **120**, 1526–1531.
24. Kubagawa, H., Vogler, L., Conrad, M., Lawton, A., and Cooper, M. (1978) *Fed. Proc., Fed. Am. Soc. Exp. Biol.* **37**, 1765A.
25. Hammerling, U., Chen, A. F., and Abbott, J. (1976) *Proc. Natl. Acad. Sci. U.S.A.* **73**, 2008–2012.
26. Raff, M. C. (1977) *Cold Spring Harbor Symp. Quant. Biol.* **41**, 159–162.
27. Rosenberg, Y. J., and Parish, C. R. (1977) *J. Immunol.* **118**, 612–617.

28. Grossi, C. E., Lydyard, P. M., and Cooper, M. D. (1977) *J. Immunol.* **119**, 749–756.
29. Melchers, F., Andersson, J., and Phillips, R. A. (1977) *Cold Spring Harbor Symp. Quant. Biol.* **41**, 147–158.
30. Balch, C. M., Dougherty, P. A., Vogler, L. B., Ades, E. W., and Ferrone, S. (1978) *J. Immunol.* **121**, 2322–2328.
31. Kearney, J. F., and Lawton, A. R. (1975) *J. Immunol.* **115**, 577–681.
32. Kubagawa, H., Vogler, L., Lawton, A., and Cooper, M. (1978) *Clin. Res.* **26**, 517A.
33. Vogler, L. B., Pearl, E. R., Gathings, W. E., Lawton, A. R., and Cooper, M. D. (1976) *Lancet* **2**, 376.
34. Hayward, A. R. (1978) *Lancet* **1**, 1014–1015.
35. Lydyard, P. M., Grossi, C. E., and Cooper, M. D. (1976) *J. Exp. Med.* **144**, 79–97.
36. Cairns, J. (1975) *Nature (London)* **255**, 197–200.

Index